ESSAYS IN HONOUR OF MICHAEL BLISS:
FIGURING THE SOCIAL

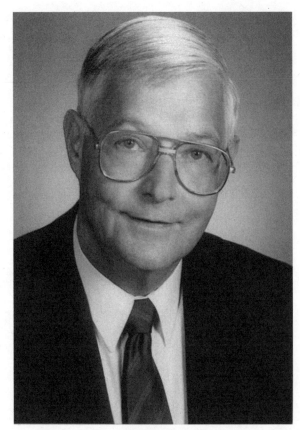

Michael Bliss

# Essays in Honour of Michael Bliss

## Figuring the Social

*Edited by E.A. Heaman, Alison Li,*
*and Shelley McKellar*

UNIVERSITY OF TORONTO PRESS
Toronto Buffalo London

© University of Toronto Press Incorporated 2008
Toronto Buffalo London

www.utppublishing.com

Printed in Canada

ISBN 978-0-8020-9097-3

Printed on acid-free paper

**Library and Archives Canada Cataloguing in Publication**

Essays in honour of Michael Bliss: figuring the social / edited by E.A. Heaman,
Alison Li and Shelly McKellar.

Includes bibliographical references.
ISBN 978-0-8020-9097-3

1. Canada – Social conditions – 1971–1991.   2. Canada – Social conditions –
1991–.   3. Canada – History – 1963–.   4. Medicine – Canada –
History.   5. Bliss, Michael, 1941–.   I. Heaman, Elsbeth, 1964–   II. Li, Alison
I-Syin, 1963–   III. McKellar, Shelley, 1967–   IV. Bliss, Michael, 1941–

FC149.E88 2008      971.064      C2007-906327-6

University of Toronto Press acknowledges the financial assistance to its publishing program of the Canada Council for the Arts and the Ontario Arts
Council.

University of Toronto Press acknowledges the financial support for its publishing activities of the Government of Canada through the Book Publishing
Industry Development Program (BPIDP).

# Contents

# Foreword

JOHN FRASER AND ELIZABETH MACCALLUM

## The College Man / John Fraser

Massey College is not in any way an ordinary place, not at the University of Toronto, not in Canada, not ordinary anywhere in fact. It is both strange and wonderful – by design. The original concept, then as now, was to show, academically, the interconnectedness between all things. Vincent Massey, the first Canadian-born governor general, conceived the College in 1960; and the first Master, Robertson Davies, made it a reality two years later. Though nestled in the bosom of the U of T, it is not of it. Massey is, as it were, connected (all its young scholars must, by statute, be enrolled at the U of T), but administratively detached. The College never hesitates to let the world know this salient fact even if the world, for the most part, couldn't care less.

Officially, it is an interdisciplinary graduate resident college, with senior and junior scholars elected from the three great streams of the academy: the humanities, the sciences, and the professions. In a sense this is also Michael Bliss's entry point as a Senior Fellow of the College, starting in 1994 when he was first elected on the College's governing Corporation, but considering many of his own professional and personal propensities (anti-elitist, anti-monarchical, etc.), it requires some further explanation of collegiate irregularities to understand just how important the place became to him, and how important he became to the place.

From its earliest days, Massey was mocked as being 'pseudo-Oxford' thanks to its gowns and the instant tradition of High Tables and 'Gaudy Night.' In fairness to the mockers, there really was an undeniable whiff of end-of-Empire academic snobbery that was Oxbridge-centred. But if there was some justice in the mockery over superficialities, and still is, a few salient points were missed along the way.

First, the College had a further mandate beyond encouraging 'scholars of great worth,' and that was to be 'a bridge community' between town and gown, bringing – or trying to bring – the two spheres together through a variety of means. These ranged from its great public lecture series (The Massey Lecture, presented in conjunction with its partners, the Canadian Broadcasting Corporation and the House of Anansi publishers; and the Walter Gordon Symposium on Public Policy) to the mid-career journalism fellowship program modelled on Harvard's Neiman Fellowships, which brings working journalists into the university for an academic year.

Second, the Oxford (well, Balliol College, to be more precise) that Vincent Massey and Robertson Davies attended in the 1920s and 1930s simply didn't exist anymore. Balliol College's gownless Left-leaning politics, along with a volubly anti-authoritarian and anti-elitist rhetoric (except where its own privileges were at stake) would have horrified both men. Also it was and remains very much an undergraduate English place, replete with undergraduate English themes, undergraduate English pranks, and the necessity for undergraduate discipline. Massey, from its first conception, was almost the polar opposite, yet out of their Balliol experience, Massey and Davies managed to create something altogether different and original: a repository for Canadian academic altruism tricked out in the engaging theatrics of Oxford nostalgia.

At the same time, and here is a third point missed by most people when they observe Massey College from the outside: this seemingly elitist establishment is remarkably anti-hierarchical and far more open to the wide world around it than most of the other institutions of the university. 'Those who try to educate must be prepared to be educated often by the very persons they seek to enlighten,' observed one of Massey's most illustrious Senior Fellows, Professor Ursula Franklin, about the proper code of conduct for all members of her college. 'Those who seek to help have to accept help equally willingly.'

Indeed, the whole point of putting 'junior' and 'senior' scholars together is to give both sides the chance of meeting each other on friendly, neutral territory, to mutual benefit. The goal of reaching out is further abetted by the reality of urban geography. Since Massey College is situated in the heart of a great metropolis, it hasn't a hope in heaven or hell of standing aloof from the swirling life around it, nor does it try to. Programs like the Junior Fellows' mentorship initiative with neighbourhood high school kids, the Scholar-At-Risk initiative with the U of T's School of Graduate Studies, and The Quadrangle Society that brings together various non-academic members of the community outside the university all testify to this reality.

So this was the world Professor Michael Bliss was elected to, or rather agreed to be elected to, in 1994. This came well into his extraordinary career both as an academic and as a public intellectual, honoured at his university and often in demand in the media and on the podium. The College has never shied away from riding on illustrious coat-tails! Given his own perceived political sensitivities (republican and right of centre), one senses Professor Bliss was initially curious in a wary sort of way of Massey with its vice-regal foundation and academically centre-leftist propensities.

But it is never wise to pigeonhole him. First and foremost, he has trained himself professionally to take an unsentimental look at both political action and governing institutions in whatever sphere happens to be under his critical scrutiny: business, academia, the medical establishment, or government. Early on, he must have realized that whatever pomposities attended Massey College, it was at heart an inspiring place that had somehow escaped many of the presiding evils of contemporary university reality and necessity. Clearly, he appreciated the proximity to both academic colleagues and young scholars spread across the full spectrum of scholarly endeavour. He also liked the way the college reached out beyond its own borders because it reflected his own scholarly impulses in both the business and medical professions. Most of all, Michael Bliss liked Massey's formally instituted collegiality, a rare enough commodity on the campus to be found memorable and worthy of commendation.

The year before I was elected Master of Massey College, Professor Bliss had begun his Massey career on the twenty-six-seat governing Corporation. Already, he was in hot water over some typically strong views. *Blissian views*, we could say. Chief among them, it soon became clear, was the growing dismay at some of the 'necessities' associated with academic money-grubbing. His irritation at universities grovelling before the lure of large gifts from tycoons who wanted their names emblazoned on anything on the campus which didn't move (and later even on those things that did move, such as professorial chairs) was growing apace and threatening to be profound. Massey College – being independent – wasn't nearly as caught up in the frenzy of courting both government and private-sector financial support as most academic institutions were xii John Fraser and Elizabeth MacCallum

by the time he signed on. That was one of the reasons it was facing an economic crisis. Imagine his chagrin, therefore, when, at one his early meetings with Corporation, he found this hitherto seemingly worthy body of academic custodians ready to sell their souls (well, just the names of its dining hall and libraries) to the highest bidder.

Something must have triggered an interesting intervention at that Corporation meeting. I wasn't there, although I already had been given responsibility for fund-raising by the third master, Professor Ann Saddlemyer. The first I knew there was trouble was when the Master phoned me and asked me how well I knew Professor Bliss:

'Only too well,' I replied, lightly. I did not bother to tell her that when he was a much younger man and working his way through to his doctorate, Michael was a history teacher at Lawrence Park Collegiate, where he was an inspiration to my wife, Elizabeth MacCallum. He had been a family hero ever since (one treated with a certain brusque familiarity, but a hero nonetheless – see Elizabeth's account following).

'Well I'm worried about him,' said Master Saddlemyer. 'Some rough things were said at Corporation. Maybe you might give him a call and see if everything is okay.'

Rough?

It seemed to me Bliss has always been able to give as good as he gets, especially in an academic wrangle. What was going on here?

Soon enough, it became clear he had got into a wrangle with one member of Corporation in particular over the business of naming principal College venues after benefactors. It was a theoretical wrangle, mind you, as no one at Massey in more than three decades had managed to raise more than a few *sous* beyond the original Massey endowment. An outsider would have said there wasn't enough loot around the place to justify the heated rhetoric. It was heated, though. To give you the flavour of the wrangle, the new boy on Corporation (Professor Bliss) took on one of the longest-serving worthies and, in effect, accused him of selling the College's honour for the proverbial mess of pottage. This had brought about a ferocious riposte that concluded with the memorable utterance: 'Now we all know where the famous phrase "ignorance is bliss" comes from.'

By the time I got to him, Michael was in that steely, ice-cold sort of mood those who know and love him absolutely *dread*. The tone of voice, the long silences, the staccato statements: all this bespoke a mounted warrior whose feet were already in the stirrups, whose helmet visor had already been lowered, whose lance was at the ready, and whose horse was impatiently pawing the ground in sympathetic harmony with its master's innermost resolve. To this day, I believe only friendship held him back from a blistering public attack on the sale of academic principles. I think he considered the fact that I had only recently been elected Master-Designate and that my wife – that young, idealistic high school student who adored and fought him all those years ago – would soon be moving into the Master's Lodging. Considering all this, I believe he decided to give us the benefit of doubt and the gift of time.

As it turned out, all this was merely a prelude to one of the most productive and contributing senior fellowships the college has ever seen in its near half-century of existence. Other senior fellows have contributed as much, but none more than Michael Bliss. Initially, it helped that he was prepared to compromise on the fund-raising front, for, in truth, the College was terribly strapped for funds in those days. Its endowment was inadequate to its needs and other sources of revenues could not come close to making up the difference. Staff was being let off, services were being cut back, and the fabric of the building was being worn thin. Compromise on the fund-raising front was matched by stalwart stewardship on Corporation and personal commitment. Ultimately, Michael Bliss's best instincts to protect the College from undue influences outside academia served it well and bolstered my own efforts at governance. If he was always there to keep me on the mark, he was also always there as Protector and Enthusiast, and as Recruiter-General, for some of the College's best Junior Fellows came to us with his encouragement. It was the College's good luck that at the apogee of his academic and writing career, Professor Bliss chose to make Massey College, and its progress, a hugely important personal commitment with all the energy, altruism, generosity, and wisdom that this entailed.

Let me deal with the energy first. Michael not only served a decade on Corporation (two successive terms of five years), he also served on its Standing Committee (which has to deal with tricky matters of inner-College conflict and debate), and its Nominating Committee (which advises Corporation on all matters related to the election of College fellows and Quadrangle Society members). He has been a hugely crucial member of the journalist selection committee, which each year sifts through dozens of applications for the prestigious Canadian Journalism Fellowships (jointly sponsored by the College and the university, and administered and hosted by Massey). All this energy constituted the formal, upfront activity of an industrious Senior Fellow who at the same time continued his busy schedule of lecturing to undergraduates, supervising graduate theses, burnishing an increasingly important role of public intellectual in the national media, and getting on with his scholarly research and highly regarded books. This energy was also deployed to realistic goals, and no doubt a large part of Michael Bliss's professional success had to do with his common sense and practicality in choosing what to go after. At Massey College, we have been grateful for some time that his practicality took us in tow.

For altruism and generosity, I am going to have a break a confidence, but I think I will be forgiven. Six or seven years ago, Michael came to me and said he wanted to do something special for the Junior Fellows. He pointed out that in his student days he had won a number of honours and prizes, but the one that resonated most to him was an achievement that was marked with a book prize. Furthermore, the book had been specially inscribed inside to mark the occasion. Each time he had cause to look something up in that book, he was reminded not only of the past achievement, but the happiness, hard work, and good memories associated with those days. He would like to share that experience, said Professor Bliss, with any Junior Fellow of the College who made it over all the hurdles to a doctorate. But he wanted to do it anonymously so that the focus would remain on the recipients rather than the donor. These book prizes are now a big feature of the final Fellows' Gaudy at Massey College, much coveted and appreciated. All that is wonderful and typical of the man's generosity, but what I particularly loved about this gift was the thoughtfulness behind it, the intertwining of his own youthful academic experience with that of the Junior Fellows, and the desire to fuel the Massey College experience with a concrete, deeply appreciated symbol. I hope I will be forgiven for blowing his cover, but it seems appropriate under the circumstances and it also underscores the central *leitmotif* of Massey College that all things are interconnected.

And finally a brief word on the wisdom of Professor Bliss. We are talking here about a deeply committed 'gentleman and scholar,' a concept so far gone from contemporary academic life – or contemporary society for that matter – it is almost a shock to be able to deploy this once familiar cliché. Anyone who knows the man personally knows his commitment to and pride in his family. Anyone who knows the man professionally will know of his engaged loyalty towards his colleagues and students. I wonder, however, if even his family or his professional colleagues know the depths of his careful concern and watchfulness when someone he has taken responsibility for encounters trouble. From the sidelines, I watched Michael Bliss carefully monitor the ups and downs of one of his students for which we shared joint responsibility and who was having some serious academic problems. I watched how astutely he assessed the problems, how adroitly he provided assistance from a careful knight's move remove – never hesitating, for example, to deploy me if he thought I could be useful even when I didn't know the entirety of his game plan – and how faithfully he stood by her through all academic vicissitudes.

All this, I know, is second nature to the man. I know this because I am married to someone he tended to long ago, under quite different circumstances, with equal astuteness, adroitness, faithfulness, and wisdom (and not a few *Blissisms*). Our lives are part of a great continuum which encompasses events and encounters both great and small, vividly recalled and dimly remembered, hugely appreciated and taken for granted. Michael Bliss is now a 'Continuing Senior Fellow' of Massey College. This is a kind of collegiate valhalla, a special category reserved for the brightest and best of its Senior Fellows who have devoted long periods of their lives and considerable efforts to our collective cause and benefit. But that's not where I want to leave him. I want to leave him back at the beginning of my true awareness of his extraordinary gift for academic inspiration and loyal friendship, and to do that I must hand over this tale to my wife and his former high school history student, Elizabeth MacCallum.

*What's past is prologue*: the Shakespearean observation was also the title of Vincent Massey's autobiography and Michael Bliss, of all people, will appreciate the interconnectedness of an essay on him that lands him right back in Lawrence Park Collegiate. He is, after all, a historian.

### The High School Teacher / Elizabeth MacCallum

'10K' doesn't sound like anything special. For me, though, it was more than the name of a classroom. It meant a whole new world where learning was exciting and high school didn't leave my stomach in knots. I don't even remember the letter of my grade 9 class, but it was The Dumb Class I can assure you. Bedridden for six months during grade 8 the year earlier, with a plaster body cast after back surgery, I had been required to complete elementary school with visiting teachers based at Sunnyview School for handicapped children. I may have graduated with A's, but when my mother phoned Lawrence Park Collegiate to register me, she was told to contact the local 'tech' school. Whoever it was only said that once.

Grade 9 at Lawrence Park – in the aforementioned 'dumb' class because I had come from a school for 'crippled' children – was one of the worst years of my life. Most teachers thought we were stupid and probably deaf too. Our history teacher yelled at us the whole time and I was the only one who seemed to notice. Fortunately, my grades were good enough to promote me into a smart grade 10 class (dear old 10K). In those days equity was not an issue.

Our homeroom teacher was new. A short, full-faced guy who was getting his teaching diploma the fast track way because of teacher shortages: teacher's college for two summers while teaching during the year. He might have come straight from heaven.

I don't even remember if Mr Bliss had finished two summers or not, but he sure knew how to teach, not always easy with a bunch of bright, but definitely smart-aleck kids from deepest North Toronto. He made us want to do well. Marked tests were returned starting from the top, beginning at the front left desk, moving down that row, then over to the next row to the right. So, with each exam and test we changed seating arrangements, and we all knew where we stood. It drove me crazy being only part-way up that left-hand row looking out onto Lawrence Avenue.

His teaching was laced with his own share of smart-aleck one-liners and, being from a small town in southern Ontario, he loved razzing us for being smug, well-off, Toronto kids. As a son of a doctor, he certainly should have understood our attitude first-hand – small town or not. Those of us who cared loved his rough-and-tumble repartee and the serious arguments about Canadian history and current issues that were a trademark of his discussions.

'But sir,' I remember myself whining with frustration at Mr Bliss's right-of-centre politics as he stood leaning against the blackboard, one knee bent to allow his foot to lean on the wall. He toyed with us affectionately, like an amiable cat lover playing with a toy mouse on a string as we challenged whatever thesis he was pushing. At the end of class there was always a line of students to ask him questions, and if he were walking into the main school building from the portable classroom where he taught us, there was usually a lively crowd of 'pseuds' (as we were called) surrounding him. He encouraged us, of course, making it no shame to work hard or to do well. He also listened with respect, as I remember very well, because on one of these 'walking seminars' I let forth with some vigour on the subject of Pope Pius XII and the persecution of Jews during the Second World War, having just seen Rolf Hochhuth's controversial play *The Deputy*. He himself had not yet seen the play, and he allowed me a lot of licence to ramble over Hochhuth's version of history.

His respect for us was also clear when Mr Bliss initiated a philosophy club and started us off with Plato, and he had the courage to admit to us that he himself had forgotten how difficult *The Republic* really was (particularly in explaining it to fifteen year olds, I suspect). At a time when high school trips were not a given, he organized one for the brighter students to go to Ottawa. He even arranged for us to meet his hometown Member of Parliament, appropriately enough a Tory stalwart in a three-piece pinstriped suit. At the end of the year, he invited the students exempted from final exams because of good marks, to his house for dinner with his wife, Liz. We were dazzled by such privilege, so generously offered.

A blissful lifetime of arguing with my respected history teacher continued even after he left Lawrence Park to return to full-time graduate work – an act of desertion we were sure would lead to intellectual death at the school, and certainly less fun. In grade 12, I was once more back in a body cast recovering from corrective spinal surgery, completely bedridden. By this time, Lawrence Park Collegiate was certainly on my side and allowed me to do my junior matriculation with only French, Mathematics, Latin, and History. A nice but rather deaf old lady from the Board of Education taught me languages. Nurses would prop me up on one side before the teacher came so I could see, and it was only after weeks of lessons that the poor discomfited woman told me that this was her deaf side and would they be able to put me onto the other side. Bruce Porter, a wonderful teacher from Lawrence, came for math, and out of the goodness of his heart, Mr Bliss came every *Saturday* morning to do a week's worth of work. You will be reassured to learn that he had no mercy on me just because I was in bed. I am pleased to report also that the 'But sir's continued apace.

Later, while I convalesced at home, the Saturday morning sessions continued, and my mother at ninety still remembers how startled she was opening the door to that 'pink cheeked young man, who looked just like a boy and it was Mr Bliss!'

That husband of mine likes to put it around that 'Mike Bliss turned my wife into a Leftist.' Not so. I was already well on the Left of the classroom in grade 10, and certainly wouldn't give Mr Bliss such credit. However, he did influence me profoundly, as he did so many other high school students, giving me the confidence to go to university to prepare for a life as an academic historian or work in current events at the CBC. Not being quite as bright as Mr Bliss credited me, it took me almost three years to notice that all my worst marks were in history and political science, and more time to realize I didn't have the stomach for the rough and tumble of daily television, and I eventually found myself working at a much more stately pace doing medical and soft science shows for *The Nature of Things*.

My first summer at Arts and Science at the CBC as a trainee producer, I found myself really excited by a documentary Professor William Saywell was making on China, on which I was allowed to participate. Mr Bliss and I had stayed in touch, and he invited me over to watch it at home with him and wonderful Liz. I was completely startled as he laced into the show, arguing that it had nothing new to say and was almost completely dependent on old footage. He was right too. This was around 1969, when hardly anyone knew what the hell was going on in China. Hell is the correct adjective for those years of the Cultural Revolution, when all TV producers had was stock shots of happy peasants working for the good of the people, and Mr Bliss's instincts for ideological fraud were – at least on this occasion! – impeccable. Like any well-tutored Bliss protégée, I was always encouraged to argue back forcefully.

Our lives turn in curious circles. When Michael was fifty-five and I was considerably less, we found ourselves together again at Massey College, he having been elected to it, myself being somewhat bemused to discover I had apparently married into it. In an early encounter at this new arena for our relationship, I accused him of wrongly pushing me into history. He looked at me in shock and amazement: 'Liz!' he said, 'I never thought I could convince you of anything.'

How little did he know.

# Preface

This volume has been compiled in honour of Michael Bliss, who retired in 2006 from the University of Toronto, where he taught in the Department of History from 1968. His eleven books and numerous articles have received many honours, including prizes awarded by the Canadian Historical Association, two City of Toronto Book Awards, two Jason Hannah Medals for medical history from the Royal Society of Canada, the Welch Medal of the American Association for the History of Medicine, and the National Business Book Award. Michael Bliss is one of Canada's foremost public intellectuals: he writes often in Canadian periodicals, comments on national radio and television, and lectures in Canada and abroad on a wide variety of topics. He is Professor Emeritus and a Fellow of Massey College. He adorns the Order of Canada and the Royal Society of Canada, which has awarded him its Tyrrell Medal 'for outstanding work in the history of Canada.' In his thirty-eight-year career, Bliss weighed in on national debates, wrote path-breaking books in many fields, and shaped the ideas and directions of students.

In an age of narrow professional specialization, Michael Bliss is a Renaissance man, with important monographs on the history of business, politics, public health, medicine, and surgery, and important articles on religion and social history, among other subjects. He has helped to shape public debate in these areas and he has also had a considerable influence on the writing of their histories. One way to measure and examine that influence is through the writing of the many historians who studied under him at the University of Toronto. He supervised nearly two dozen dissertations to completion, on subjects that spanned the whole range of his own scholarly works and beyond, into areas that Bliss himself hardly imagined as fields of serious inquiry. His students fill positions across the country, from Vancouver and Calgary through London, Toronto, and Montreal, to Halifax and Fredericton. Many of those he has supervised now teach in history departments, others work in the private sector, administering and writing public history projects or writing for national newspapers. Some are junior scholars just beginning to make their way in academia and the private sector; others are senior scholars who fill departmental and national research chairs or belong to the Royal Society of Canada. Together they represent a cross-section of the history profession as it has evolved over the last four decades.

This volume is a collection of representative essays from former students of Michael Bliss. Taken together, they constitute an important reflection on the writing of social history in Canada from the 1970s to the early twenty-first century. Their disciplinary span is considerable, reflecting the range of Michael Bliss's interests. An initial section provides some perspective on the business of being a scholar in Canada in the late twentieth century – both in and out of the university. It situates Michael Bliss as a public figure, as a scholar, and as a teacher. It also provides the groundwork for the scholarly essays that follow by interrogating the formation of professional historians in modern academe and the relationship between teacher and student. Of Bliss's students represented here, roughly half follow him here in writing about the history of medicine; the other half have chosen to write about business, politics, the state, religion, and the family. In fact, there can be no simple division into medical and non-medical topics: business, politics, the state, religion, and the family have all shaped the development of modern medicine, and the essays in this volume reflect that broad overlap in purportedly distinct fields. Essays that ostensibly deal with medical topics are just as concerned with issues of business and public policy as those dealing with commercial ventures and tariff legislation. In organizing this collection, we have grouped the contributions under four headings to underline the interplay of the public and the private: politics and business, family and religion, health and public policy, and medical science and practice. In each of these areas, the authors tease out the dynamic relation between the individual and society in the shaping of bodies, affections, and beliefs.

The authors here show their common debt to social history. Michael Bliss wrote sweeping works of history that spanned centuries and he wrote biographies of individuals that were explorations of social context as much as of individual choice within that context. His students have been equally concerned to relate the public to the private and to preserve the individual in the social, and in this they reflect the core concerns of social history. Susan Pederson remarks in the *London Review of Books* in October 2006: 'The real trick of social history is to grasp the link between the whole and the part, the public and the private: to understand the connection between statistics on the decline in fertility and Mrs W's puzzling ability to limit her children to three when her mother, too, had wanted three children but in the end had six. Social history's master narratives grew from the attempt to understand just such connections, to show how seismic social change and millions of tiny tremors linked up.'

In creating this volume we are striving to display the broad sweep of subjects pursued by the generation of Bliss's students and, moreover, to demonstrate that, despite the variety of topics, these authors are fellow travellers in social history, sharing common questions, concerns, and methods. Medical history is not a reified field distinct from national or social or political history, but is deeply embedded in all of these fields just as they too owe something of their modern shape to science and medicine. And, as in Bliss's work, the individual life often serves as a unifying factor.

We chose the title 'Figuring the Social' to represent the dynamic relationship between social history and the subdisciplines of history represented here. Oxford defines the verb 'to figure' as 'To give figure to; to form, shape; to bring into shape.' We do not follow Margaret Thatcher's reduction of the social to the individual, but rather celebrate the ways that society is given concrete form and figure through local studies, sometimes of an individual, sometimes of a cohort, sometimes of a political or institutional entity. Keeping one's eye on society, trying to *figure* it out, while writing about the particular is one of the great challenges of doing history. We also have in mind other aspects of that rich and dense word 'figure.' The reference to numerals, *figures*, invokes a concern with economics and business, with financial pressures, that underlies many of the papers in this collection, many of them haunted by the question of to what extent financial concerns have conflicted with conceptions of the public good, with the 'society' that Thatcher so vehemently denied; in short, whether the 'social' can be translated or transfigured into the economic, into figures. We also invoke the literal meaning of 'figure' as a reference to the human body, with the reminder that people are inescapably physical as well as spiritual and social beings, and that, therefore, the history of society and the history of medicine can never stray very far from one another.

The essays in this volume demonstrate the intellectual vibrancy and coherence as well as the public relevance of Canadian history today. In this way, Michael Bliss's influence endures.

# Acknowledgments

The editors would like to express their gratitude towards the Hannah Institute for the History of Medicine, a branch of Associated Medical Services. Over many years, more lately in conjunction with the Canadian Institutes of Health Research, it has provided substantial funding for research in medical history. As well as funding graduate and postgraduate research for many scholars represented here, it also sponsored the lecture that Michael Bliss delivered as a 'Hannah Happening' in Kingston, Ontario, in 2002, reproduced here as chapter 1. It provided essential funds for the publication of this book.

The editors would also like to thank all those connected with the preparation of the book, including the anonymous referees and the editors at University of Toronto Press, particularly John St James, Richard Ratzlaff, and above all Len Husband, who encouraged us from the beginning.

ESSAYS IN HONOUR OF MICHAEL BLISS:
FIGURING THE SOCIAL

# Introduction:
# Michael Bliss and the Delicate
# Balance of Individual and Society

E.A. HEAMAN

Michael Bliss was in on the early development of social history in Canada, and it was something that drew students to him. His was not the social history of large bodies of statistics, impersonality, and the Annales school, but the social history of ideas, events, activities, people's lives. Social history initially was a promise of opening up areas neglected by constitutional and national historians – it would explore the history of all of society, all members of society, and where it touched on politics, or diplomacy, or constitutionalism, it would be a social history of these political activities. While purists might trace the lineage of social history from leftist intellectual traditions and from sociology, for many, social history served primarily as a banner or rallying point for those not interested in high politics and without any particular political or methodological leanings. If the category 'social history' lacked definition from this perspective, it was also unclear just what distinguished politics from society. If politics was defined in the narrow sense as constitution-making in the backrooms by the boys, that wasn't social history, but if politics was more widely defined as the things that are politicized in social relationships and formally debated about the way that peoples hang together or fall apart, or even simply as a concern for power and inequality, as political historians began to argue, well, perhaps political and social history weren't so far apart.[1]

Bliss's earliest work was in the social ideas of the Methodist Church.[2] This was the topic of his major research essay during his MA studies, done for a seminar with Donald Creighton, and it was his initial PhD project. But after he had completed his courses and reading work, he found he no longer wanted to study churchmen and was more interested in the new American work on business history. It was not a big shift: both the churches and the businessmen were grappling with the same sorts of problems, including the rise of organized labour, the emergence of social science, and the First World War. There was also a one-off paper, published midway through his PhD thesis, on pre-Freudian sexual ideas in Canada. The piece amounted to an exploration of public discourse about the intimate self, but Bliss definitively turned away from this sort of analysis and more squarely towards the business history that made his reputation: his doctoral dissertation, published as *A Living Profit* (1974), which surveyed the ideas of businessmen around the turn of the century (and earned him a tenure-track position at the University of Toronto even before its completion) and then a more focused examination of the ideas and practices of one businessman, Joseph Flavelle, pork butcher extraordinaire (*A Canadian Millionaire*, 1978). This was an important transition. The developing scholarly work on public discourses about the intimate self tended to identify an invasion of the self and discourses about the self by experts and authorities. It is exemplified by the work of Michael Foucault and Ian Hacking, whose studies of psychiatrists – and other experts – amounted to an attack on the autonomy of the liberal self, an attack that has laid the foundation for much of postmodernity's war on certainty.[3] If there isn't a solid, grounded self, then it would seem to be discourse, not people, who are in control of events.

But this was a conclusion Michael Bliss had already rejected in his philosophy studies: he didn't like the reflexivity of modern philosophy. He distrusted the certainties of the old grand narratives, but he didn't want to discard them wholesale either. He moved from philosophy into history because he liked history's matter-of-fact empiricism, its interest in particular historical problems rather than grand sweeping generalizations about humanity. So, it was entirely in character that he would move from intellectual history – first of psychosocial discourses, then of the discourse of businessmen – to the study of individuals who had actualized their discourses in some important fashion. And more than actualized: who had actually done something useful with them. Flavelle was a fascinating character because he was somehow bigger and better than either business or religious discourses of the day. He rose to the top because he never let himself be fooled by comforting complacencies. He wasn't lulled into professional or religious certainties, but rather eyed the market with his own canny eye, his own formula for success, one that could not be reduced to some sort of generalizeable formula, to the consternation of other investors who kept losing money where he kept making it, even in the face of the stock-market collapse of 1929.

The biography of Flavelle was good social history because one learned a great deal about the times as well as the life of the man. The account was rooted in profound knowledge of local Ontario and international business, of the local and national nature of Ontario politics, of Methodism, of the First World War, and so on. Bliss told the tale easily and expansively, but the hero was never dissolved into his context and he was a quintessential Bliss hero in this respect. Even when unfairly made a pariah, Flavelle remained the master of his fate, the captain of his soul. Notoriously, Flavelle damned wartime profiteering and was then discovered to have prospered rather handsomely during the war. Flavelle did not immolate himself, as some soldiers were indeed immolating themselves at the front, and so perhaps self-immolation wasn't too much to ask for in the midst of a total war, but beyond that extremely high standard, Bliss implied, Flavelle behaved well. The lesson here, perhaps, was that prophets are without honour in their own country, and if you must rely on the popular press to do your work, you are well advised not to let it influence your sense of self, and not to let public disagreement and disapproval make any difference either way.

Bliss next turned to insulin, producing his most successful and famous book. *The Discovery of Insulin* (1982) brought the story of insulin to a worldwide audience both in and out of the academy. This was something of a new departure, but as we have seen, he had already broached medical history in his earliest writings and he was, moreover, very familiar with early-twentieth-century Canadian medicine, having watched his father practise it. He read a book on exploration that traced the explorers' steps almost one footfall at a time, and wondered if the same could be done for a medical discovery – each advance, each regression recorded and described almost as if Michael Bliss himself had been in the lab watching each move. In this book, as in the Flavelle book, Bliss drew on an extraordinarily rich collection of sources: the lab notebooks, as well as letters and interviews, conveyed all the steps and missteps, the collaboration and the quarrels.

This was a fascinating story – four very imperfect human beings, with greater or lesser mastery of the science needed to make the famous discovery, and the famous discovery itself – one of the greatest triumphs of modern medicine, saving many, many people, most of them children, from slow and agonizing death. Bliss liked writing about the redemption of humanity.[4] Amidst all the uncertainties of intellectual discourse, here was certainty with a vengeance. Insulin was a good thing that even the most postmodern contrarian, even the vivisectionist, could hardly deny had a positive cost-benefit ratio.

How these flawed humans ever managed to come up with it – there was the other fascination of the tale. There was Banting, a man who, it would be fair to say, had far less mastery of science than Flavelle had of pork-butchering, aided by a student assistant and a junior biochemist with a 'bathtub chemistry' style of brewing extracts, while the one knowledgeable and experienced scientist, J.J.R. Macleod, stood back and radiated disapproval most of the time. The kinds of things that social historians of science primarily focus on – transmission of a discovery across space and time – in this case study were all but ignored and made to seem almost frictionless. But the discovery itself recapitulated all the difficulties of human beings in society, trying and failing to get along most of the time. While Bliss bypassed the explicit theoretical discussions that preoccupied historians and sociologists of science, this book made its way onto bibliographies and syllabi as a powerful and highly readable illustration of the social negotiations that shape laboratory life. And that same fascination propels the reader through the biography of Banting that followed in fairly short order (1984). Again, here was a man who made his own history, more or less by the seat of his pants. He never became a great scientist, but still Bliss saw much to admire in the transition that Banting made from dyslexic rural kid to Nobel laureate to national director of medical science.

The next three books were all of larger scope: a survey of five centuries of Canadian business (*Northern Enterprise*, 1987), a study of the smallpox epidemic in Montreal in 1885 (*Plague*, 1991), and a survey of Canadian prime ministers from Confederation (*Right Honourable Men*, 1994). The first and the last were nation-building books, attempts to describe the formulation of a Canadian national community. Like Donald Creighton, Bliss told the story in two stages, first describing the epic of nationhood through an examination of Canadian business and businessmen, then producing a top-down, biographical, history of politics.[5] Like Banting, the businessmen had as many failures as they had successes, but nonetheless theirs was a success story. And if businessmen were successful, it was because they made their own success. The conclusion of *Northern Enterprise*, like that of *A Living Profit*, expressed a sympathy and respect for his subjects, the businessmen, that seemed greater than his respect for his contemporaries: 'Many Canadian businessmen, who lived in a world of constantly changing

*Right Honourable Men* was a book poised midway between the individual and society – it was national history organized around a series of biographies, but the formulation was not intellectually satisfactory. It conveyed the rise of popular agency, but the biographical focus prevented any serious discussion of how that transition occurred. Trudeau, he argued, transferred power to the people while discovering for himself the limits of government action – but there was little on the extent to which Trudeau's hand was forced by the emergence of gay rights, second-wave feminism, growing aboriginal militancy, and the like. Nor could Bliss properly explore the full capacity for choice and agency among the prime ministers themselves – not in anything like the depth he had enjoyed in his biographies, and without that depth, there really wasn't more than the skeleton of an argument about agency. And perhaps Bliss was somewhat repelled by the demands of public life on his subjects and, conceivably, on himself. People who sought to direct the public, and to save it from itself, found themselves too dependent on its whims. If there were a model for authentic human existence, it would not be found among public men. And neither, perhaps, would it be found among public historians; perhaps specialized scholarship was a better way of conveying the claims of history to the public. After all, Bliss had never had any difficulty selling his specialized studies to the wider or at least the educated public.

After *Right Honourable Men*, Bliss turned from public and political history to the study of men who achieved greatness in their own field of medicine and became public figures only indirectly. They were more sheltered from the fickleness and fashions of the public than were politicians because they had, first and foremost, the admiration of educated professional men whose opinions in these matters were worth having. His next two books (and final ones to date) were biographies of heroic men who had helped to usher in medical modernity: Sir William Osler (1999) and Harvey Cushing (2005).

One important observation to be made of these books is their place in the overall trajectory: Bliss describes them as forming part of a quadrilogy that recounts the history of modern medicine. First, we have the pre-modern world of smallpox, a world, one is tempted to say, lit only by fire, and not yet enlightened by modern medicine. Second, the reader sees the development of sound general medicine in North America in the person of Osler, a man who learned the best of old-world medicine in Europe and brought it to North America, ending his days as Regius Professor of Medicine at Oxford. Then there was Cushing, a

markets, accountability, and relentless measurement of success or failure, seemed more aware of these challenges than either politicians or the public at large. With exceptions, Canadian businessmen supported the lifting of the dead hand of past policies, so they could be free to compete, expand, and maximize the wealth and opportunities available to the Canadian people.'[6] And so did Michael Bliss, who came out strongly in support of the free trade agreement of the late 1980s, unlike most intellectuals.

Businessmen like Flavelle were comparable to scientists like Banting: when they got it right, they improved the lot of mankind. So too did the politicians – politicians whom Bliss surveyed in his one work of political history, *Right Honourable Men*. But often they did not get it right. Some were incompetent, others were too far removed from public opinion, still others too much in thrall to it, so that they gave in to demands like those of ethnic nationalism that could only weaken national politics. The story was one of the descent of politics, by which Bliss meant the descent of agency, from the backroom boys to the general public, increasingly broadly defined as the whole community of people in Canada, regardless of race or gender. There was also some suggestion of creeping incompetence (Brian Mulroney, he declared, would have made a good mayor of Boston), but Bliss also testified to the enormous competence of such twentieth-century prime ministers as Mackenzie King and Trudeau.

This was not his best or most convincing book. It was the product of a fit of bad conscience. Bliss's Creighton Lecture of 1991 had identified a crisis of Canadian political nationality (subsequent to the failure of the Meech Lake Accord) that was, at least in part, due to the abnegation of Canadian historians who tunnelled into their own specialist molehills and ignored the comings and goings of Canada writ large. The book was Bliss's attempt to remedy the crisis identified in his Creighton Lecture. It was meant to make people a little more familiar with and hopeful about Canadian politics at the top, and most certainly was not written for Canadian academics, who were, largely, deaf or hostile to his observations. Bliss suggested that the academics had permitted the country to drift towards imminent collapse. In fact, for many, this was a principled position. At the conference on the history of the Department of History at the University of Toronto held earlier the same day as the Creighton Lecture, invited speakers representing regional, labour, and gender history among other approaches, some of them trained at Toronto, delivered papers that pre-emptively criticized national history and defended their varieties of social history. This was as much a debate about pedagogy as it was about the writing of history – some speakers recalled their experiences as students in developing fields and others surveyed the overall performance of the department in these fields. Following one such paper that criticized the conservative tone of the history taught at Toronto, Michael Bliss stood up and observed that the students had probably taught one another more than they had ever learned from the faculty, and that this was in the nature of things.

Some greeted the confrontation and the debates that it set off as signs of healthy disagreement; others were deeply disturbed by them. The message of some leftist speakers – better that historians abandon nationalism altogether than social history – was greeted with nodding approval by many of the current graduate students in the audience, but with open dismay by the department's alumni who had been invited back to their old school to reflect on its past and future and who raised trembling hands in the air to register their concern for history and for the nation. Bliss's paper was published in the *Journal of Canadian Studies* alongside two papers taking a critical view of the call for a return to national history; all remain staple readings in the Canadian field for comprehensive exams.[7]

While Bliss carefully did not repudiate social history in his lecture, there were grounds nonetheless for seeing his larger intellectual argument as a repudiation of social history. That lingering distrust of public opinion found in *Northern Enterprise* also permeated *Right Honourable Men*. It was also fully and squarely expressed in the book he published between these two: *Plague*. There was some surprise and even shock at Bliss's insistence, in that book and in papers he gave at the time, that many leaders of opinion in French-Canadian Montreal – politicians and priests as well as unreconstructed physicians – were wrong in opposing vaccines. While sympathetic towards the victims of the epidemic, most of them children, Bliss blamed their culture for the recalcitrance shown towards scientific modernity. This view was unexceptionable in scientific and medical circles, but it defied a generation of history writing on the left hostile to the totalizations and abstractions of scientific modernity and sympathetic to peoples who had resisted it even at such high costs. Bliss's business history had always put him on the side of capitalism and modernity, against the leftists who saw these as causing more problems than solutions for marginalized peoples, but now the attack was more frontal and it was well understood to be such. Bliss became

something of a pariah in progressive academic circles, and if, Flavelle, he wasn't entirely blameless, again like Flavelle he simply ried on with his work and interests. The national newspaper-read public devoured Bliss's writings and arguments enthusiastica throughout the 1990s and he became a prominent public commentat while at the university undergraduates flocked to his classes and, for t most part, listened enraptured.

Bliss was unsympathetic to leadership – be it regional or national when that leadership led the public astray. A similar indictment for resis tance to economic modernization could be found in *Northern Enterpris* where Bliss condemned the 'billions' poured into 'dying industries an firms … particularly in Quebec and the Maritimes.'[8] Likewise, in *Righi Honourable Men*, Bliss seemed discomfited at the extent to which discourses – of ethnic nationalism, regionalism, and all the other isms that the Canadian nation is heir to – seemed to get the better of just about everyone, even men like Pearson or Trudeau, who had begun from promising internationalist or anti-nationalist and liberal positions and had descended into impotence or populism. To some, Bliss's histories and above all his national history came close to sharing the Ontario-centric view of his early teacher, Donald Creighton. In a paper addressing the continuing debate raised by Bliss's Creighton Lecture, John Dickinson, a professor at the Université de Montréal, observed that 'the existence of a universally accepted national vision of Canada's past is the figment of southern Ontario's imagination.'[9]

Bliss seems to have come to something like the same conclusion from different grounds. He was rapidly losing enthusiasm for the theme of pan-Canadian nationalism. *Right Honourable Men* was not fully successful because Bliss had lost faith in the subjects of the book – the prime ministers – and he didn't really like to write books about subjects he didn't like. Yes, some people came out well, like Mackenzie King, but mostly for his shiftiness and prevarication – this was hardly a positive model for action, hardly an example of the spirit that won Nobel prizes or built up national wealth. Politicians hadn't come out well in the previous books and they could hardly come out well now. The message was even clearer in the book's second edition, which concluded (Bliss generally shows his hand in his conclusions) that, in contemporary Canada, everyone was simply going on with their private lives. Bliss had set out to write the history of some sort of common public and national identity in Canada and had found, as with Oakland, there was no there there.

virtuoso neurosurgeon who turned his back on the old world and transformed the new in his own image, so that ambitious European surgeons began to come to America for training. Finally, there was the discovery of insulin, which, even more than Cushing's neurosurgery, exemplified the best that modern medical science could offer.

Osler was an immensely appealing character to write about for someone like Michael Bliss. For several years he urged students to take up Osler as a thesis topic, and when none did, Bliss finally took on the task. Osler's importance was, above all, as a teacher. Bringing students into the wards, he made teaching practical and he fused more closely together pathology and medicine, which had remained all too separate in the curriculum and in ordinary practice. Osler was one of the greatest physicians and greatest writers in the medical-history canon. His most important publication, *The Principles and Practice of Medicine*, did not advance medical science so much as it codified what was known and frankly admitted all that wasn't known. Osler was not an important laboratory scientist, but he was an important popularizer of science, mediating between the laboratory men, the general practitioners, and the general public. He was to medicine as Santa is to Christmas: a genial public face, and in Osler's case an enormously humanist one, with deep and affectionate knowledge of history and literature, something that he conveyed to his devoted students. Equally important, I think, was the fact that Osler was a teacher. Like all good social historians, Bliss remains interested in the transmission of ideas, models of behaviour, and practices from person to person, but Bliss's interest is primarily in intentional acts of communication and reception, like that of teaching, rather than the unintentional ways that we imbibe and transmit popular discourses.

Good students can and eventually do defy their teachers, and that was Cushing's genius: to know that he was better than what European teachers had to offer him and to set new standards of surgical investigation and boldness that created that most difficult and specialized medical field, neurosurgery. Here, at last, was the finest model that Bliss could find of someone who made their own history on their own terms. Like Banting, he was a flawed human being, more flawed than Osler, on whom Bliss could find no flies or warts, but nonetheless Cushing was the greater scientist and, therefore, the greater model of human freedom – in the sense of both individual self-determination and also the self-determination of the human species to overcome physical constraints. Freedom is one way to define this trajectory;

authority is another. Science has more moral authority in the world than business or politics, and it deserves respect, respect that Michael Bliss pays to it and urges upon readers. This might be the final answer that Michael Bliss would give to postmodern scholars who claim that there is no certain knowledge: yes there is, and those who repudiate it are no better than the uneducated, misled Montrealers who denied their children vaccination at the height of the smallpox epidemic.

So, here we have a certain way of doing history, Michael Bliss's way: the beginnings marked by a concern for the social, for questions about how behaviour occurs in society, the later years marked by a greater fascination with the way that behaviour is not constrained by society but transcends its context and achieves some sort of self-determination. Bliss isn't the first to undergo this sort of intellectual voyage – it is Rousseau's, for example, from early discovery that society reshapes men's natures to the later works on education and solitude as avenues to personal freedom.

The delicate balance of individual and society was tipped, ultimately, in favour of the individual. This is not to say that social history disappears from the tale – but it becomes subordinate to biography as a ruling framework. It is also subordinate to biography as a way of making sense of the life. In this respect, Michael Bliss's use of biography is very different from, for example, Brian Young's in his biography of George-Étienne Cartier, a man primarily understood through his status and engagements as a Montreal bourgeois.[10] Nonetheless, Bliss has continued to write books that are very much of the 'life and times' and convey a great deal of rich social history – albeit primarily the social life of the medical school or the university or the hospital, with decreasing attention to social relations radiating out from those core institutions.

What does 'social' mean here? It is impossible not to conclude, from the writings of Michael Bliss, that 'the social' is not a rigorous explanatory category. In so far as it is a rigorous explanatory category for scholars, including some published here, it must provide adequate determination for action. Flavelle or Banting or Cushing or Osler went to grade school because that's what small children did – that's the sort of explanation that social historians seek and that Michael Bliss eschews in his accounts. The kinds of decisions that interest him are precisely those least likely to be determined by what the general mass of humanity might do in the same circumstances as those of his subject. And that same reluctance to relinquish exquisite individuality is also, perhaps, central to his lifelong disinterest in national history. Michael Bliss does, on occasion, develop or draw upon generalizations about how Canadians behave (for example, he has observed several times that they tend to show respect for constituted authority) or about people living in one region of Canada rather than another, or people living in one century rather than another. But this kind of generalizing is more likely to be found in his occasional pieces.

If social history occupied a diminishing role in the oeuvre of Michael Bliss, what of the profession at large, and what particularly of his students, many of whom were drawn to work with him precisely for his early reputation as a social historian? The history of social history in Canada has been roughly sketched by historians like Carl Berger and A.B. McKillop,[11] but it has not been told in any sort of chronological fashion with reference to teaching, even though most historians are taught to do what they do. The editors have collected these essays by former students of Michael Bliss, in a festschrift, as a contribution to the continuing debate about the extent to which the advent of social history has led to intellectual fragmentation and incoherence. This is a practical question relating to patterns of education, but it has not been so analysed by Canadian historians. Traditional intellectual history, after the model of Arthur Lovejoy's history of ideas, tended to trace the development of an idea from a previous one. Under the influence of Thomas Kuhn and Michel Foucault, many intellectual historians currently emphasize rupture and discontinuity between ideas. This approach would tend to emphasize fragmentation and incoherence among different subdisciplines of history. But what precisely is meant by incoherence has not been seriously explored in terms of Canadian history.

The complaint of intellectual impoverishment through specialization is a venerable one, with many extant versions. It is found, for example, in Adam Smith, who deplored the intellectual effects of concentration on narrow tasks in urban factories; in nineteenth-century humanists, who decried the narrow, self-interested scope that practical education and a practical life of business gave to the middle classes; and among the great generalist physicians of Osler's day, who were perplexed and repelled by new medical and surgical theories and practices emerging from specialist hospitals outside of their spheres of influence. The first kind of narrowness relies on an almost physical understanding of the process of cogitation. The second is primarily a moral criticism. The third approaches epistemological theory and can be assimilated with Thomas Kuhn's 1962 argument for scientific paradigms that reflect scholarly communities and that are mutually incomprehensible to one another.

Kuhn rejected the notion that scientific improvements occurred through the improvement of existing knowledge and instead argued that important new discoveries required new ways of thinking, ways that could not be translated to scientists outside of that paradigm.[12] Without following the philosophical debate that continues to rage over the meaning of 'incomprehensible' and 'translation' in this context, I will note the attention Kuhn pays to the role that textbooks and pedagogy play in creating distinctive styles of scientific thought. Textbooks, Kuhn argues, tend to erase alternative or prior modes of thinking and to teach students to reason or to solve problems only in one particular way. Other forms of pedagogy such as exams – including comprehensive examinations for doctoral students – could conceivably perform much the same function for advanced history students and could, therefore, serve as the gateway to broad or narrow conceptions of what counts as good history.

Michael Bliss taught and wrote upon a few basic historical themes – medicine, business, and politics – in analyses that were alternatively framed as large-scale societal events or as individual life stories. In his own academic career, he moved from one special subject to another, showing a certain defiance of narrow academic boundaries. Was this defiance sustainable in the next generation of historians whom he taught? I would suggest that if we approach the writing of social history from a biographical perspective – through the life writings of Michael Bliss and his students – the limitations of the 'incoherence' model quickly become apparent. It is entirely possible to write the history of a subdiscipline, such as medical history or military history, as an autonomous area of inquiry, not uninfluenced by broader trends in social history, but nonetheless possessing an internal coherence, a set of problems, methods, and a vocabulary, all its own. One could also point to key textbooks as helping to formulate that special set of characteristics. Timothy Cook's recent history of authorized war histories in Canada provides an outstanding example of just such an inquiry into a special field.[13] But such an approach cannot prove incoherence or even fragmentation: it cannot prove that the fields and the scholars within them are alienated from one another. Some scholars do follow narrow trajectories all their lives. But most do not. Most read widely and write for diverse and multiple audiences – sometimes serially, and sometimes simultaneously. A historiographical survey that eschewed textbook formulations and instead followed the intellectual trajectories of individual scholars, through the choices they make from one year and one decade to the next, would be far more likely to prove intellectual continuity and coherence rather than alienation. In this collection, which brings together some recent writings by Michael Bliss's students, it becomes possible to assess the extent to which some of the different branches of Canadian history continue to 'speak to' one another by sharing techniques, problems, and vocabularies, even as they may differ enormously in their choice of subjects or their political orientation or their targeted audience. Such a collection can show moral and intellectual continuity even as its contents branch into such ostensibly discrete fields as medical history, business history, and religious history.

Ultimately, 'all the chickens come home to roost.' This phrase is borrowed from Charles Taylor, the foremost philosopher of the modern self, who has used it to counter the arguments from postmodern scholars in favour of a fragmented series of selves and the absence of a core being. Here, the chickens are the students of Michael Bliss, all trained at the University of Toronto and then fanning out to the different regions of the country. In this collection, the roost is not the sheltering wings of their old professor: Michael Bliss does not, himself, lend personal coherence to the work of his students. Rather, all are sheltered in the 'roost' of history, even of social history, albeit a social history that has acquired new techniques, concerns, and languages from some of the subfields that it has helped to spawn.

The remainder of this introduction will say a few words about the intellectual trajectories of Michael Bliss's students, drawing upon the essays published here and also upon past works and especially their PhD dissertations. While I cannot do justice to their full range of scholarly concerns, I hope to outline some general lines of development and to formulate some conclusions as to what their work tells us about the way Canadian history has developed over the last three decades. The scholars published here may not be representative of the full range of Canadian historiography, but they are not far off that breadth either.[14] They do not represent any one school of history – Michael Bliss wasn't that sort of a teacher – but rather the richness and complexity of historiographical choices made during the 1970s, 1980s, and 1990s.

Not all the contributors here write as social historians. Some – including Michael Bliss himself – provide personal reminiscences. Another assesses Michael Bliss's performance on the contemporary journalistic scene. Such contributions do not stray from the path of objectivity and analysis, but rather bring to bear on their diverse topics analytic skills honed at the University of Toronto. Good history-writing, indeed good writing of any sort, requires a certain amount of common sense and psychological insight, a recognition as to how the personal and the public relate to one another in past and present lives, as well as the more obvious need for facility with factual information. These investigations of personal agency and scope share subject and method with some of the investigations into family and biography also presented here. But most contributors provide historical studies, on topics relat-. ing to their scholarly interests. And just as Michael Bliss displayed a range of political engagements and voices during his varied career, so do the scholars represented here. Political stripes are more or less prominently on display, as authors weigh economic influences against political ones, public opinion against elite leadership or specialized knowledge, and survey the collision of states, experts, and families. These are the sort of big questions that underpin public debates about 'whither the nation,' and authors give them their due, albeit in a style and a language that reflect their years of sober training in the fashioning of knowledge.

Doctoral training is a complex process, intended on the one hand to maximize independence of judgment, on the other to ensure that candidates meet strict disciplinary standards of rigour. At the University of Toronto, throughout the period from the 1960s to the end of the century, students completed a year of course work and then spent months preparing for comprehensive examinations, both written and oral, based on their mastery of about two hundred books. Only after this gruelling preparatory work was completed were they sent off to research and write their dissertations on the topic of their choosing. The history department at the University of Toronto was proud of its tradition of leaving students to develop their dissertations largely by themselves, to find their own level and place in the profession.[15] Michael Bliss appreciated having so much latitude in his own intellectual development, and he tried to give his students the same latitude or 'benign neglect.' Students were left to sink or swim. Not all of them saw the process through to completion; several fell by the wayside. Where there was no useful meeting of minds, the student either went off to work with someone else (and some of his successful students worked informally but intensely with other professors) or they dropped out of the program entirely. Thus, though the process permitted diversity and disagreement, there were also considerable pressures in favour of conformity, consensus, and self-censorship on the part of students.

The preparation for the comprehensive exams required the student to read through a canon of Canadian historical writing. The contents of the canon changed considerably over the years – when Bliss was a student, the students mostly read political and constitutional history. This was true even in the seminars and fields done with the younger teachers in the department, Ramsay Cook and Robert Craig Brown, because there was little else to read, although these men encouraged their students to investigate a broader range of research topics for their own writings. Michael Bliss recalled attending an extremely vibrant seminar led by Ramsay Cook in 1966–7 with brilliant and engaged fellow students, including Mary Vipond, Paul Rutherford, and David Bercuson. By the time he began teaching and supervising senior students himself, Bliss was thoroughly receptive to the wider possibilities of reading and writing Canadian history. As the editor for the Social History of Canada series, he was seen to be at the forefront of social history in Canada, and that proved a powerful draw to students. Remembering and approving of his own supervisors' openness to novelty in history, Bliss invited his students themselves to suggest the kinds of topics they would like to investigate for seminars. At one such seminar, when a young Veronica Strong-Boag suggested a week of readings on women, he added it to the curriculum. These advanced seminars continued to resonate with palpable excitement, according to Strong-Boag, as extremely strong students, including Gregory Kealey, John Dickinson, Bruce Tucker, and Craig Heron, debated the pros and cons of the old history and the new. Notoriously, when she proposed to take up a topic relating to women for her PhD thesis, he advised her that there was 'no future in women's history.' But he also told her plainly that he was willing to supervise any topic she chose and, consequently, did supervise to defence her thesis on the National Council of Women of Canada.[16] Strong-Boag made a brilliant future for herself in women's history: she was a pioneer of the field and remains one of its most prominent, exacting, and readable practitioners.

For Veronica Strong-Boag, the raison d'être of history is, first and foremost, social justice. History is, for her, an act of reparation. In writing history, one is exercising power, a power traditionally monopolized by elite white men to the considerable benefit of elite white men. But enlightened and conscientious historians should write history that includes the oppressed and the vulnerable and that explains how the lines of power and influence have been drawn. Strong-Boag's presidential address before the Canadian Historical Association in 1994 was directed in part to Michael Bliss's Creighton Lecture, in part to other nationalist historians, particularly Jack Granatstein, who had been rather more hostile to social history. She complained that established history was still dominated by the old traditions and that it failed 'to interrogate power relations and address the reality of oppression within Canadian society,' a failure particularly manifest in its treatment of women, race, class, and also of children. She summed up her positive conclusions as follows:

> When historians expand their vision, through an acknowledgement of privilege and the creation of a pluralistic community of scholars, we will be a good deal closer to coming to terms with Canadian life. This is the first step towards constructing ways of living together, whatever their exact constitutional form, that no longer require some voices to be disadvantaged while others are allowed to monopolize decision-making about what constitutes truth, citizenship and identity.[17]

Both Bliss and Strong-Boag saw a role for history in reconstructing the Canadian polity to make it more informed and tolerant, but their sense of the immediate priorities were apparently very different, with Bliss concerned to save some sort of a master narrative and Strong-Boag arguing that, based on past evidence, master narratives marginalized large groups of Canadians and so should probably be sacrificed in favour of pluralism and egalitarianism. Her primary concern is with the history of power – relationships of power determine who should be studied and how, and the goal of the historian is to identify and correct imbalances and abuses of power. By contrast, Bliss's concern has always been with authority rather than power. Here authority might be defined as earned power: that is, the particular combination of knowledge, skill, and judgment that particular individuals developed and that, along with action, earned them a wider hearing. Imbalances of power reflect, to some degree at least, imbalances of ability, reason, judgment. Bliss probably would not deny that there is also a great deal of unearned power at large in the world, but his actions suggest he doesn't feel personally obliged to address it as a problem. One can account for one person's earned authority by writing their biography; one cannot address their unearned authority without undertaking a sociological treatise full of the kind of generalizations that Bliss has sought to eschew in his scholarly writing. I suspect that he views these sorts of generalisations in much the same light as the grand political narratives of yore: both require too much faith in the scholarship of one's colleagues.

Strong-Boag has been one of the leading scholars to disseminate the message for social justice, but she is far from bearing the message alone. Another early leftist student of Bliss who has spent a lifetime writing progressive political . arguments is James Struthers, who, in 1979, defended a thesis, later published as a book with the same title, 'No Fault of Their Own: Unemployment and the Canadian Welfare State 1911–1941.'[18] Both Bliss and Struthers seem to recall with some fondness arguments raging back and forth across the seminar table about the extent to which the state could or should be called forward to redress economic inequalities within society. Qua pundit, Michael Bliss has always taken a conservative position on these questions, though it is not one that features prominently in his historical monographs and articles. Struthers, by contrast, is particularly concerned to make the argument for state protection for the economically disadvantaged – in this collection, for veterans, who serve here as a synechdoche for the elderly in Canada. Should the state be cleaning peoples' curtains? The question may sound beyond the realms of public discourse, but Struthers's careful analysis of the program of home-care for veterans shows that there was once a lively public debate on exactly this question. The piece might further seem to suggest that politicians should seriously consider extending such services to an aging population more generally. As one might expect of a student of Michael Bliss, Struthers pays close attention to the respective claims of economic efficiency and social concern, suggesting that they may not here be in competition.

Where Strong-Boag's attention has come to focus on the young, Struthers's concern has been transferred to the elderly, especially the dependent elderly. Between them they analyse both the earned entitlements and the unearned, natural needs of Canadian peoples. Their essays in this collection provide outstanding examples of progressive, politically inspired social history. Both pry into the private life of Canadians, a private life that can be described, for the most part, as 'hidden from history,' because of the difficulty in finding sources not only about domestic life, but also about the most shameful and private acts of that domestic life. Thus, Bliss, Struthers, and Strong-Boag all investigate private life, but where Bliss focuses on one or two exceptional and ungeneralizeable examples, Struthers and Strong-Boag want to know what kinds of norms and practices govern ordinary behaviour throughout the population as a whole, throughout the country as a whole. Both, therefore, write national history, but a *social* national history that completely reverses national history's focus on the known and public actions of the few.

If the dearth of good, analytical writing about a given subject amounted to a political argument for its reconsideration, then there was a good political argument to be made in favour of the social history of business in the 1970s. Businessmen, unlike the dependent elderly or children, had a loud and indeed perhaps monopolistic voice over the mainstream, national media at the time, but searching historical analysis of their arguments and claims were lacking. One did not have to be a leftist intellectual to take up a neglected topic, and Michael Bliss has drawn a wide variety of students to business history. In 1978 Bruce Wilson wrote a thesis, later turned into a monograph, 'The Enterprises of Robert Hamilton: A Study of Wealth and Influence in Early Upper Canada, 1776–1812.' Wilson had done most of his work with Michiel Horn, but when Horn departed for Dalhousie University, Michael Bliss supervised the dissertation in its final stages. This was a well-rounded investigation into the connection between commerce, politics, and personal influence on the early frontier.[19] Wilson produced more historical work as well as archival resources before his death in the late 1990s. In 1982 Ben Forster defended a thesis on the development of the Canadian National Policy, that is, John A. Macdonald's protectionist tariff of 1879. Like Bliss, he cast a sceptical eye on the clamourings of the businessmen and industrialists, and argued that the tariff reflected not their self-professed weakness but rather their political and economic strength.[20] In this collection Forster takes up the prehistory of the tariff again in order to demolish the nation-building arguments that, he suggests, have distorted economic and political history. Scrutinizing the policies and politics of A.T. Galt in particular, he finds scant evidence for economic nationalism before Confederation and, rather, a more universalist ethos tempered by a streak of opportunism. The article exemplifies the best of the new national history: in exploring high politics, it rejects Creightonesque teleologies that would have some sort of preformed Canadian essence shaping the development of the nascent political community.

In her dissertation (deposited in 1988 and published in 1990), using an approach that owed much to Bliss's work on Flavelle, Joy Santink analysed the techniques that made Timothy Eaton a successful business-man.[21] Also written in the spirit of objective investigation of the relations between businessmen and politicians were the dissertations defended by Gene Allen in 1991 on 'The Origins of the Intercolonial Railway, 1835–1869' and John Turley-Ewart in 2000 on 'Gentlemen Bankers, Politicians, and Bureaucrats: The History of the Canadian Bankers Association, 1891–1924.' While the latter two dissertations remain unpublished, taken all together these productions add up to an impressive collection of writings about the development of Canadian business and its invariably close connection to politics. They share the stage with a number of other historians writing about the history of business, and particularly the more overtly Marxist school around Peter Baskerville at the University of Victoria and Graham D. Taylor at Dalhousie University, co-authors of a rival *Concise History of Business in Canada*, published in 1994.[22]

Both Turley-Ewart and Allen have moved from business history to journalism, being involved in the national media. Turley-Ewart remains passionately devoted to the public sphere in Canada, writing for the *National Post*, and on the occasion of Michael Bliss's retirement he penned a passionate apologia for his teacher's contribution to the national public interest. For this collection, he provides a more searching inquiry into how Bliss became a public writer of stature and influence, a development that he locates within a particular concatenation of political and professional circumstances during the 1980s. Michael Bliss wrote his books for the wider public and, as Turley-Ewart shows, he defended the wisdom of that wider public against the scornful and scandalous rhetoric and practices of political pundits.

Gene Allen has gone on to teach the history of the Canadian media at Ryerson University. The work he presents here seeks to identify the influence that business, in this case through the commercialization of the Canadian media, has exercised on public discourse. While he acknowledges his intellectual debt to Michael Bliss, his work is nonetheless strikingly different from Bliss's early investigations. He identifies his field as business history overlapping with *cultural* history. Where Bliss treated newspapers and journals as largely transparent vessels for ideas, Allen investigates the content of the form: the ways in which information has been 'gathered, organized, and made available,' all of which features emerge as coequal with the actual ideas expressed. This kind of investigation is not unrelated to the approach Veronica Strong-Boag advocates, with its concern for access to and control of discourse as something to be studied in its own right.

Other students who came to work with Bliss were drawn by his very earliest work on the Methodist Church, the only piece of his ever published in the *Canadian Historical Review* (still the first place to which an ambitious young student sends his or her work). While George Rawlyk at Queen's University remained, into the 1990s, a powerful attraction for students interested in the history of religion in Canada, Bliss did attract two students, Brian Hogan and David Marshall, defending dissertations in the mid-1980s on the history of religious ideas – variations on the 'social history of Methodist thought' that had initially interested Bliss. Hogan was interested in Catholic social thought and action in Ontario, while Marshall wrote about Protestant secularization.[23] These were two sides of the same coin: explorations of how the churches responded to modernity, how they sought 'social relevance' within a secularizing society without themselves secularizing. While the two scholars came to different conclusions as to the success of the churchmen's endeavours in that direction, both emphasized social history. As Hogan remarked in his abstract: 'Throughout, attention is directed towards trade union, credit union and co-operative activities.' Both their contributions to this volume represent further development of their thought along these lines. Hogan continues his ambitious survey of religious thought into the twentieth century, insisting on the convergence of critical thinking about history and society and critical religious inquiry and self-inquiry. His exploration of the tension between the relentless rationalism of modern scholarship and the ineffability of religious thought seems distinctly reminiscent of Bliss's effort to find the irreducible within a field founded on reducibility. Where the concept of 'myth' haunts national history, here, in Hogan's survey of the history of religion, it is rather the concept of 'error' that haunts historians who resist notions that knowledge is, ultimately, socially constructed. Like Michael Bliss in the autobiographical essay included here, Hogan seeks a terra firma for historical knowledge, somewhere between positivism and the scorched earth of symmetry thesis. Both defend something akin to humanism.

All three authors in the section on 'Family and Religion' address love, but where Hogan is concerned about the figure of the Father, David Marshall and Veronica Strong-Boag address the father-figure and the place of love in the social construction of that figure. Strong-Boag's essay reveals that, in public and state records, love was almost invisible and that, instead, as Cynthia Commachio has observed, fatherhood 'came to be associated almost exclusively with its material aspects.' All the more valuable, therefore, is David Marshall's reliance on private correspondence for his contribution here, namely, a revealing set of letters written by the clergyman and author Charles Gordon to his much-loved son. Marshall contrasts the tortured construction of father-hood that results when historians rely on such public sources as advice manuals with the much more subtle and indeed very moving portrayals that can emerge from personal correspondence. A beautifully accomplished investigation of father-and-son relations that simultaneously illustrates and explains how one family experienced a kind of secularization, the essay represents perhaps the greatest continuity found here with the kind of history that Michael Bliss himself writes – the history of modernity refracted through intimate personal relations.

Meanwhile, Bliss's growing interest in the history of medical science was drawing students interested in the history of Canadian science and medicine. First among these was Suzanne Zeller, whose PhD thesis, defended in 1985 and published in 1987, described the role that science played in the construction of the transcontinental nation. Zeller painstakingly surveyed the development of the 'inventory sciences' in Canada: geology, botany, and meteorology, and showed how they simultaneously inhabited public and private space in Canada, forcing politicians and scholars to come to mutual terms of recognition.[24] This was a pioneering work in an undeveloped field, and her forthcoming book on the physical sciences in Canada is certain to make an even greater mark in an even more undeveloped field.

Medicine followed by business remained the dominant themes for nearly all the subsequent students of Michael Bliss. During the mid- to late 1990s came a slew of dissertations written squarely within the emerging specialized discipline of the history of medicine. The field had long been dominated by medical professionals, who were gradually sharing and then ceding place to professional historians turned out by history departments writing for other historians in departments around the world. A specialized journal for Canadian medical history was founded in the mid-1980s, and a series of Hannah professorships were established at universities around Ontario, with a few beyond Ontario. The Institute for the History and Philosophy of Science and Technology had always remained a valuable resource for students interested in science, but Bliss himself had no particular relationship with it; he formed closer working relations with the Hannah professors named to Toronto, especially Edward Shorter, who also held a position in the history department. But while the history of medicine was a growing field in Canada, many students still preferred a base inside a mainstream history department that would provide them with wider access to employment opportunities. So Bliss attracted many of these students, some of whom had done earlier undergraduate or graduate work in the history of medicine with Hannah-funded professors elsewhere; others were Canadianists drawn by Bliss's own seminar in Canadian medical history; still others owed little to academics and everything to personal experience for their interests in medical history.

In 1992 Alison Li defended her thesis on 'J.B. Collip and the Making of Medical Research in Canada'; in 1994, it was Barbara Clow's turn, defending her thesis on 'The Problem of Cancer: Negotiating Disease in Ontario, 1925–1945'; in 1995 Christopher Rutty defended his thesis 'Do Something ... Do Anything: Poliomyelitis in Canada, 1927–1967'; in 1997 Geoffrey Reaume won plaudits from examiners for his '999 Queen Street West: Patient Life at the Toronto Hospital for the Insane, 1870–1940'; in 1999 Shelley McKellar deposited her thesis 'The Career of Gordon Murray: Patterns of Change in Mid-Twentieth-Century Medicine in Canada'; and finally, in 2005 Sasha Mullally defended her thesis 'Unpacking the Black Bag: Rural Medicine in the Maritime Provinces and Northern New England States, 1900–1950.'[25]

All of these dissertations were self-confidently medical history, more specialized in that respect than that of Zeller with its bridges to high politics. Their questions and methods were overwhelmingly drawn from the growing literature in that specialized field. Under what conditions did medical research emerge? How much professional authority did doctors wield in the fight against polio or cancer? How far could a surgeon's authority carry him when he took up controversial new operations? What would a patient's history of cancer look like? What of a patient's history of an insane asylum?

Some of these historians were interested in social history; others were more interested in the way that events unfolded inside the laboratory and the university department. As medical historians sought to establish their discipline, they often brandished the label 'social historian' as a kind of battle-axe to lay waste to the internalist histories of medicine written by doctors that amounted to whiggish tales of heroic struggle, culminating in a success that followed naturally from experiments and trials done correctly and wisely. Social historians in Canada and beyond argued that social factors should be considered at every stage of the history of an invention. There were many aspects to this argument. Thomas Kuhn's definition of a scientific paradigm amounted to a social description of scientific communities with emphasis on the cultural and social reasons why a given group of scholars adopted or discarded a given hypothesis.[26] In 1982 the spokesmen for the Edinburgh 'strong' school, Barry Barnes and David Bloor, carried the argument to logical conclusions when they objected to the tendency of historians to argue that true theories were accepted for scientific and rational reasons while false theories were accepted for social reasons. Barnes and Bloor insisted that all theories should be treated symmetrically, with attention paid to social factors.[27] Classic examples of these social factors were famously provided by studies of Louis Pasteur: on the one hand by Bruno Latour, one of the founders of science studies, who examined how Pasteur managed to produce such conclusive experiments and, further, to sell those experiments as genuinely reflecting quite different events outside the laboratory, in the real world; on the other hand by Gerald Gieson's *The Private Science of Louis Pasteur*, which suggested he fudged the data, hiding unfavourable results.[28]

Michael Bliss did not respond particularly favourably to this body of literature. During an undergraduate seminar, when a graduate student tried to interject Thomas Kuhn's name into a conversation about Canadian medicine, Bliss barked, 'I won't have that name mentioned in this classroom.' Kuhn was at the forefront of the relativism and sociologization of philosophy that he had rejected early on. The Gieson book did not seem to him as scandalous as it was made out to be: similar accusations could be made of the insulin discoverers, Bliss mused, but that didn't amount to a serious debunking of their accomplishment. Bliss's work, which had never been quite squarely in the history of science and never quite found an appreciative audience among historians of science, tended to diverge from the iconoclastic accounts that were becoming mainstream in departments of medical history. During a 1994 conversation between Michael Bliss, Jacalyn Duffin, and J.T.H. Connor, published in the *Canadian Bulletin of Medical History*, Duffin observed that the 'debunking' abstracts were generally accepted for the forthcoming conference of the American Association for the History of Medicine, and the hagiographical ones rejected, while Bliss emphasized the extent to which he had 'worked very hard to counter' debunking tendencies in his recent *Banting*.[29]

Just as Bliss's students of social and business history reflected a range of political and historiographical positions, so too did those working in the field of medical history. Some were generally respectful of medical authority in the way that Bliss himself was generally respectful of medicine's accomplishments; others were unabashed iconoclasts. But it would be a mistake to characterize these theses simply along a leftist/rightist pole, because the arguments were more complex than that.

On the one hand, it is easy to identify a certain amount of respect for the hard accomplishments of medicine in the work of Alison Li, Christopher Rutty, and Shelley McKellar. All described the early history of scientific research in Canada, the laborious attempts to establish research laboratories at McGill and Toronto and to confront with science and compassion some of the most horrifying diseases and epidemics that Canadians have ever known. Rutty's work, for example, trumpeted the success of the polio vaccine, and he also insisted that effective state intervention in the early polio epidemics created expectations that led to the development of a national system of health insurance. The modern state and modern medicine mutually constituted one another, and this was, on the whole, a good thing for patients. The story of the founding of the Connaught laboratories in Toronto, which Rutty narrates here, is a one of successful accomplishment: all sorts of social and political factors went into its founding, but the fact that social factors were crucial didn't mean that the project was reducible to mere politics, as the more extreme leftist historians of science might suggest.

Li's work on Collip, later published as a monograph, was neither hagiographical nor debunking: it painstakingly described his career as reflecting the transition in Canada from little to 'big' science, with large-team investigations and expensive laboratories, quite different from the conditions in Toronto in the early 1920s. Li's was solid social history that explored the conditions for big science in such features as the modernization of the university, growing collaboration between academics and the pharmaceutical industry, and the development of research-funding agencies, as well the creation of a 'social identity' for the budding medical research community.

McKellar's study of Gordon Murray took note of Murray's many successes and talents – the lives that his inventions saved, the medical research community that he created in Toronto – again as part of a chronicle describing the early development of scientific research in Canada. She then dispassionately charted Murray's claim to have reversed spinal paralysis, an unsubstantiated claim that provoked colleagues and the public to turn against him. McKellar's account is of surgical hubris, but if Murray comes out badly, the profession as a whole comes out relatively well: his Toronto colleagues investigated the facts of the case rather than covering up for him. The press, perhaps, behaved rather badly by first exaggerating his claims and then exaggerating the critiques; Murray, perhaps, abused his professional authority in this one instance; but his colleagues reined him in. In a similar vein, in the essay that she publishes here, McKellar describes Willem Kolff's work on the artificial heart as a not unadmirable balance of humanitarianism, professional ambition, and professional caution. But she also suggests that, pace Michael Bliss, men like Kolff cannot be understood on their own terms: the success or failure of the artificial heart is bound up with broader patterns of the industralization and commercialization of modern medicine and also of the greater public's fascination with and fear of technology, especially as it invades the concept of the human and especially after such disappointments and tragedies as lobotomy, thalidomide, and rejuvenation surgery. The article exemplifies John V. Pickstone's recent argument that modern medicine is best understood as *production*, and as industrial production, rather than as skill or knowledge.[30]

To some extent, these studies were post-revisionist: when the last generation of historians has debunked, there is a certain amount of academic credit to be obtained by debunking the debunkers and taking science seriously. But there was also a more nuanced argument at work in the writings of these scholars, namely, that medical authority occurred in a wider medical marketplace shaped as much by popular and professional conceptions and misconceptions of science as by the scholarly papers and practices that once bore the burden of the hagiographic history of medicine. There was always some degree of cultural tumult around early medical science in Canada. There were alternative polio healers who flourished during the epidemics and who served a useful purpose by countering some excesses of the medical profession (such as the insistence on immobility). The endocrinology that Collip helped to found in Canada was bedevilled by popular fantasies of sexual rejuvenation and feverish interest in the possibilities of 'making fat ladies thin and old men virile.' Murray and his colleagues were themselves bedevilled by the difficulties of distinguishing between good and bad science.

The argument was made more explicitly and expansively in the work of Barbara Clow, who discovered that while '"scientific medicine" commanded considerable respect in the 1920s and '30s, regular doctors were not able to dominate the management of cancer.' Patients shopped around in what Roy Porter called the 'medical marketplace'[31] and, with scientific medicine often helpless in the face of advanced cancer (a fact that the scientific doctors themselves were loath to admit publicly), alternative healers offered much that the physicians could not, but that patients needed. Clow questioned the very idea of professional authority, arguing that the irregular 'quacks' had a share in its construction and its popularity, such as it was, with the general public. Scientific modernity didn't look so scientific or so modern, according to this account. In the essay published here, Clow shows how medical authority, and the state's precipitate rush to reliance upon it, led to a profoundly inadequate response to the disaster of thalidomyde that delayed the drug's recall and seriously underestimated the extent of the problem. In the articles by Rutty, Clow, Li, and McKellar in this volume, the ties between medical history and business history are made explicit: commercial considerations vied with patient and practitioner interests in the shaping of medical research and therapeutics.

Like the work of Clow, that of Geoffrey Reaume suggests problems that are 'hard-wired,' so to speak, to the exercise of medical authority. A psychiatric survivor himself, Reaume was, on the whole, more respectful of patient testimony than of doctors' utterances. In the face of critics who insisted that the mad, being mad, had no coherent voice to recover, Reaume defended the ultimate coherence and reasonableness of patient discourses, mad or not. He insisted that scholars must listen to these people and incorporate their concerns into a total understanding of the place of madness in society. As well as his own experience and that of his friends, Reaume also drew upon leftist theorists, particularly Karl Marx (he used to run an informal class on Marx during his PhD years) and Michel Foucault, theorists whom Bliss largely distrusted, and so Bliss's seminar rooms and offices continued to ring with lively scholarly debate. Reaume's contribution to this collection reflects his very early entry into medical history under the tutelage of Michael Bliss; his later profile includes a growing interest in disability studies, a field in which he now lectures. Reaume can be put in the same camp as Strong-Boag and Struthers as a scholar whose single greatest motivation is to identify and aid the vulnerable and the marginalized.

In 1995 and 1996 there appeared two dissertations that squatted across the disciplines of business history, the history of technology, and social history, both of them turned into monographs that grace the Engineering Library at the University of Toronto.[32] Richard White defended his thesis on 'The Civil Engineering Careers of Frank and Walter Shanly, c. 1840–1890,' and, as with many students of Bliss, immediately turned it into a monograph. This was a close case study of railways as business, and as a state-sponsored business, refracted through the intellectual, social, and economic structures of the time, but more particularly through the relationship between two brothers. In method and in general approach, this was a work that closely approximated Bliss's own work, though the coincidence was as much a reflection of particular taste as of any pedagogical plan on Bliss's part, as White's contribution here reveals. In describing his relationship with Michael Bliss, White provides a rare, candid glimpse into the transmission of knowledge and values, both overt and tacit, that occurs in the modern university.

The other dissertation, Elsbeth Heaman's 'Commercial Leviathan: Central Canadian Exhibitions at Home and Abroad during the Nineteenth Century,' was a slightly more contrarian account of agricultural and industrial fairs, taking as its central theme one not dissimilar to that of *Right Honourable Men*: the descent of historical agency from social elites to the generality of the public through such mechanisms as growing commercialism. Heaman lent some dignity to the exhibitions by linking them to such high political events as the rebellions and Confederation, but the form of analysis owed more to Foucault's models of discourse analysis than to the collective biography of *Right Honourable Men*. Both the thesis topic and the approach were met with initial (and more than initial) disapproval, but in the final days Michael Bliss could be heard reassuring a quailing ABD[33] that the results were suitable for defence. And however distinct the methods, an interest in the relations between economic and cultural history, along with the comparison of English- and French-speaking Canadians, was common to both scholars and continues to mark Heaman's work, even as she extends her investigation back into the eighteenth century.

For Heaman, as for Gene Allen in their papers submitted here, a central concern is with the materialities of communication. Newspapers (like exhibitions) were both discrete forms of communication that shaped, to no small degree, the content of the message that they were intended to convey. Indeed, all three of the essays in the 'Politics and Business' section, though they investigate different periods, squarely confront a myth, that is to say, a fictional identity or norm projected onto the public sphere and part of the fabric of 'national' history. Forster, the leading historian of tariffs in early Canada, takes on the myth of a grand 'national' policy of protectionism in the mid-nineteenth century – a myth that has helped to project the notion of an economically and ideologically connected nation back before Canadian confederation – and shows it to be a misreading of the sources, the product of hindsight. Allen also reveals a certain romanticization of the nineteenth-century public sphere when he disproves any dramatic shift from politically partisan to commercial newspaper content between 1870 and 1930. And Heaman examines the ethnic stereotype of 'ignorance' that was attributed to French Canadians in the mid-eighteenth century. She unpacks its meaning at that time by contrasting how the press and pamphleteers wrote about British and French citizens' capacities and by asking to what extent historians and philosophers conceived of a knowledgeable citizenry. All three authors carefully disentangle the relationship between politics and economics. For Heaman, the British contrast between British commercialism and French valour helped to construct the stereotype of French-Canadian ignorance. Foster and Allen likewise insist on the greater importance and pervasiveness of pragmatic economic ways of thinking at the expense of more traditionally ideological visions of politics and the public sphere. In keeping with Michael Bliss's Creighton Lecture, therefore, all three investigate national history, but their findings tend more to deconstruct it than to prop it up, and all three are rather closer, in spirit, to the early work of Michael Bliss, *A Living Profit*, with its investigation of the romantic and liberal mythologies that early Canadian businessmen foisted upon the public sphere, albeit with updated theoretical and methodological apparatus and a greater suspicion of the very notion of a public sphere.

Sasha Mullally's work on medical biography also investigates the public construction of mythological stereotypes. Her identification of substantial differences between an unpublished and a published memoir addresses the ways in which commercialization affects professional discourse, and it adds a subtle note of cultural analysis to the ongoing dissection of medical authority. Publishers excised those aspects of medical experience that they thought undermined medical authority; ironically, Mullally suggests, they excised precisely those sorts of authority – make-do bricolage – that rural doctors probably most excelled at. Medical authority here emerges as a kind of empty construct that undermined the form it actually took in the countryside.

Mullally's work is social history, but it is also cultural history. It reflects the linguistic turn in historical analysis – the discovery that the texts most historians use are inherently fictitious and made-up in important ways. Diaries aren't more reliable sources than published memoirs – they just organize their fictions differently. Whereas social history tends to look at historical subjects as physical bodies in space to be acted upon, cultural history tends to focus on the text-like qualities of people's activities and utterances, bringing all the tools of highbrow intellectual analysis to such ordinary objects as commonplace books or a patient's admission record.

Social history is far from obsolete – but increasingly shares pride of place as a central organizing field with cultural history. Both approaches enable historians to interrogate the larger cultural and social context for the local activities and practices that they investigate. Under these circumstances, it seems difficult to understand how 'social history' could be seen as a force for fragmentation. Rather it provides a set of master narratives that help new historians converge with the previous generations. No serious scholar investigating the history of business or science or politics in Canada, for example, can ignore such social factors as the industrial revolution, the growing commercialization and commodification of domestic artefacts and the media, the development of the interventionist state, the rights revolution, or the emergence of sovereign professions and academic disciplines. These are important causal factors, far more important than the national categories like 'confederation' that used to dominate explanations, to the neglect of serious analysis of cause and effect. National history insisted that science, medicine, business, and other fields all be subordinate to a certain kind of political analysis. Social history does not impose any such hierarchy, so the relations of priority can emerge from the analysis itself. Where Bliss and his students have approached national breadth, it has generally been with the utmost scepticism about the utility and truthfulness of grand national narratives.

The title of this introduction paraphrases a chapter of Carl Berger's *The Writing of Canadian History,* 'William Morton: The Delicate Balance of Region and Nation,' which argued that the relationship between these geographical categories provided a powerful tension animating W.L. Morton's prose. Similarly, the juxtaposition, contrast, and continuity between the individual and the collectivity, the self and society, animated the work of Michael Bliss and continues to animate the work of his students. In their dissertations and subsequent work, in the essays collected here, most of the authors have shown a concern with explaining large social trends through the perspective of individuals, or vice versa. Strong-Boag, for example, has collaborated on wide-ranging textbooks and a popular biography of the Mohawk poet Pauline Johnson.[34] This is not to suggest any lack of tension between the self and the social as organizing concepts. The essays tend to waver between the kind of exquisite specificity that Michael Bliss has invested in his biographies and broad generalizations about people who are all too often anonymous or identified in such fleeting terms as to be mere caricatures. Anonymity remains a profound problem for social historians – the more people one encompasses in one's study, the less about them one can convey, and so the determination to write encompassing and inclusive history can lead to a certain amount of depersonalization and objectification.

But perhaps this remains the greatest lesson that Michael Bliss has for his students and for historians generally. The most important part of history remains human beings who, justice demands, should be represented as fully as possible. Pursuit of that exquisite specificity and individuality must be, like the pursuit of objectivity, a core concern for history, one that it can never quite attain, we all know, but one that it can never quite abandon either. The original conservative historian, David Hume, responded to the whigs – who had previously dominated the writing of history and had told the story as one of freedom and the perfection of civil society – that in authority he was upholding something even more basic and 'essential to its very existence.'[35] To some extent, this might be said of Michael Bliss's contribution to the canon of Canadian historiography. Without some deeper psychological insight, social history can never produce more than a shopping list of alternatives open to people without much serious exploration of psychological compulsion. In general, history has tended to rely on fairly crude models of human behaviour in order to explain decisions in mass. So the best explanations of human motive and the best examples of full and authentic humanity have largely come from historical biographies. From this perspective, Michael Bliss has upheld standards for rigorous, socially contextualized investigations of human beings of a sort that we should aspire to in expanding the range of human subjects, as so many of Bliss's students have done in their own, very diverse analyses.

But this 'delicate balance' is not simply a tension between the centripetal force of the individual and the centrifugal force of society. Michael Bliss, like David Hume, was always concerned with the nature of authority. The intellectual interest in authority also generally marks the works of his students, even those who don't subscribe to the project of reinforcing it. Authority here means something more than simply some sort of societal super-ego. It is always grounded authority: it exists quite concretely in the state, the media, the family (or father), and in the profession (whether that of engineers, physicians, surgeons, general practitioners, or historians themselves). There is no one use of 'authority' among the historians represented here and the potential range is wide, from a form of charisma to a form of the discursive 'power' that underlies the theories of Michel Foucault. What does seem clear is that authority is a central gateway between individuality and society, that the forms of authority listed above overlap considerably, and that they can sometimes dissolve into something quite different, as perhaps happens when a father raises a child or a professor trains a student and launches him or her towards independence. Authority was once, perhaps, understood naively as a *substitute* for reason, but in recent writing it is now better understood as a complicated constituent *of* reason and one that has some sort of promise of freedom because – in the world of Michael Bliss at least – it is something that human beings can themselves grasp, master, and become.

To some degree, this promise of freedom through enlightenment seems to take us back to the real Enlightenment, the one that toppled kings and bishops, not to mention corrupted universities, in the name of reason and the people. Michael Bliss seems to convey a degree of optimism about society coupled with a certain degree of pessimism regarding the management of that society by politicians and the reflection upon that society by historians and other self-styled experts. And perhaps it is to some degree true that Bliss's knowing subject is pre-Foucault, and even pre-Hume: a stable and transcendant figure who can know himself and know the past *as it really was*, 'wie es eigentlich gewesen.' But perhaps it can also be said that Bliss, in his studied distrust of generalizations and his growing refusal to accept or construct surrogates for individual choices and freedoms made within a complex social matrix, somewhat resembles that great modern sceptic, Michel Foucault, whose rejection of 'Enlightenment' (as reason triumphant over authority) and whose denial that there was such a thing as 'man,' was once described, by Ian Hacking, as not pessimism but something else: a refusal to give a 'surrogate for whatever it is that springs eternal in the human breast.'[36]

Michael Bliss's work is hopeful because his subjects pursued justice for their fellow human beings, understanding justice to be something more than just good to one's friends and evil to one's enemies, but better conditions for all people. They didn't always get it right; they didn't always do justice as we would see it done today. But nonetheless it is perhaps helpful to understand both Bliss himself and the dead white men that he studied as forming vital parts of an ongoing project to find and serve truth and justice to the world, and as having more in common, perhaps, with the radicals and progressives than he might concede.

NOTES

Thanks to the other authors in the collection for their comments on this piece, and thanks also to Michael Bliss and Suzanne Morton for their helpful remarks.

1 For early and late examples, see Jacques Le Goff, 'Is Politics Still the Backbone of History?' *Daedalus* 100 (1971): 1–19 and Larry A. Glassford, 'Conflict, Power and Influence through Time: Challenging the Orthodoxy of Social History,' *National History* 1 (2000): 307–20.
2 See the Bibliography of Michael Bliss at the end of this volume.
3 Greatest hits would include: Michel Foucault, *Madness and Civilization: A History of Insanity in the Age of Reason* (New York: Vintage, 1965, 1973); his *Discipline and Punish: The Birth of the Prison*, trans. Alan Sheridan (New York: Vintage, 1979); and his multi-volume *History of Sexuality* (reissued, New York: Vintage, 1990); and Ian Hacking, *Rewriting the Soul: Multiple Personality and the Sciences of Memory* (Princeton: Princeton University Press, 1995).
4 See chapter 1.
5 Donald Creighton, *The Commercial Empire of the St Lawrence* (Toronto: Ryerson, 1937; later reissued as *The Empire of the St Lawrence*) and *John A Macdonald* (Toronto: Macmillan, 1952, 1955).
6 *Northern Enterprise: Five Centuries of Canadian Business* (Toronto: McClelland and Stewart, 1987), 584.
7 The essays are published together: Michael Bliss, 'Privatizing the Mind: The Sundering of Canadian History, the Sundering of Canada,' *Journal of Canadian Studies* 26, 4 (Winter 1991–2): 5–17; Gregory S. Kealey, 'Class in English-Canadian Historical Writing: Neither Privatizing, Nor Sundering,' *Journal of Canadian Studies* 27, 2 (Summer 1992): 123–9; Linda Kealey, Ruth Pierson, Joan Sangster, and Veronica Strong-Boag, 'Teaching Canadian History in the 1990s: Whose "National" History Are We Lamenting?' *Journal of Canadian Studies* 27, 2 (Summer 1992): 129–31.
8 Bliss, *Northern Enterprise*, 572.
9 John Dickinson, 'Canadian Historians – Agents of Unity or Disunity?' *Journal of Canadian Studies* 32 (Summer 1996), 150.
10 Brian J. Young, *George-Etienne Cartier, Montreal Bourgeois* (Montreal: McGill-Queen's University Press, 1981).
11 Carl Berger, *The Writing of Canadian History: Aspects of English-Canadian Historical Writing since 1900*, 2nd ed. (Toronto: University of Toronto Press, 1986) and A.B. McKillop, 'Who Killed Canadian History? A View from the Trenches,' *Canadian Historical Review* 80, 2 (June 1999): 269–99.

12 Thomas S. Kuhn, *The Structure of Scientific Revolutions*, 3rd ed. (Chicago: University of Chicago Press, 1996)

13 Tim Cook, *Clio's Warriors: Canadian Historians and the Writing of the World Wars* (Vancouver: UBC Press, 2006).

14 The editors approached all students of Michael Bliss who were currently writing.

15 Three sources on this: Martin L. Friedland, *The University of Toronto: A History* (Toronto: University of Toronto Press, 2002); Claude Bissell, *Halfway up Parnassus: A Personal Account of the University of Toronto, 1932–1971* (Toronto: University of Toronto Press, 1974); and Robert Bothwell, *Laying the Foundation: A Century of History at University of Toronto* (Toronto: University of Toronto Press, 1991). I have also relied, here as elsewhere, on personal communications by Michael Bliss.

16 See the appendix to this Introduction for a list of dissertations defended under Bliss.

17 Veronica Strong-Boag, 'Contested Space: The Politics of Canadian Memory,' presidential discourse, Canadian Historical Association, 1994: http:// www.cha-shc.ca/bilingue/addresses/1994.htm.

18 James Struthers, *No Fault of Their Own: Unemployment and the Canadian Welfare State 1911–1941* (Toronto: University of Toronto Press, 1983).

19 Bruce G. Wilson, *The Enterprises of Robert Hamilton: A Study of Wealth and Influence in Early Upper Canada, 1776–1812* (Ottawa: Carleton University Press, 1983).

20 J.J.B. Forster, *A Conjunction of Interests: Business, Politics, and Tariffs, 1825–1879* (Toronto: University of Toronto Press, 1986).

21 Joy L. Santink, *Timothy Eaton and the Rise of His Department Store* (Toronto: University of Toronto Press, 1990).

22 Graham D. Taylor and Peter A. Baskerville, *A Concise History of Business in Canada* (Don Mills, ON: Oxford University Press, 1994).

23 David B. Marshall, *Secularizing the Faith: Canadian Protestant Clergy and the Crisis of Belief, 1850–1940* (Toronto: University of Toronto Press, 1992).

24 Suzanne Zeller, *Inventing Canada: Early Victorian Science and the Idea of a Transcontinental Nation* (Toronto: University of Toronto Press, 1987).

25 Published monographs that resulted are Alison Li, *J.B. Collip and the Development of Medical Research in Canada: Extracts and Enterprise* (Montreal: McGill-Queen's University Press, 2003); Barbara Clow, *Negotiating Disease: Power and Cancer Care, 1900–1950* (Montreal: McGill-Queen's University Press, 2001); Geoffrey Reaume, *Remembrance of Patients Past: Patient Life at the Toronto Hospital for the Insane, 1870–1940* (Don Mills: Oxford University Press, 2000); Shelley McKellar, *Surgical Limits: The Life of Gordon Murray* (Toronto: University of Toronto Press, 2003); others are forthcoming.

26 Kuhn, *The Structure of Scientific Revolutions.*
27 Barry Barnes and David Bloor, 'Relativism, Rationalism and the Sociology of Knowledge,' in M. Hollis and S. Lukes, eds, *Rationality and Relativism* (Oxford: Blackwell, 1982), 21–47; see also *Social Studies of Knowledge* 26, 2 (May 1996): passim.
28 Bruno Latour, *The Pasteurization of France*, trans. Alan Sheridan and John Law (Cambridge, MA: Harvard University Press, 1988); Gerald L. Geison, *The Private Science of Louis Pasteur* (Princeton: Princeton University Press, 1995).
29 Jennifer J. Connor, 'Life Writing in Medical History,' *Canadian Bulletin of Medical History* 13, 1 (1996): 134.
30 John V. Pickstone, *Ways of Knowing: A New History of Science, Technology, and Medicine* (Chicago: University of Chicago Press, 2000).
31 Roy Porter, *Health for Sale: Quackery in England 1660–1850* (Manchester: Manchester University Press, 1989).
32 Richard White, *Gentlemen Engineers: The Working Lives of Frank and Walter Shanly* (Toronto: University of Toronto Press, 1999) and E.A. Heaman, *The Inglorious Arts of Peace: Exhibitions in Canadian Society during the Nineteenth Century* (Toronto: University of Toronto Press, 1999).
33 PhD students who have passed their coursework and comprehensive exams are known as 'ABDs,' which stands for 'All But Dissertation.'
34 Veronica Strong-Boag and Carole Gerson, *Paddling Her Own Canoe: The Times and Texts of E. Pauline Johnson (Tekahionwake)* (Toronto: University of Toronto Press, 2000); with Margaret Conrad and Alvin Finkel, *History of the Canadian Peoples*, 2nd ed. (Toronto: Copp Clark Pitman, 1993); and the collection, co-edited with Anita Clair Fellman, *Rethinking Canada: The Promise of Women's History*, 3rd ed. (Don Mills, ON: Oxford University Press, 1997).
35 The remark appears both in his essay 'Of the Origin of Government' and at the end of volume 2 of his *History of England*.
36 Ian Hacking, 'The Archaeology of Michel Foucault,' *New York Review of Books* 28, 8 (14 May 1981), and see Michel Foucault, 'What Is Enlightenment?' in Paul Rabinow ed., *The Foucault Reader* (New York, Pantheon Books, 1984), 32–50.

APPENDIX: DOCTORAL DISSERTATIONS SUPERVISED BY MICHAEL BLISS

1975    Veronica Strong-Boag, The Parliament of Women: The National Council of Women of Canada, 1893–1929

1978    Bruce Wilson, The Enterprises of Robert Hamilton: A Study of Wealth and Influence in Early Upper Canada, 1776–1812

1979    James Struthers, No Fault of Their Own: Unemployment and the Canadian Welfare State 1911–1941

1982    J.J. Benjamin Forster, Tariffs and Politics: The Genesis of the National Policy, 1842–1879

1985    Suzanne Zeller, Inventing Canada: Victorian Inventory Science and Canadian Nation Building, 1830–1880

1986    Brian Hogan, Salted with Fire: Studies in Catholic Social Thought and Action in Ontario, 1931–1961

1987    David Marshall, Secularizing the Faith: Canadian Protestant Clergy and the Crisis of Belief, 1850–1940

1988    Joy Santink, Timothy Eaton and the Rise of the Department Store

1991    Gene Allen, The Origins of the Intercolonial Railway, 1835–1969

Linda Rae Steward, A Woman of Courage: A Biography of Agnes Campbell Macphail

1993    Alison Li, J.B. Collip and the Making of Medical Research in Canada

1994    Barbara Clow, The Problem of Cancer: Negotiating Disease in Ontario, 1925–1945

1995    Richard White, The Civil Engineering Careers of Frank and Walter Shanly, c. 1840–c. 1890

Christopher Rutty, 'Do Something … Do Anything': Poliomyelitis in Canada, 1927–1967

1996    Elsbeth Heaman, Commercial Leviathan: Central Canadian Exhibitions at Home and Abroad during the Nineteenth Century

38   E.A. Heaman

1997   Geoffrey Reaume, 999 Queen Street West: Patient Life at the
       Toronto Hospital for the Insane, 1870–1940

1999   Shelley McKellar, The Career of Gordon Murray: Patterns of
       Change in Mid-20th-Century Medicine in Canada

2000   John Turley-Ewart, Gentlemen Bankers, Politicians, and Bureau-
       crats: The History of the Canadian Bankers Association, 1891–1924

2005   Sasha Mullally, Unpacking the Black Bag: Rural Medicine in the
       Maritime Provinces and Northern New England States, 1900–1950

# The Career and Influence of Michael Bliss

# 1 Growth, Progress, and the Quest for Salvation: Confessions of a Medical Historian

MICHAEL BLISS

Not so long ago it was still fashionable to expect little boys to be able to say what they wanted to be when they grew up. In my case, from the time I could talk I would automatically say I wanted to grow up to be a doctor like my dad, a general practitioner in our little town of Kingsville, Ontario.

When I was twelve or thirteen my father started showing me a bit about the medical life. For years I had often gone along for the ride when he was making house calls in the country. Of course I couldn't get to see the living patients, but Dad was also the township coroner, so he began taking me to emergency calls, to car accidents and drownings, where I got to see the dead, the very fresh cadavers, which I found I viewed with much the same equanimity as Dad or any other budding medical student. There was no problem with squeamishness, and the whole experience was an unusual story of father–son bonding that I mean to write about at more length some Father's Day.

But there came a limit. A year or two on, when I was about fourteen, there was a Sunday afternoon when Dad's and my Scrabble game was interrupted by the appearance at the office door of a policeman with a drunk in tow, the drunk having been in a fight and suffering a badly slashed face. Dad had to sew him up, suturing both inside and outside the cheek, and invited me to watch what would be a demonstration of his surgical skill. I did, and as I sat and watched on that Sunday afternoon in

This essay was originally published in *Ars Medica: A Journal of Medicine, the Arts, and Humanities* 1, 1 (2004): 4–14. We are very grateful for permission to reprint it.

his consulting room, with blood and alcohol fumes everywhere, reflecting on my own complete disinterest in and lack of all manual skills, I decided that this was not what I wanted to do in life. And that was the end of my ambition to be a doctor.

I went to the University of Toronto a few years later, in 1958, with the vague idea of becoming a scientist, probably an astrophysicist. After a year of studying math, physics, and chemistry, I switched to philosophy, because I realized that I was interested in more fundamental or perhaps higher questions, the ultimate issues about the purpose of life and the possibilities of transcendence or salvation. For the next three years at the University of Toronto I was privileged to experience a rigorous, structured, and truly excellent honour course immersion in the main currents of philosophic thought and method. By the end of it I had reached some working conclusions that, whether or not they were well thought out, have more or less guided my intellectual life.

My philosophy training left me inclined to a deep-seated skepticism. Part of the skepticism was methodological, as I doubted the possibility of reaching more than highly tentative knowledge in most fundamental or sweeping matters. Influenced by British analytic philosophy, I concluded that the concepts and language of most traditional metaphysical inquiry were either meaningless or impossibly complex, and that for me these inquiries were dead or irrelevant ends. It also seemed clear that much traditional social theory, which tended to deal with vast generalizations about the course of history or the nature of man, or the evolution of communities, was based on shoddy use of evidence, shoddy definition, and shoddy language, and bordered on intellectual quackery.

My skepticism in the 1950s partly reflected a fairly widespread suspicion of almost all ideologies in those years, not least the old nineteenth-century liberal idea of progress, of the upward march of humanity towards a happy destiny characterized by ever-finer moral, intellectual, and technological achievement. In the aftermath of the two world wars, and especially the Holocaust, and living in the shadow of nuclear annihilation, it seemed impossible, even risible, to talk about human progress. If the twentieth century had demonstrated anything, it seemed to be the human capacity for unspeakable evil. Most traditional faith and hope also seemed irrelevant or illusory in a secular, scientific world. The most fitting description of the human condition seemed to involve existential absurdity, and about the only feasible prescription for handling daily life, exemplified for some of us in those days by the French intellectual and activist Albert Camus, was to get on with it in an attitude of constant doubt, provisional commitment only, and questioning of authority.

Of course one had to make a living in the real world. After a bit of toing and froing, I settled on teaching and. writing history. Because I lived in Canada and was married and had no prospect of doing graduate work outside of Canada, and had no strong feelings about the subject of my work, I chose to teach and write Canadian history. The first area that curiosity happened to lead me into was economic or business history, a field in which I spent the first third of my professional life and wrote three books. My work was characterized from the beginning by large dollops of the scepticism I've mentioned. I liked to stay close to my sources, eschew generalization, and see the historian's quest as fundamentally humanistic rather than as a social science. I have always identified with R.G. Collingwood's suggestion that the historian's job is to recreate as closely as possible incidents, events, human lives in their existential (or Aristotelian) uniqueness. My sense of doing biography, for example, has always been modelled after Walt Whitman's injunction to the poet, to 'drag the dead out of their coffins and stand them again on their feet ... He says to the past, Rise and walk before me that I may realize you.' My biographies are attempts to resurrect dead subjects, an image I'll return to.

About 1978, I decided to indulge my curiosity in a new area and explore the history of the discovery of insulin – writing the biography, as it were, of a highly controversial and poorly understood medical discovery. My interest in this subject came in large part out of my family's medical background. It was also stimulated by my very early background in science (that first undergraduate year in math, physics, and chemistry hadn't been a total waste after all) and some reading I'd been doing in, of all things, the history of polar exploration, which raised for me a methodological interest in the possibility of very detailed, day-to-day recreation of past discrete events. If you could virtually retrace the footsteps of Arctic explorers could you virtually redo the insulin experiments?

I published two books on the insulin story, *The Discovery of Insulin* in 1982 and *Banting: A Biography* in 1984, and at first thought of my medical history excursion as just a kind of mid-life change of pace. I returned to previous interests in Canadian history, which by then also included a heavy emphasis on Canadian politics, which has always interested me as part of any citizen's or scholar's civic obligation.

Nonetheless, the history of medicine proved to have a magnetic appeal, not least because of the response of students and readers to *The Discovery of Insulin*. By the late 1980s work in the history of medicine was taking control of my scholarly time. I've now written a total of four books in medical history, am working on a fifth, and consider that this area of history is my final scholarly resting place. (While I keep a hand in Canadian history and especially in writing about Canadian politics, I see my political and policy commentary as a different genre: it's journalistic, polemical, tentative, and intentionally controversial; also, in a phrase of Margaret Atwood's, a kind of intellectual knitting.)

It did not at first occur to me that three of my books in medical history would form a coherent body of work, supporting certain propositions about the modern history of medicine and its relationship to older ideas of progress. The books were not written for that purpose, or so I thought at the time; nor were they written according to any notion of logical or chronological design. Each was a study of a limited, discrete event or a single human life. But they now appear to me to form a trilogy in which key ideas about medicine and the human condition are developed.

*Plague: A Story of Smallpox in Montreal*, which I published in 1991, is a grim story of a terrible public health disaster. It recounts how smallpox raged out of control in Montreal in the summer and autumn of 1885, killing about three thousand people in the city and another three thousand in its suburbs. It is a story of huge ironies – the ravages of a horrible, loathsome, disfiguring, and often fatal disease that doctors were helpless to treat in patients, yet had the potential to completely prevent, even eliminate, thanks to the marvellous breakthrough associated with Edward Jenner: the technique of vaccination. But in this year in Montreal the possibilities of vaccination were overcome by fear, ignorance, and fatalism in certain sections of the population, who did not allow their children to get vaccinated, and who, when the children died of smallpox, accepted the visitation as God's will – indeed, they were so terrified of vaccination and the public health authorities that they rioted against it, and sick patients had to be removed to hospital by force.

Mostly through devices highlighting the ironies of the epidemic, the pages of *Plague* are meant to convey contempt for that religious turn of mind that saw the spread of smallpox as a decision by the Divinity, for reasons good, bad, or mysterious, to take to Himself so many of the little children of Montreal. This is a book about death being able to ravage a city because of the overpowering of medical knowledge by other factors, religious ideology in particular, but also the fanaticism of ethnic nationalists, and the stupidities of those who challenge the rigour of scientific method. (It happened that the book ended on a hopeful note, with the apparent total elimination of smallpox in the 1970s through vaccination and quarantine. After being assured in 1991 that the last two strains of the virus, held in Moscow and Atlanta, were to be destroyed in just a few months, I ended the book with what has turned out to be a stunningly ironic sentence: 'For smallpox, history has come to an end.' *Plague* went out of print a few years after publication. This year my publisher is issuing a new edition, with a new preface.)

*William Osler: A Life in Medicine*, published in 1999, is, among many other things, a story of the empowerment of medicine, a story of the coming of what can still usefully be called modern medicine. *Osler* is the life of a minister's son, who abandoned his first thought of a churchly vocation like his father's, embraced medicine instead, had a spectacular career, which included writing a textbook that became the Bible of early modern medicine, and came to see medicine and its practitioners as offering to suffering, sinful humanity about the only form of salvation it could hope for – relief from the ills that plague us.

Young Osler gave up his faith in the supernatural and invested such hope as he had in the possibility of what he called 'man's redemption of man,' which was basically the improvements in the human condition held out by medical progress – instancing not only the conquest of smallpox by vaccination (his first hospital appointment was as a smallpox doctor in Montreal in the 1870s), but such marvellous developments as the use of asepsis and anaesthesia in surgery, which led to a vast lessening in human suffering, and the gradual conquest of many infectious diseases through sanitation and other public health measures. Osler really did believe in medicine's ability to bring about progress (he thought it was just about the only profession that could), and in this sense he celebrated medicine as the hope of humanity – in effect preaching the good news, the gospel of what medicine and doctors could do: man's redemption of man.

'Some of the brightest hopes of humanity are with the medical profession,' Osler said in 1891. 'To it, not to law or theology, belong the promises. Disease will always be with us, but we may look forward confidently to the time when epidemics shall be no more, when typhoid shall be as rare as typhus, and tuberculosis as leprosy ... What has been done is but an earnest of the things that shall be done ...'

Brave words, which only partially disguised the embarrassing fact of the ineffectiveness that beset Osler and his colleagues at almost every turn. In the 1890s and early 1900s there were not many disease conditions that doctors could treat with much hope of success. Much of medicine was still more promise than payoff, and there were times when about the best that Osler could do was to predict the great things that would be done in the future. He was able to do this on the basis of the proven, measurable progress of medical science. One glorious instance of this in his career was the introduction in the mid-1890s of thyroid extract as a replacement therapy for the thyroid secretory deficiency that causes myxoedema or cretinism. Osler liked to show before-and-after pictures of the amazing ability of this area of medicine to transform the lives of desperately ill children. He would go on to predict that the study of the secretions of other organs, such as the pancreas, would one day make it possible for medicine to treat other deadly diseases, such as diabetes.

Osler, who was a great and good man, died in 1919, so he just missed seeing his prediction about diabetes come spectacularly true in 1922. Here I come to the third in my trilogy of medical books – the detailed description of the events surrounding the discovery of insulin at the University of Toronto, which produced results in diabetic children so spectacular that observers fell back on their spiritual heritage to use words like *miracle* and *resurrection*.

No wonder. The before-and-after pictures of the diabetic little children who had their lives saved by insulin are about as visually spectacular as any in the history of medicine, and the stories of the children's literal salvation immensely moving. It was an extraordinary personal experience to write *The Discovery of Insulin*, an odyssey that included meeting two of the original Toronto patients still alive some sixty years after they were first treated by Fred Banting. They're dead now, but twenty years after that book's publication I find myself still giving lectures on historical events that amount to an intensely moving story of salvation/redemption through medical research.

The merging of the old prophetic supernaturalist religion into the new secular humanism, the old imagery into the new reality, becomes deeply beautiful and poignant, I think, when we consider Elliott Joslin, a gentle diabetes doctor and Osler protegé, telling of how by Christmas of 1922 he had seen so many 'near resurrections' that it reminded him of the chapter in the Bible where the prophet Ezekiel goes into the valley of dry bones:

And, behold, there were very many in the open valley; and, lo, they were
very dry.
And he said unto me, Son of Man, can these bones live?
And ... lo, the sinews and the flesh came upon them, and the skin covered
them above: but there was no breath in them.
Then said He unto me, Prophesy unto the wind, prophesy, Son of Man,
and say to the wind, thus saith the Lord God: Come from the four winds,
O breath, and breathe upon these slain, that they may live.
So I prophesied as he commanded me, and the breath came into them,
and they lived, and stood up upon their feet, an exceeding great army.

Sometimes after I give my talk on the discovery of insulin – or its
new version, a talk called 'From Osler to Insulin' – I reflect on the ways
in which this celebratory story, which I know can have a profound
inspirational effect, is misleading. Everyone with a smattering of
knowledge of the history of medicine knows that discoveries like insulin don't happen very often; they hardly ever happen; they're atypical
of how research proceeds. The whole idea of medical 'progress' is very
tricky. Medicine, both in theory and practice, moves very erratically,
never in a straight line. As Osler perfectly well understood, sometimes
it appears to go backwards, or in circles, or into dead ends. Medical
'truths,' like so many other kinds of truths, often turn out to be socially
constructed, contingent, friable, and evanescent, which helps to
explain why relativist, skeptical, cynical approaches to the study of
doctors and disease are currently so much in vogue among graduate
students in history of medicine programs – indeed perhaps also among
medical students.

A certain amount of this cynicism and skepticism is sensible. One
understands perfectly well the perilousness of turning physicians into a
new priesthood, and investing blind faith in their rituals, and encouraging them to indulge further their temperamental inclination to infallibil-
ity. Like all other forms of science, medicine is very far from being a shield
against mistake, against harm, against real evil – a lesson that, insofar as
we needed to learn it (one imagines how horrified Osler would have
been), was another of the many taught to us in the Nazi death camps. In
the more mundane world of everyday practice, doctors have often
screwed up very badly. (Indeed Osler himself made a major error in his
lifetime in failing to foresee his own profession's ability to make inroads
on what seemed to be old age, and compounded the error by proclaiming, only partly tongue-in-cheek, the virtues of euthanizing retirees.)

But still ... A few years ago I was a member of a panel of historians put together by CBC Radio to discuss an apparently fascinating proposition: when in all of human history was the very best time to be alive? If you could choose any century, any era, when would you most prefer to live? What terrific scope for discussion this will be, the producers must have thought to themselves, only to find themselves completely discombobulated when all four members of the panel instantly agreed: each of us would prefer to live in the present. Why? Because of health care, we all instantly agreed, because in the present you stand a better chance of leading a long, pain-free, healthy life than at any time in the past.

Osler was right. Here in health care is human progress, literally the improvement of the human condition. And while historians and others may deny the fact of progress, they belie their ideas when asked to choose when they would prefer to live, just as the great historian Roy Porter belied his fashionable cynicism by entitling his general history of medicine *The Greatest Benefit to Mankind* after a remark about the profession by the great man of common sense, Samuel Johnson.

While understanding perfectly well the shortcomings of medicine and health care, and the problems of garnering real knowledge in the realm of medical history, I have no trouble with the basic notion that at times in looking at the history of medicine we are studying, revealing, and, when it is appropriate, celebrating human achievement aimed at the redemption and salvation of humankind. This is the great satisfaction I find in doing medical history. If, as another historian once put it, most of what we do is hold a damn dim candle over a damn dark abyss, sometimes the light shines on truly beautiful formations. It ought to be even more satisfying to be doing medicine itself – unless, of course, one does it badly, as I would have done trying to sew up bleeding drunkards on a Sunday afternoon. And even at its best, at its most triumphant, whether in micro- or macrocosm, medical progress leaves us less than satisfied. There is the immensely frustrating fact that health care offers only temporary salvation. It buys time, but the time always runs out – even for those virtually resurrected children who outlived every one of the discoverers of insulin. They're all dead now. We can assault morbidity, we can postpone mortality, but we can't change the absolute mortality rate, which is permanently stuck at 100 per cent. Which means, of course, that the deal Osler offers us, of salvation through physical health and health care – he called it a 'ministry of health' – is hugely unsatisfactory compared to what Osler's father peddled, which was life everlasting.

Profound historical insights may be in short supply, but I think one of them is the proposition that the secularization of our societies in the last 150 years has meant a collapse in human life expectancy, from eternity to less than a hundred years. That's why, like snowmen desperate to stave off melting, the more successes we have with health care, the more of our resources we are determined to devote to it. It's not the Reverend Featherstone Osler's game, but in postmodern, post-Christian societies it's the only game in town, and it remains existentially absurd.

Osler also taught us, however – doctors, historians, and laypeople as well – that the best way to handle all of the absurdities of life – medical, sacred, and secular – is to do the best we can to maintain our equanimity. When we grow up, we probably should want to be like Osler.

# 2 Inspiration as Instruction: Michael Bliss as a Graduate Adviser, 1989–1994

RICHARD WHITE

I do not remember exactly when or where I first heard the name Michael Bliss. I know it was in Edmonton in the mid-1980s, while I was an undergraduate student at the University of Alberta – evidently he had something of a national reputation by that time – and I recall my impressions being favourable, but that is as much as I can say with complete certainty.

What I particularly wish I could recall more precisely is whether it was at the university that I first heard the name. I suspect it was not – a recollection that might surprise those who think of Michael Bliss primarily as an academic. Perhaps it would even surprise Michael Bliss himself. The University of Toronto did have a fairly high profile at the University of Alberta at that time, among those in Canadian history at least. Several of the most active Canadian history professors had Toronto PhDs – Doug Owram being the best known, but also David Hall, Paul Voisey, and John Eagle – so one did occasionally hear talk of the University of Toronto. But I have no memory of hearing Michael Bliss's name being mentioned by either the faculty or students, inside or outside of classes.

This should not really be all that surprising. For one thing, the Toronto connection should not be overdrawn. Notwithstanding that so many of the Alberta Canadianists had received their PhDs from the University of Toronto, I do not recall them talking up the place, or pushing it as the best choice for graduate studies. If anything, one got the impression that the days of Toronto's dominance in Canadian history had passed. They certainly presented staying in Edmonton for graduate work as a serious option, and I remember being advised to consider studying at York University with Viv Nelles. Moreover, none of these men had studied with Michael Bliss, so he, personally, was not an essential part of the connection. If one name embodied that relationship it was Carl Berger, who had supervised Doug Owram's thesis on Western expansionism and of whom Owram, I do recall, spoke highly.[1]

I think it was probably through the media that I first encountered Michael Bliss. These were years when his face and voice frequently appeared on CBC television and radio, offering opinions on constitutional matters and free trade. I certainly saw and heard him more than once, and remember being intrigued by his cogent and pleasantly contrarian views. That is not to say that his academic standing was unimportant. He was always presented in media interviews as a university man, and I always thought of him as such when he spoke. But it is to say that it was as a *public* intellectual, engaged by present-day issues, rather than as an expert just down from the ivory tower, that I likely first encountered the man who would in time become my academic adviser.

Intellectually, I first met Michael Bliss by reading his book *A Living Profit*, which Doug Owram included on a Canadian Intellectual History reading list I worked through in my final months in Edmonton as I prepared for graduate school.[2] So before long the name did become an academic author for me. That book captivated me, but it was its readability that gave it such power, not its argument. There seemed nothing startling in the conclusion that businessmen carried on their affairs in pursuit of a *living* profit rather than some mythical exorbitant one – I knew half a dozen people of whom that was true. But as so many others have remarked, reading Michael Bliss was such a pleasure. The book could be breezed through without the slightest effort, a stark contrast to some of the other works on Owram's list. It seemed to be in keeping with the non-academic intellectual I had encountered on the CBC.

In fact, there was something rather unusual about the argument in that book which might well have contributed to its appeal, although I certainly did not realize it at the time. That an author in the early 1970s should take as inspiration a book published in the heyday of 1950s consensus history – E.C. Kirkland, *Dream and Thought in the Business Community, 1860–1900* – was a bold and quite unorthodox thing to do. By 1974 the New Left had already pretty much swept away that short-lived consensus school (which had itself been a fairly conscious challenge to the critical stance of 1920s progressive historians – Peter Novick nicely terms it 'counterprogressive' history).[3] Bliss was undoubtedly aware of the contrarian position he was taking in *A Living Profit*. He reveals this in his introduction by noting, rather dismissively, that the view of businessmen as evil robber barons was 'still common among humanist intellectuals, media personalities, and arts students in universities.' What is especially illuminating in that passage, however, is the word 'still,' for it reveals that his budding opposition to 1960s anti-establishmentism was taking shape not because of an aversion to radicalism but because this supposedly new mind-set was, to him, little more than a surviving strand of the old 'robber baron' critique made in the 1920s. An open-minded empirical study such as he was offering in his book would cut through this long-lived anti-business prejudice, as Kirkland's study had a generation earlier, and demonstrate that 'neither the past nor the present is quite that simple.'[4] The progressive fly needed one final swat.

Reflecting on this now, it seems surprising to find New Left history being dismissed as just a return to 1920s progressivism.[5] Few now would make such a claim. Behind the new history lay not only the enormous momentum of 1960s counterculture, but also a whole new school of Marxist theorists. It was to prove both new and permanent, and one would think that both the strength and the breadth of this new current would have been evident to all. At the same time, though, it is important to be reminded that voices were raised to challenge the historiographical revolutionaries of the New Left who, to anyone who did not join their club, might have seemed a little overly self-important. One way to discredit revolutionaries, of course, is to reveal their radical solutions as nothing more than retreads, and such was Michael Bliss's rhetorical tack. It might seem a little out of step now, but it was a bold and quite defensible line of argument at the time.

To pursue this a little further, one might ask how far along and how well understood the historiographical revolution of the 1960s was in Toronto in the early 1970s. It is easy for the British historiographer Willie Thompson to write that by the early 1970s 'the western historiographical landscape had been transformed,' and that a decidedly leftist social history had 'taken centre-stage,' but Willie Thompson did not live in Toronto.[6] Michael Bliss once recalled that he had first learned about American progressive historians and their views of 'robber barons' in the 1960s from Ken McNaught, who was still carrying the progressive movement's torch at the University of Toronto at that time – the counter-progressive 'consensus' school of the 1950s, in other words, had barely arrived in the 1960s, let alone the New Left's challenge to that school. Moreover, Michael Cross, the series editor for the Canadian Social History Series, in which A Living Profit was published, opens his preface to the book declaring, 'Social History is about people.' Such a statement, in

1974, seems almost quaint when put up against Eric Hobsbawm's seminal essay on social history, already several years old, in which he calls for social history to move beyond the old-fashioned history of people to a more rigourous, social-science inspired 'history of society.'[7] Perhaps Michael Bliss's being slightly out of step with international historiographical trends derived, at first anyway, as much from the intellectual world he lived in as from his own inclinations.

In any case, by the time I arrived at the University of Toronto to begin graduate studies in 1989, Michael Bliss had become, tentatively at least, my supervisor of choice. That is not to say I came to Toronto to study with him. That would be going too far. I still knew very little about this man, having neither seen nor spoken to him. I had read *A Living Profit*, but none of his other work, and thoughts of New Leftists and Progressives and where he fit on the spectrum had not even entered my mind. It was to the institution that I came, to the place where so many of the Canadian historians I had read over the previous few years in Edmonton worked and resided – Berger, Eccles, Van Kirk, Brown, Silver – and where the Canadian history tradition was so strong – Careless was the name I knew best. But there was undoubtedly something about Michael Bliss that had begun to appeal to me, at least the Michael Bliss I had come to know before leaving Edmonton. I remember being on the university campus in Toronto with a few hours to spare after some registration tasks, anxious to start familiarizing myself with the library, and finding myself searching the catalogue and shelves for, of all things, Michael Bliss books – just some random name that popped into my head.

I have no clear memory of our first actual meeting, which is telling in that Michael Bliss was always very approachable, and never made you feel that meeting him was a memorable event in your life. We probably first met in his office when I asked him to supervise my MA research paper, which he was happy to do, and then a few more times that fall to talk about the paper. I do not recall discussing much of importance in those early meetings, or of Michael Bliss revealing many things about himself or his thinking. What I do remember is a routine that would continue for all my years as his student. Our meetings always occurred during his weekly three-hour block of office hours, and often involved waiting in the hall outside his office for other students to finish their meetings – rather like sitting in the doctor's waiting room, without the benefit of chairs and magazines or the convenience of set appointments. He allotted only so much time to see students, and he kept to this strictly. One might think this would have bothered us, but I have not a single recollection of feeling slighted myself or of hearing other students complain. Quite likely, if necessary, he would have accommodated us at other times, but who felt the need? This is what one got working with a busy man, and his busyness reflected his importance, which in turn made his tutelage that much more valuable. Once in his office, meetings would occasionally be interrupted by a phone call from an editor or agent, a distraction that added even more to the meeting's value.

When we did get to discussing my research paper, it quickly became clear that his approach to supervising students, in my case anyway, was more to urge on than to guide or advise. I had decided to study the introduction of electricity to London, Ontario – my hometown and the home of Adam Beck – in the early years of Ontario Hydro, just before and after the First World War. Ontario Hydro, the great public provider of electricity in Ontario, had intrigued me even before I began to study history, and my interest had been spurred and focused by the argument that the businessmen behind the public power movement were acting more in self-interest than in a true public spirit – an interpretation I had found in Viv Nelles's *The Politics of Development*.[8] But nobody I read had actually studied how this early electricity had been used. Did it power the factories of the businessmen who lobbied for its cheap public supply? This historical question was right in line with Bliss's earlier work on businessmen's ideas – some thorough empirical work would uncover 'what really happened' in one incident in the history of Canadian business, and it would be done with an open, not unsympathetic, mind. Despite this common ground, however, Michael Bliss's approach was to leave me intellectually on my own. There was not a mention of the recent historiography of business and how my study might fit into it, or any suggestions of what I might read in the field. I was discovering what I later came to understand was a central tenet of Michael Bliss's graduate teaching – let students find out for themselves.

It was in the second term, in his seminar in Canadian medical history, that I came to know Michael Bliss a little better. This experience, perhaps more than his supervision of my research paper, encouraged me to continue at the university with him as my adviser. Admittedly, the material we read in the seminar was probably not at the leading edge, but that did not in any way lessen its value. Medical history has now become an appealing subject for those exploring how power is manifest in the construction of knowledge and institutions, for the medical world has long been ruled by the notorious false kings – men, modernity, and science – that such historiography seeks to topple and expose. And even then, in the late 1980s, such an approach would have been ascendant elsewhere. But we saw none of it in our readings. I do not recall the words 'power' or 'Foucault' being uttered or read even once. But the intellectual climate of the seminar was by no means backward. This was no study of the march of scientific progress. The guiding principle for us was the blending together of medical and social history, in which was embedded a fair amount of relativism.[9] We considered disease transmission and native contact, cholera and political unrest, public health and urban reform, medical professionals and the welfare state. The readings satisfied me well enough as an introduction to the field, and in fact seemed rather current in their integration of medical history into the mainstream and their bringing into question, at least to a degree, the notion of progress.

What mattered at least as much, though, was the seminar itself. Michael Bliss had an ability to be interested in everyone's comments, and to respond by refining or reinterpreting them to stimulate further discussion. This made the class meetings very 'inclusive' – to use a neologism that would never have passed his lips – and relaxed. Even more, he allowed us, as his students, into his own life ever so slightly. We read Anne Collins's *In The Sleep Room*, and then discussed it, with her, at a lunch he arranged at the Arts and Letters Club, where he was a member.[10] And to conclude our term, he held our final seminar at his home one weekday evening, the gathering ending with an offer of cognac. What we were experiencing, it seems clear now, was the last gasp of an old university tradition in which professors and students share something of a social life. Paternalistic some might see it now, but I found it generous and encouraging. University life looked appealing enough to sign up for another four years.

Entering the doctoral program was a fairly routine administrative matter, but for Michael Bliss the decision to accept one as his student was an event with some formality. We met at his house for lunch late in the summer, after all my MA work had been completed. I made a pitch of sorts, explaining what I wanted to study and hoped to accomplish, and he agreed to take me on. He was welcoming, but at the same time quite forthright in admitting he would not have much to do with me. I was made to understand that my PhD would not be a joint project in the manner of some sciences, where the professor and student work together in the same lab and lunch together in the same common room. He would keep to his office hours, and be available for appointments, but beyond this I should not expect to see much of him. I knew what he meant by this time, and it suited me fine. We shook hands to close the deal.

So began four intense years of reading, research, and writing from the fall of 1990 to the fall of 1994. As is probably the case for all who have gone through long periods of study, my PhD program has become one big blur of memory with the passage of time, and the sequence of events nearly forgotten. I do not think I actually saw much of Michael Bliss in the early years. I had no seminars with him, and my Canadian field reading was supervised by Carl Berger (as was the case for all 'Canadianists'). But we did meet from time to time, during his set office hours as before, to discuss one thing or another.

One thing I do recall is that I had a difficult time finding a thesis topic. This was the subject of several meetings, at more than one of which Michael grew impatient. I also know I felt particularly helpless. It seems to me now that mature students returning to academia after a time away – which was my case – do so with a substantial disadvantage, usually being unfamiliar with current academic concepts and problems, and that this handicap is most noticeable in their slow and uncertain selection of thesis topics. Students who enter graduate school straight from undergraduate studies appear to have an easier time of it, arriving with ready-made historical problems to explore and approaches to follow. Those from outside come either with fading memories of older, abandoned paradigms or with interests and views developed from experience and independent reading – neither of which serve one well in academia. But more to the point, Michael Bliss seemed to offer me little help in solving this problem. He did suggest a few topics, none of which seemed right to me. He did emphasize that what I chose to study would define me in the scholarly world – that one's thesis became one's intellectual calling card – but he gave no advice on what topics might engage the academic community, or what sort of calling card certain topics would make. Here, again, was his laissez-faire teaching philosophy.

So what was it that made a student choose to study with Michael Bliss? His commitment to being a public intellectual stands out as one of the reasons. His being such a non-academic academic, a man of letters rather than a university professor per se, held appeal to someone who was re-entering academic life. But I can also see now, though I did not recognize it at the time, that I was attracted by his distance from 1960s radicalism, a thread in his thinking I had first glimpsed and been somewhat tantalized by in *A Living Profit*. I, myself, had been substantially affected by the counterculture earlier in my life. But by the 1980s, like most of my friends, I had moved on, a response partly to a yearning for satisfying work and partly to the demands of parenthood. Not that I had turned traitor entirely. I looked back fondly, and it was with a touch of regret that I had reconciled myself to a destiny in the dreaded middle class. But that regret was always lightened – again, as it was for many I knew – by a little self-deprecation for our having been so fanciful and by a sincere desire to do well on our newly chosen paths. With these thoughts in mind I entered academe in the late 1980s and found myself, rather surprisingly, falling in not with academics of my own generation but with professors of the earlier generation who, like Michael Bliss, had not even participated in the counterculture. The academic staff of my own age, with whom I had at first expected to feel some kinship, seemed rather alien. Still busy distancing themselves from and critiquing the institutions of society, these historians of the aging New Left (which everyone my age seemed to be) struck me as rather dated, and their ideas even a little stale. By contrast, with Michael Bliss and other older professors, although they and I inhabited thoroughly different worlds, I could establish a comfortable teacher–student relationship that would last through my entire time as a graduate student.

Probably the aspect of Michael Bliss that attracted me more than any other, however, was the quality of his work. He wrote good history. I had not read much of his work when I began to study with him, but after reading two of his best books, *The Discovery of Insulin* and *A Canadian Millionaire*, during my time as his student I became a fan.[11] The former gripped and carried one along with the narrative power of a mystery, offering a reading experience quite unlike most others for a student working through a list of academic monographs for the PhD examination, yet it still offered some insight (some would say not enough) into the process of scientific research and discovery. But the latter work impressed me even more – a portrait of one person's life so rich that the background of the picture is as full of detail as the subject himself. I learned as much about Methodism, business management, pork packing, and artillery shell manufacture as I did about Sir Joseph Flavelle, which was of course the point. I had never before realized why 'the life and times' appeared so often in the subtitle of biographies, but here was the genre defined. As well, though both books were firmly rooted in historical sources, they were much more than archival lab reports. They were creations of their own; they had people with motivations and sentiments, a shape and flow to the chapters, and always enough context to be fully understandable.

They also represented a very traditional historiography, the fact and significance of which occurred to me slowly, and not fully until after I had completed my studies and moved on. In choosing to study with Michael Bliss I had placed myself under the tutelage of a 'conservative' historian.

When and why this label came to be applied to Michael Bliss – and whether it is even accurate – is an intriguing question. The roots of it undoubtedly lie in his distancing himself from the counterculture of the late 1960s. I later learned from conversations with him (in response to my questions; he never reminisced unasked) that he had been appalled by 1960s radicalism. To him it just lured students away to drugs and ill-discipline and placed ideology in the way of open intellectual inquiry. His political sympathies had been with the left in his young adulthood – his first intellectual mentor had been Ken McNaught – but he had baulked and kept his own ground when the academic herd stampeded off towards radicalism. That his well-known 1970 article on branch plants was published in a collection of leftish essays, compiled by the University League for Social Reform, reminds us of his intellectual origins (although he once recalled that the other contributors to that volume might have been a little disquieted by his argument once they saw the article in print).[12] Not joining the radicals will get one labelled conservative soon enough, regardless of where one actually stands. But Michael Bliss's growing interest in business history in the 1970s, where by he acquired sympathy for such matters as secure markets and open trade, probably gave some substance to the image.

In terms of electoral politics, he had been an early supporter of Trudeau and the Liberal party, so his roots are not Conservative in the party sense of the word either. He drifted away from Trudeau to the Joe Clark Conservatives in the 1970s. He once said this had been mostly on account of the growing deficit and Trudeau's views on the Constitution, but that he had not remained in the Conservative camp once Brian Mulroney became party leader. Whether this all amounts to being a political conservative is hard to say. But once he became a public figure, in the 1980s, he was certainly viewed as a Conservative, mostly because of his position in the free trade debates of 1986 and 1987. He spoke strongly and openly in support of free trade with the United States on the grounds that Canada's dependence on trade made such an agreement next to essential. As he put it in the closing section of his comprehensive history of Canadian business, published during those debates, Canada should emulate the Scandinavians: 'Specialize, find and exploit comparative advantage, look outward, choose quality instead of quantity, let culture grow in the fresh air of economic freedom.'[13] This was a view he advocated repeatedly in newspaper columns and media interviews. To be called 'conservative' for urging the country to break free from a long-standing policy, especially if that policy is protectionism, is to distort the essential meaning of the word. But free trade was advocated by a Conservative government, and largely supported by the business lobby, so to line up on its side was to be conservative.

Probably better known and more fully considered, at least among his academic colleagues, was Michael Bliss's historiographical conservatism, a label that came to be attached to him over the very years I spent as his student. Several events stand out clearly in my memory.

The first phase of a PhD program was to read – 'master' was the word commonly used – the literature on one's subject under the tutelage of an adviser. Joy Parr's *The Gender of Breadwinners* was on my Canadian business history reading list, a book that at the time (1991) was new and highly regarded.[14] One day on my way to meet Michael Bliss to discuss the book I had a chance encounter with a fellow student who had just finished reading it herself. She spoke highly of it, explaining that it was the first really good example of post-structuralism in Canadian history. I took this seriously, and once seated across the desk from Michael asked him if he could explain it to me, and help me understand, the concept of post-structuralism. The question was met with a burst of laughter. My first reaction was relief – evidently I would not have to grasp this abstruse concept to receive a PhD.

Around the same time I witnessed a somewhat more public declaration. Michael Bliss had been writing a book on the 1885 Montreal smallpox epidemic throughout the time I was his student. He rarely spoke about his work, but somehow we all knew. It was no surprise, then, that he appeared on the schedule of presenters for the departmental research colloquium in the winter of early 1991 giving a talk on his new book. His presentation took the form of a reading from a nearly finished manuscript, and quite a surprise it was to those of us attending. What he had crafted was a 'non-fiction novel'[15] narrating the dramatic events of the 1885 epidemic, in which large numbers of poor French Canadians in the unhealthy wards of east Montreal died of smallpox largely on account of their refusal to allow themselves to be vaccinated by the city's mostly English-speaking doctors. (Jenner's smallpox vaccine was in use by this time, and smallpox was a fairly controllable disease.) The writing was rich with the sights and smells of old Montreal, and enlivened by dialogue among the participants, much of it in the historical present. It struck me as a splendid thing to do with historical sources. I was won over.

Bliss's talk was followed by questions and discussion, as was the custom, and one question and response I remember well. A faculty member in the room, a European historian, pointed out that this work seemed to be going against present-day historiographic currents by showing so little sympathy for the French Canadians. Should he not have some sympathy for their folk medicine, their suspicion of author-ity, and their resistance to modernization? Where, in other words, was the cultural relativism? No, said Michael Bliss, sympathy of that sort was uncalled for. This was a case of tragedy being caused by ignorance and superstition.[16]

The declaration of historiographic conservatism that drew the most attention by far was his now notorious Creighton Lecture, delivered at the University of Toronto in April 1991.[17] Speaking to a hundred or so insiders in a small two-tiered lecture theatre in University College, Bliss took Canadian academic historians to task for being unable, and perhaps worse disinclined, to offer perspective and vision to the consti-tutional renewal process then under way. As he saw it, this lack of interest in constitutional affairs among historians was rooted in a com-paratively recent turn away from *Canadian* history towards a whole range of historical specialties. 'We are business historians, labour histo-rians, Western, Maritime, Ontario, Quebec historians, intellectual histo-rians, historians of women, education, law, cities, culture, crime, smallpox – historians of almost anything but Canada.'[18] What was most regrettable about this turn away from national history in the 1970s and 1980s, he went on to argue, is that it occurred when the coun-try and its citizens – deeply immersed as they were in constitutional debates – were most in need of knowledge about their country's consti-tutional history. Yet contemporary historians, himself included, had lit-tle to offer. Having abandoned their role as interpreters of national experiences, they left the public (and the drafters of Meech Lake) 'both historically blind and prisoners of long-dead historians.' 'I think we should try harder to help,' he concluded.

Negative reaction began even before the lecture was delivered, and continued for months, even years, both formally and in the form of 'buzz' throughout the profession.[19] His opponents construed the lecture as a reactionary screed against new directions in social history; it was said to blame the new history for the decline of national unity and to call for a return to 'good old national history.'[20] But such criticism misrepresented Bliss's argument. As a member of the audience that night, I certainly heard nothing of the sort. For one thing, he included himself among the culpable – this was unmistakable in the delivery – something his critics seem not to have noticed, or perhaps found incomprehensible. But more important, he explicitly rejected a return to the old national history of Creighton, Lower, and Underhill. It was a *new* national history he was calling for, a history that included Canadians 'whose integration into our historical and national consciousness is the finest achievement of our history writing since the 1960s.'[21]

Admittedly, the lecture could be challenged for leaving a string of big questions unasked and unanswered (What, if anything, is the causal connection between the decline of national identity and the decline of national history? Can we really have a new *national* history? Is the notion of a conventional national identity even tenable in a culturally diverse society?). But Bliss's basic point, that historians were not equipped or inclined to contribute to the national constitutional debate, and his plea for historians to somehow add historical perspective to the constitution-making process, struck me as hard to deny and beyond reproach. Criticism of his views seemed to be aimed at a lecture that did not happen, or perhaps at a lecture that his opponents imagined had happened, revealing a deep and rather disturbing ideological division in academic Canadian history.[22] Michael Bliss, however, seemed to pass through the whole affair unfazed. Being a man of action, he left his critics unanswered and moved on to do his bit by writing a popular history of Canada's political traditions.[23]

Does all this add up to Michael Bliss being a conservative historian? Initially, I resisted the description. True, Bliss followed humanist principles in his writing, but in doing so he was challenging new orthodoxies and thus being forward-thinking, not conservative. True, he was doggedly empiricist and had no interest in what was then called 'theoretical' history, but surely this was an indication that he valued clear

accessible writing and wished to reach the public, not that he was reactionary. True, he was more willing than most to retain a faith in
progress – but only on the strength of evidence, not dogma. And true,
he showed a somewhat old-fashioned concern for national history, but
he certainly had moved well beyond the *grand* national narratives of
the previous generation. As a teacher he seemed remarkably open to
people and ideas of all types – more so than many 'non-conservative'
professors – and he never preached conservatism either in the sense of
party allegiance or political ideology.

But in the end, the word conservative, for me anyway, came to seem
not inapt for the writing of Michael Bliss. This is not to disparage his
work in any way, but simply to say that much of its strength lies – along
with his personal abilities and insights – in Bliss's retention of ideas and
techniques that others have abandoned. As the philosopher of conservatism Russell Kirk reminds us, conservatives 'ought not to be judged just
by what they failed to avert, but more by what they preserved.'[24]

Even this needs some qualification, and the place to begin is with the
point made by recent historiographers that history writing has in fact
undergone two revolutions since the 1960s.[25] The first, running from
the 1960s through to the 1980s, is the profound revolution in both the
scope and sympathies of historical research brought about by the rise
of social history. The historical canvas was vastly and irrevocably
expanded, as a host of previously marginalized people entered the picture.[26] The impetus for this reform came mostly from the left, and as
time passed this political orientation seems to have grown to the point
that the appellations 'social historian' and 'conservative historian'
were mutually exclusive. But the reform had had a wider ideological
base at first. Virtually all academic historians, regardless of political
stance, had been affected by it. Though admittedly reflecting the shift
in scope much more than in sympathies, Michael Bliss's *A Living Profit*
(1974) shows this change to a degree, concentrating on the ideas of
ordinary businessmen rather than on the great industrialists, as does
*Plague* (1991) in its exploration of everyday life among the common
people. This revolution Michael Bliss had not resisted.

The next revolution, the turn to postmodernism – with its emphasis
on relativism and constructionism,[27] and its insistence that all research
findings be put into the paradigms of certain European philosophers –
Michael Bliss showed not the slightest sign of taking part in, or even
taking notice of, in the early 1990s. Here, perhaps, is his conservatism.
Before making too much of this, though, one should note that although

several of postmodernism's tributaries had been flowing for over a decade, the concept was not accepted as an over-arching paradigm, even by leading intellectuals, until the 1980s.[28] And it was certainly not yet the 'one best way.'[29] Several other historiographical avenues seemed possible as a way of building on, or moving beyond, the earlier revolution.[30] Thoroughly researched micro-historical portraits of communities or events, inspired by European work, seemed possible. So too a new kind of historical narrative, built up from meticulous, Rankean research but free from association with progress and *grand* narratives, and covering a wide social spectrum, seemed an option. Both of these appealed in that they re-introduced individual human motives and sentiments into historiography. As it turned out, these other avenues petered out in Canadian historiography, but they had at one time seemed viable, even vital. Thus, Michael Bliss's work in the early 1990s was not as traditional when it was written as it looks now.

Nor was he usually aggressive in his historiographical conservatism. He did not actively oppose or subvert the new trends – he laughed at post-structuralism but did not demand that it be ignored. Notwithstanding the critics of his Creighton Lecture, he never became a preachy neo-conservative writing poison-pen tracts about how historiographic novelty was leading us to damnation.[31] And his work does, in fact, show a willingness to experiment. But it is also true he took his models from older traditions, that he doubted the new intellectual fads, and that he had a humanist's 'affection for the proliferating variety and mystery of human existence' that Russell Kirk notes has been among the basic tenets of conservatism for over two hundred years.[32] The word conservative might not be such a bad fit after all.

As for what his conservatism, qualified though it is, meant for his students, I can of course only speak from my own experience. I felt not the slightest pressure to conform to any political position or to take on a topic of national scope or significance. These were his views, and they stayed with him. His historiographical conservatism no doubt discouraged us from exploring contemporary cultural and social theory, although those of us who resisted most fully were likely more than a little complicit in the act. Perhaps it also permitted students, such as myself, to write theses that ended up taking a rather traditional form. But if these are shortcomings – and I'm not sure they are – they are more than counterbalanced by his expecting the traditional qualities of solid empiricism and clear writing, and it seems to me that no matter where one chooses to go as a historian there is no better place to begin.

Looking back at my years with Michael Bliss, I admit that at times I have felt some modest regret that I did not receive more academic advice from my academic adviser, for his style was remarkably hands-off. But much more often I feel otherwise, realizing that in truth I benefited from that lack of guidance. With guidance comes prescription, whether one wants it or not, and as I ponder the discoveries I made while researching and writing my dissertation, I believe that many of them I simply would not have made had I been following a prescribed path. For me, and I'm sure for others, Michael Bliss was more of a model than an adviser, and what he provided was more inspiration than instruction. Though he expected a certain standard, his style was not really to tell one what to do. But he worked hard, finished what he started, and did excellent work, and in doing so was a constant inducement for completing and improving my own work. That was his way, and it meant that, for good or ill, my way was mine.

NOTES

1 Later published as Doug Owram, *Promise of Eden: The Canadian Expansionist Movement and the Idea of the West, 1856–1900* (Toronto: University of Toronto Press, 1980).
2 Michael Bliss, *A Living Profit: Studies in the Social History of Canadian Business, 1883–1911* (Toronto: McClelland and Stewart, 1974).
3 E.C. Kirkland, *Dream and Thought in the Business Community* (Ithaca: Cornell University Press, 1956); Peter Novick, *That Noble Dream: The 'Objectivity Question' and the American Historical Profession* (Cambridge: Cambridge University Press, 1988), 332.
4 Bliss, *A Living Profit*, 13.
5 The thesis on which the book is based was already a few years old in 1974.
6 Willie Thompson, *What Happened to History?* (London: Pluto Press, 2000), 49.
7 E.J. Hobsbawm, 'From Social History to the History of Society,' in *Essays in Social History*, ed. M.W. Flinn and T.C. Smout (Oxford: Clarendon Press, 1974; essay originally published 1971).
8 H.V. Nelles, *The Politics of Development: Forests, Mines, & Hydro-electric Power in Ontario, 1849–1941* (Toronto: Macmillan, 1974); this is not to suggest that Nelles follows this interpretation.
9 The main readers we used were *Health, Disease and Medicine: Essays in Canadian History*, ed. Charles G. Roland (Toronto: Hannah Institute for the

History of Medicine, 1984); and *Medicine in Canadian Society: Historical Perspectives*, ed. S.E.D. Shortt (Montreal: McGill-Queen's University Press, 1981).

10  Anne Collins, *In the Sleep Room: The Story of the CIA Brainwashing Experiments in Canada* (Toronto: Lester & Orpen Dennys, 1988).

11  Michael Bliss, *The Discovery of Insulin* (Toronto: McClelland and Stewart, 1982); Michael Bliss, *A Canadian Millionaire: The Life and Business Times of Sir Joseph Flavelle, Bart., 1858–1939* (Toronto: Macmillan, 1978).

12  Michael Bliss, 'Canadianizing American Business: The Roots of the Branch Plant,' in *Close the 49th Parallel etc.: The Americanization of Canadian Business*, ed. Ian Lumsden (Toronto: University of Toronto Press, 1970).

13  Michael Bliss, *Northern Enterprise: Five Centuries of Canadian Business* (Toronto: McClelland and Stewart, 1987), 583–4.

14  Joy Parr, *The Gender of Breadwinners: Women, Men, and Change in Two Industrial Towns, 1880–1950* (Toronto: University of Toronto Press, 1990).

15  Published as *Plague: A Story of Smallpox in Montreal* (Toronto: HarperCollins, 1991); Bliss used this label in the preface of the book, but later told me he thought it ill-advised and a little pretentious.

16  I believe these were his exact words, but since I am relying only on my memory I have not employed quotation marks. Bliss offers a brief, compelling explanation of his views on medical progress in a recently published article 'Growth, Progress, and the Quest for Salvation: Confessions of a Medical Historian,' *Ars Medica: A Journal of Medicine, the Arts, and Humanities* 1, 1 (Fall 2004), reprinted in this volume as chapter 1.

17  Subsequently published as Michael Bliss, 'Privatizing the Mind: The Sundering of Canadian History, the Sundering of Canada,' *Journal of Canadian Studies* 26, 4 (Winter 1991–2): 5–17.

18  Bliss, 'Privatizing the Mind,' 9.

19  Gregory Kealey, speaking the afternoon before the lecture, as part of a weekend of events commemorating the hundredth anniversary of the history department, criticized what he expected Michael Bliss to say. Three responses to the lecture, one of them a version of Kealey's talk, were published as 'Point-Counterpoint: "Sundering Canadian History,"' *Journal of Canadian Studies* 27, 2 (Summer 1992): 123–35. The lecture was cited as an example of neo-conservative reaction in the outgoing CHA presidential addresses of 1992 (Gail Cuthbert Grant) and 1994 (Veronica Strong-Boag). In 2000 a group of graduate students asked me, in an academic job interview, which side of the Michael Bliss controversy I was on.

20  Gail Cuthbert Grant, 'National Unity and the Politics of Political History,' *Journal of the Canadian Historical Association*, new ser., 3 (1992): 6.

21  Bliss, 'Privatizing the Mind,' 16.
22  Reaction to the lecture was complicated by the fact that Jack Granatstein had published *Who Killed Canadian History?* at about the same time; despite differences between the two, Bliss's lecture was at times lumped together with Granatstein's book by critics.
23  Michael Bliss, *Right Honourable Men: The Descent of Politics from Macdonald to Mulroney* (Toronto: HarperCollins, 1994); Bliss took as his inspiration, once again, a book from the U.S. post-war consensus school, Richard Hofstadter's *The American Political Tradition and the Men Who Made It* (New York: Knopf, 1948); see also Novick, *That Noble Dream*, 323–4. One might note that, interesting and valuable though that book is, it took us no closer to defining our national identity or agreeing on national constitutional principles.
24  Russell Kirk, *The Conservative Mind from Burke to Eliot*, rev. ed. (Chicago: Regnery, 1986), 293.
25  I am following primarily Thompson, *What Happened to History?*; Georg Iggers, *Historiography in the Twentieth Century, From Scientific Objectivity to the Postmodern Challenge* (Middletown, CT: Wesleyan University Press, 1997); Terry Eagleton, *After Theory* (New York: Basic Books, 2003); and the excellent introduction to the *Encyclopedia of European Social History from 1350 to 2000*, vol. 1, ed. Peter Stearns (New York: Charles Scribner's Sons, 2001), especially the section 'Proliferation and Growth: The Boom Years, the 1960s to the 1980s,' 12–24. The notion of the two revolutions, a line of interpretation being advanced primarily by Marxist critics, is explored in Thompson's chapter 3, 'Continuing Revolution or Counter-Revolution' and Eagleton's chapters 1 through 3.
26  Carl Berger, *The Writing of Canadian History: Aspects of English-Canadian Historical Writing since 1900*, 2nd ed. (Toronto: University of Toronto Press, 1986), chap. 11, 'Tradition and the New History.'
27  A fine elucidation of constructionism is Ian Hacking, *The Social Construction of What?* (Cambridge, MA: Harvard University Press, 1999).
28  Perry Anderson, *The Origins of Postmodernity* (London and New York: Verso, 1998), chap. 3, 'Capture.'
29  I am lifting this from the title of a recent book on F.W. Taylor, of scientific management fame: Robert Kanigel, *The One Best Way: Frederick Winslow Taylor and the Enigma of Efficiency* (New York: Viking, 1997).
30  Iggers, *Historiography in the Twentieth Century*, 97–117.
31  In this he can be contrasted with the conservative historians described by Novick, *That Noble Dream*, 462–5.
32  Kirk, *The Conservative Mind from Burke to Eliot*, 8.

# 3 Michael Bliss in the Media

Michael Bliss sells newspapers. Editors court him because readers buy the broadsheets that publish him. This is a rare accomplishment, for Bliss successfully bridged the gap between Canadian historians and the media. In so doing he enhanced the national profile of the University of Toronto, to the delight of university administrators, and simultaneously provoked ridicule from colleagues wary of newsprint and television journalism, which they dismissed as unsatisfactory mediums that dumb down complicated ideas, quash nuance, and ultimately distort by means of simplification. Such reservations about journalism are neither uncommon nor unjustified. The Organization of American Historians observed that 'scholars are sometimes reluctant to speak freely with those from the media, in part because they fear the intellectual, personal, and political consequences of seeing their complex, and often subtle forms of historical interpretation reduced to a fifteen-second "sound bite" or to a short quotation taken out of context.'[1] Bliss recognized the risks and biases of the genre. In a 1985 letter to the editor, for example, Bliss took aim at a *Financial Post* news report and editorial lamenting what editors perceived as the growing problem of corporate concentration in Canada:

> As you know, or should know, the Royal Commission on Corporate Concentration did not find the problem was getting worse. Most of the statistics used by alarmist journalists to buttress what is really a hoary old Marxist chestnut about monopoly capitalism are selective and misleading. Anyone who reflects on the growing diversity and complexity of the Canadian economy as it has developed over time will realize that growth has, in the

long run, led to a dilution of economic power. Why are the reporters and editors of *The Financial Post* parroting ignorant left-wing rhetoric?[2]

Bliss's use of 'alarmist' is noteworthy. Among their shortcomings, journalists tend to encourage exaggeration as a marketing device. This is evident on television and surfaces on the front pages of newspapers, which are designed both in content and presentation to do more than catalogue the day's significant stories. They are also sales tools, used to coax readers to the news-box, where proprietors hope their front page will persuade consumers to part with their money and pick up a copy. Front-page headlines are sometimes 'torqued'[3] to this end, while the advent of colour print in the 1980s, combined with the influence of television on media consumption, surfaces in larger, eye-catching photographs that are stories onto themselves.[4]

While historians have valid concerns about the media's fallibility, editors and producers are often suspicious of Canada's historians and are reluctant to rewrite well-known story narratives based on new historical research that isn't easily grasped or that grates against conventional wisdom.[5] Journalists who do weave new historical interpretations into their writing must find ways to resolve the risk of undoing well-known storylines that can cause larger problems when they are trying to construct a report that readers will understand. Take slavery, for example, an institution that is generally characterized in Canada's media as a phenomenon of the British Empire and later the United States, rather than a part of Canadian history itself. Afua Cooper's *The Hanging of Angelique* is a history of an African female *slave* who responded to her Montreal mistress's brutality by burning down her house in April 1734, starting a larger fire in Montreal in the process. Angelique was tried and hanged for her actions.[6] Through her book, Cooper has attempted to debunk the convention that slavery is not a Canadian issue. Her work has drawn the attention of the Canadian press and it has made its way into newspaper copy, yet most reports on the two hundredth anniversary of the abolition of slavery in March 2007 described slavery as the sin of others.[7] Canadian journalists crow about the fact that slavery was abolished in Canada in 1834, three decades before it was abolished in the United States; about the underground railroad (a message reinforced by a Historica Minute broadcast repeatedly on television that emphasizes that Canada was a beacon of freedom amidst the slave trade);[8] and that the slaves in this country never numbered anywhere near those in the United States or the southern reaches of Britian's eighteenth-century empire. Their narrative allows the Canadian press to present the country's experience as morally superior to that of the United States and Britain, a comforting view that has an audience among the reading public and that militates against revisions such as that suggested by Cooper.

Much of the unease between the media and the academy, however, is also tied to the different ways historians tell their stories and the dissimilar audiences they cater to. Whereas many historians engage in coterie writing, with its own structure and vocabulary created for a small group of specialists,[9] journalists write for a broad audience, using language that is generally universal. As part of that process, journalists rely on narrative structure because that is the most common way people organize and communicate information. Newspaper content is built on it, as is television news. Editors and producers seek out contributions from people who convey information using story narratives with wide appeal or those who add to conventional narratives on the popular debates of the day. The narrative is ultimately relied upon to explain, teach, and entertain. 'It is the bundle in which we wrap truth, hope, and dread. It is crucial to civilization.'[10] Narrative is not, however, crucial to Canadian historians who write specialized, analytical history, a genre that has become popular in the academy over the past thirty years. Analytical history tends to examine Canada's past through studies that organize historical experience around such themes as gender, race, or class, to name a few. Such writing often spends more time deconstructing elements of historical experience to flesh out as much meaning as possible, rather than locate it in sweeping political narratives that derive meaning from historical experiences in the context of a larger, shared Canadian project. Such history leans towards the personal rather than the public. Yet it is often the larger narrative, the public history of politics that emphasizes common concerns, that the media want to talk about because it draws the largest audiences. In essence, the more readers who relate to a story or opinion piece, the wider the readership it is likely to have. History written in this fashion attracts media praise.[11]

Analytical history presents impressive insight on particular issues, but at the same time can baffle the media because of the arcane academic language in which it is often written and its resistance to recasting writing in ways that open it up to a wider audience. Mark Starowicz, the executive producer of the CBC television series *Canada: A People's History*, first broadcast in 2000, reflected media apprehension when he expressed disappointment with analytical historians, suggesting that what has happened to Canadian historiography is 'narrative cleansing.'[12] Charlotte Gray argues that Starowicz and his team, in producing the popular series on Canada's history, faced a 'challenge that the history profession has ducked for [years]: they have tried to make a thrilling and coherent tale out of the past that, thanks to academic infighting and political caution, has left most Canadians bored, confused, or downright cold.'[13] By the time he had finished producing the documentary, Starowicz believed Canadian 'historians, with the exception of Pierre Berton ... are not telling the stories. History is essentially an analytical, not a narrative discipline. Narrative historians are a controversial minority. We need good storytellers.'[14]

That Michael Bliss is a member of that 'controversial minority' of narrative historians does not satisfactorily explain how he built a successful sideline to his academic career as a Canadian media personality. Knowing how to tell a story is but one factor. Having a story people want to read is another. How Bliss succeeded prompted debate in history common rooms as well as suggestions that he was part of a small, privileged group of male professors granted access to the media because he propped up the establishment. Such theories have not given way to scholarly study and the reasons for his media success remain a matter of conjecture. What brought Bliss out of the academic quad and into the public square? How did he bridge the gap between the two worlds? Did Bliss accomplish anything in his twenty years in journalism that began in the 1980s when he emerged as an informed political commentator on the state of the federation and on free trade with the United States?

This essay will focus for the most part on Bliss's print journalism, which I have become closely associated with as a writer and editor at the *National Post*, the upstart Canadian broadsheet launched in 1998. Bliss began writing for the *Post* that year (he had penned a weekly column for the *Toronto Star* previously), and continued to do so on a fairly regular basis until his retirement from journalism in 2006. In order to chronicle and explain Michael Bliss's media success, I rely on interviews with Bliss and other media personalities, as well as on newspaper and magazine archives. In addition, I use sizeable quotes from a few of Bliss's newspaper columns to illustrate his writing style and its effectiveness.

While I touch on long-standing and often heated discussions about the nature of the historical profession in Canada, it is not my intention to pass judgment on different genres of history. This essay is about how a Canadian historian, Michael Bliss, became an important media personality by writing columns on a range of subjects tied together by common themes – the merits of free-market capitalism, a strong central government, the affront of political corruption, and respect for individual rights. In so doing, it opens a window, however slightly, on the Canadian media and why they gave a Canadian historian a voice in national affairs.

The questions that Bliss's journalism provokes can only begin to be answered here. Still, it is possible to discern the wherewithal Bliss possessed to excel, the political context that helped swing the media's door his way, the reasons he took up journalism, and, to a lesser extent, the impact of his political commentary on our national debates. If there is an overarching thesis to be drawn from Bliss's media success, which took him from the letters page, when he began, to the front page in his final years writing for the *National Post*, it is that Canadians possess a strong appetite for analyses steeped in and informed by the country's history. Canadians by and large respect their historians, even when they disagree with them. If nothing else, Michael Bliss is a testament to that.

Journalism students may wish to skip the next few paragraphs. For in explaining why newspaper editors allocated precious newsprint space to Michael Bliss, it is necessary to address one of the conceits journalism schools rely on to draw eager students through their doors. Journalism schools promote classes and programs that offer the impression that those who attend them will emerge as journalists with a voice in public affairs, when in fact the students they produce more often than not end up working as copy-editors or as basic reporters. Such work is essential, yet differs substantially from that of an editor or opinion columnist, who can shape public-policy debates. Editors generally assign topics to reporters, rewrite copy, choose the headlines, decide where to place the content on the page and on what page, and settle on what news reports will and will not be published. Reporters find their voice in the scoops they dig up, but most of the time reporters toil on stories assigned by editors. Columnists have a freer hand and are given their own voice – that is, the ability to express explicitly their opinions – though editors still play an important role by hiring columnists whose opinions are aligned with the newspaper's market or spiking columns that for one reason or another don't, as it is said in the business, 'work.'[15] Editors are the invisible hand of journalism and shape the issues that are debated from behind their desks. Copy-editors do not do this. They correct grammar, check facts, and display content created by others.

Thus, a degree from a journalism school is not a ticket to winning a voice in public affairs, let alone a job in the newspaper business, despite what journalism schools would like students to believe and their efforts to offer a broader liberal education. Four years of history, English, economics, or politics enhanced by graduate work in these subjects can't be replicated in six or seven courses spread over four years of journalism school. Some schools claim to know what editors want and promote it as a means of selling their programs of study. Take Ryerson University's School of Journalism, for example. This is what the school advises students who want to be print journalists:

> The newspaper stream provides students with the skills needed to work immediately in any print newsroom. That means gaining experience with reporting, researching, interviewing, meeting deadlines, copy editing, layout and design, computer-assisted reporting, and writing for online media. Once students reach the final year, they are ready to produce their own newspaper ... What are editors looking for? As well as basic skills, they want reporters who demonstrate curiosity, persistence, and passion and excitement for the craft.[16]

Raising such expectations can lead to disappointment. Student interns show up in newsrooms full of enthusiasm and with ideas and opinions that they want to share, only to discover that excitement is not a substitute for the insight that comes with being well read and knowledgeable.

What is missing in Ryerson's claims is the demand among editors for educated observers – writers who recognize a significant story when they see it and can explain its significance to those who cannot. Journalism schools do not teach that. It comes from knowledge rooted in literature, philosophy, science, history, and politics. Robert Fulford, a grand man in Canadian journalism whose career spans more than half a century, spent several years teaching part-time at Ryerson's journalism school. In a column written some years after he left the school, Fulford observed that he 'sensed an air of mild embarrassment hanging over the whole enterprise.' Fulford offers a telling anecdote in this regard: 'One day a new part-time teacher, having been astounded to discover that his students couldn't write the English language, suggested that we needed a crash program in literacy. It was quickly decided that there wasn't room for it in the schedule and it probably wouldn't work anyway.'[17] Journalism schools are more trade schools than places of higher learning, though they appear to be the latter rather than the former because they grant degrees. Those closely associated with journalism recognize that J-schools are not 'professionally necessary (most successful journalists did not attend one) and even universities that offer the subject tend to consider it marginal.'[18]

What editors need to create a newspaper that will generate sales – for sales matter to advertisers, who pay more to reach more people – is well represented in a 1998 essay by Donna Logan, the founding director of and a professor at the University of British Columbia's Sing Tao School of Journalism. In conversing with an editor at an 'influential Canadian daily,' Professor Logan learned that the editor 'was considering not hiring any more journalism graduates: "I need people who understand how the justice system works, how public policy is formulated, how the banking system functions, et cetera. In order to do insightful reporting, one has to know the inner workings of society's major institutions, public and private. Otherwise one ends up sniffing around the edges."'[19] It is this demand for expertise, especially its skilful use in informing debates of wide interest, that gives an incentive to newspaper editors to look beyond J-schools, creating opportunities in journalism for others who can fill the void. In the 1980s editors peered across the divide between their world and the academy as Canada underwent transformative economic and political change, seeking Canadian historians who could make sense of the nation's shifting political values. Most analytical historians did not or could not answer the calls of editors. Michael Bliss did.

Two issues changed Canada in the 1980s. The first was Prime Minister Pierre Trudeau's patriation of the Constitution in 1982. While the *Constitution Act 1982* raised expectations for a more just society, one in which the judiciary would occupy a fundamental role in clarifying the country's values, it also plunged Canada into political turmoil when Quebec's separatist government objected to the proposed constitution only to have its concerns overridden by the prime minister and Canada's other provincial premiers. The 1988 Free Trade Agreement with the United States also ushered in profound change and with it came a debate about the nature of Canadian identity. Together, free trade and efforts to bring Quebec into the constitutional fold after 1982 precipitated an existential crisis in Canada.[20] Media outlets needed commentators who could draw on Canadian economic and constitutional history and make compelling arguments that would help explain and ease the insecurities of the time.

Michael Bliss could do that, as could others. What distinguished Bliss, though, may have been his well-founded determination to eschew much of the conventional wisdom promoted by the country's political elites who signed on to the 1987 Meech Lake Accord and the 1992 Charlottetown Accord, agreements crafted to accommodate Quebec separatists with special constitutional deals. Bliss argued both were bad for Canada. Nor would Bliss let protectionists throughout the free-trade debate get away with trying to dupe Canadians into believing that their national identity was rooted in trade barriers that dated from Sir John A. Macdonald's National Policy of 1879. Knowing the larger political narrative of Canada and Confederation, with all its ups and downs, was an asset in this context. It provided a perspective that seemed fresh to a public with little sense of the country's history and enabled Bliss to ride the wave of change that was remaking the country's political values in the 1980s. Political scientist Neil Nevitte captures that change most succinctly when he describes it as the 'decline of deference.'[21] Canadians were less inclined to be led by their politicians and the chattering classes supporting them. Bliss lent intellectual legitimacy to Canadians who disagreed with elites cutting constitutional deals with Quebec and supplied them with ammunition against the fear-mongering of protectionists. Consequently, his arguments had a market that gave him traction with editors.

Increasing that market took patience. Newspapers, magazines, and other media producers first looked to Bliss for sharp and short quotes to fill out stories. A close reading of *Maclean's* magazine in the late 1980s and early 1990s reflects this trend and the skill with which Bliss was able to comply. Take, for instance, his response during the free-trade debate in 1988 to news that the Liberal opposition used their majority of seats in the Senate to block the free-trade agreement and force an election. Bliss told the *Maclean's* writer that the Liberal ploy was 'deplorable. The leader of the opposition is going to tell us what issues are important enough to have an election on. It is profoundly undemocratic. It really is the old Liberal arrogance which one would have thought was beaten out of them when they were reduced to 40 seats.'[22]

Just as Bliss could highlight offences against parliamentary democracy, he also effectively put the spotlight on political absurdities. In 1992 he was asked to comment on Ontario provincial politics and a scandal concerning Shelley Martel, who, as an NDP cabinet minister in 1991, bad-mouthed a doctor at a party after allegedly using her position to obtain private information about the physician. This sparked an inquiry and the remarkable response from Martel that she had lied at the party and never had inside information. Hence she was not guilty of breeching ministerial ethics. Bliss's pithy summation? 'She's a minister whose honour depends on proving she was a liar. The idea of government as a kind of circus is something we haven't had before in Ontario.'[23] This is called 'good copy' in newspaper rooms. There is no equivocating, the words carry an authoritative tone informed by a concern for a minister's lack of integrity. Moreover, such comments improved the quality of the stories they were inserted into, bolstering the publication's brand, which can ultimately help lift readership and advertising revenues.

Yet possessing the ability to provide good quotes does not guarantee success writing opinion columns. David Damrosch captures the challenge succinctly, saying: 'Even for scholars who are elegant prose stylists, it isn't an easy matter to make the transition from writing for Milton's "fit audience, though few" to a larger but less fit readership.'[24] Writing op-eds did not come easy to Bliss, a fact he readily acknowledges.[25] He had to work at it and learn how, in a short space, to pack in enough detail to be persuasive but not so much as to be dense and unreadable. Andrew Coyne, arguably the best national-affairs columnist in Canada, notes that Bliss writes 'with great vigour, mixing righteous anger with good humour, and never succumbs to academese. The combination – impeccable scholarship and effortless readability – is devastating.'[26] The late author and journalist Christina McCall remarked once that a good 'article needs three components – research, writing and thinking. Research is hard,' she added, 'writing is harder, but thinking harder still.'[27] Bliss's articles 'provided an ideal balance of these elements' according to Fulford, who has a keen journalistic eye. What distinguishes a Bliss essay is the 'unusually fine sense of context and a serious thinking-through of subject and theme.' Laying out the context, appealing to reason, writing with authority, and presenting a clear position, all were key to Bliss's ability to build an audience among editors, decision makers, and the public.

During the debates about Quebec's role in the federation and free trade, Michael Bliss was busy writing books that garnered awards and elevated his scholarly reputation at home and abroad. He also had to contend with the onerous duties of teaching undergraduate and graduate courses while supervising PhD candidates, a task that not only demands academic finesse, but the ability to deal with the fragile sensibilities that candidates are apt to display as they make their way through their program. That Bliss would add to these responsibilities the additional commitment to do interviews and write columns for papers and long articles for magazines raises the question, Why?

The answer comes in three parts. The first entails Bliss's view of journalism; the second, what he believes a historian should aspire to be; and the third, how he defines Canadian history and its role within the debates of our times. Although Bliss does not keep his reservations about journalism to himself, he also respects its role and influence in society. Indeed, he contends that newspapers are 'some of our most important history books. When historians ... try to write authoritative history, we turn constantly to the newspapers that have provided us with the first draft.'[28] First drafts always contain mistakes, sentences that could be better and comments that reflection would reveal as intemperate. Despite such shortcomings, there are rich veins of insight to be mined in the daily press. Bliss's *The Discovery of Insulin* is evidence of that. *Daily Star* reports in 1922 and thereafter by journalist Roy Greenaway were, said Bliss, 'vitally' important to his book because Greenaway 'was able to reveal more about the intense personal rivalries among the discovery team than anyone else made public for many years.'[29] More than adding new colours to the past's palette, Bliss sees journalism making a genuine contribution to our understanding of important events. Rather than a step down for a scholar, Bliss looked at journalism as a sister profession to history. For many academics, making contacts in the media and working with them is a chore best left to university public-relations departments which, today, are called on more and more to act as a broker between professors who want to write an opinion piece and a paper's comment editors.[30]

While Bliss recognized that history and journalism had a common end, he also came to believe that historians should enter the public square, an idea that was impressed upon him by a distinguished educator and man of principle – Kenneth McNaught, author of the first biography of J.S. Woodsworth and of the popular *Penguin History of Canada*. McNaught, one of Bliss's mentors at the University of Toronto when he was completing his graduate work, taught Bliss that 'scholarship was about passing judgement.' A historian should have a good moral compass and be prepared to follow it. Most important, McNaught was interested in improving the quality of Canada's political life. Bliss remembered this lesson. In writing McNaught's obituary for the *Ottawa Citizen* in December 1997, Bliss recalled that 'Ken was for many of us a role model long before the term became fashionable. Professors should aspire to improve the world, McNaught taught us, and he professed constantly on radio, television, on oped pages, and in letters to editors.'[31]

Seeing journalism as a worthwhile endeavour, alongside the idea that historians have a public role to play, helps explain why Bliss answered reporters' queries and took to the op-ed pages and the airwaves – but not fully. His definition of Canadian history and the state of the craft during Canada's two decades of angst, the 1980s and 1990s, is as significant a factor as the first two. Bliss explained in a speech to the Association of Canadian Studies in 2001 that Canadian history is by definition about Canada, 'which means that it's about the experiences the people who call themselves Canadian recognize as Canadian, which is to say it's about experiences they have had more or less in common, which means that it's about the public history of the country.'[32] Ten years before, he had generated outrage among some of his fellow Canadian historians by suggesting they had lost sight of what Canadian history is about at a crucial time in the country's life. Bliss argued that 'from the 1970s on Canadian history had turned inward, becoming personalized, privatised, and solipsistic, and that in succumbing to these trends we were failing in our basic duty as teachers to the point where the capacity for Canadian citizenship was being imperilled.'[33] In addition to publicly unveiling how he felt about trends within his profession, Bliss revealed something else during his most talked-about lecture. Through his scholarship, writing Canadian history as he characterized it, and by extension his journalism, which reached the widest possible audience, Michael Bliss believed he was fulfilling his basic duty as a teacher.

Yet engaging the media is not seen as a basic duty by many historians. Indeed, in a conversation I had with a senior historian responsible for guiding young scholars at the University of Toronto it became clear that this professor would not encourage others, especially those seeking tenure, to write for newspapers. To do so was considered an unnecessary distraction likely to hinder efforts to win tenure and build a successful career. To that end, the senior historian suggested it was far better for scholars to write books that would win the praise of twenty-five or fifty specialists in a given field and leave journalism to journalists. That was not the view taken by Robert Prichard, president of the University of Toronto from 1990 to 2000. The university was grateful for the national exposure Bliss's journalism brought it, which increased its public profile and helped fill history department coffers by drawing large numbers of eager students to Bliss's undergraduate history course, where full-time students mixed with business professionals, civil servants, aspiring politicians, and others.[34]

Did Bliss teach Canadians anything? It is a question worth asking, though admittedly it is hard to answer. Clearer are the themes Bliss pursued through his op-eds and appearances on television. Arguing the merits of free-market capitalism, particularly free trade between Canada and the United States, in 1987 and 1988, launched Bliss into the national spotlight. The move was aided to a great extent by the publication of *Northern Enterprise* in 1987, a book that won a large readership and that excited the business community across the country. Here was a historian who knew the story of Canadian business and was better qualified and able to talk about it than most businessmen. He said much and wrote even more during one of the country's most vigorous debates that pitted protectionists and cultural nationalists on one side and those who believed in free trade and saw Canada as more than the sum of her trade barriers on the other. As the free-trade election of 1988 was heading into its last weeks, Bliss wrote an important essay for the *Toronto Star*, critical of its editorial position, which summed up much of his thinking at the time:

> Above all ... Canadians of the 1980s are not moved by the deep anti-Americanism that shaped the 1960s generation. Many of today's Canadians never lived through or have forgotten the great events of those far-off times: American imperialism in Viet Nam, riots shattering American cities, the Kennedy assassination, Watergate, Canada's coming of age at Expo '67. Our leading nationalist gurus from that time – Walter Gordon and George Grant – are dead and had little influence in their last years. Their disciples, particularly the Atwood-generation of cultural nationalists, are well over 40 and sometimes seem out of touch with well-travelled, secure, aggressive young Canadians of this generation. It seems vaguely silly to still be arguing in the 1980s that free trade means the rape of frail Miss Canada by that lecherous bully, Uncle Sam. And yet the editorial board of The Star has not changed a note in its nationalist tune in 20 years.
>
> In fact, the real conservatives in this election are Liberals and New Democrats and their followers, people who staunchly oppose free trade and virtually every other change brought in by the Mulroney government – from the privatization of Air Canada through rationalization of postal service. Canada's Expo generation has had a lifestyle so pleasant and comfortable, particularly in regions like southwestern Ontario, that Messrs. Broadbent and Turner see no reason for change, particularly in the direction of competitiveness and efficiency. The election may show that time is passing them by.[35]

Bliss's contribution to the free-trade debate was designed to persuade audiences that bringing down trade barriers was a progressive step that would make Canadians wealthier. Those who opposed it appeared in Bliss's commentaries at best to underestimate the business sector's ability to compete and the strength of the nation's identity and at worst as special interests that benefited from trade barriers at the general public's expense. In this debate and afterwards Bliss offered the proponents of free markets an advocate who could marshal knowledge about Canada's business history to demolish sentimentalist economics.[36] He could, in effect, help teach Canadians about the history of their economy and its development, and the press was happy to oblige in this effort, as editors who were free-market supporters were eager to find strong advocates for the cause while those who opposed it, like the *Toronto Star*, needed to offer some balance in their pages in order to maintain the credibility that comes with saying they gave the other side a fair hearing.

At the same time that Canadians were debating free trade, however, Bliss was also participating in quite a different challenge facing the country, one that put him on the opposite side of Brian Mulroney's Conservative government and aligned him with populists, such as Preston Manning, in opposition to the Meech Lake Accord. In the eyes of the media, supporting the Conservative government's free-trade proposal while opposing vigorously its attempt at a constitutional deal with Quebec, which it began negotiating in 1985, would have added to Bliss's credibility by laying to rest any concerns editors may have had that Bliss was a Tory partisan. It also made it harder for protectionists to attack Bliss as a Conservative stooge, and for Meech supporters in the Conservative government to write Bliss off as a university quack, for they were using his arguments to support the battle for free trade.

This confluence of circumstance kept Bliss in the middle of two national debates during the late 1980s. While his contribution to winning the public over to free trade was important, he most likely endeared himself to politically engaged ordinary Canadians through his opposition to the Meech Lake Accord. On this subject Bliss identified most readily with Canadians and encouraged them to stand up to political elites who he believed were putting the country in jeopardy by meddling in constitutional matters that they did not themselves fully understand while watering down the role of the central government. In June 1987 the *Toronto Star* published a 1600-word column by Bliss that reflects his work to rally Meech opponents:

If you are an ordinary Canadian, concerned about the country your children will inherit, you ought to be appalled that our politicians have set us up for a wild constitutional leap in the dark. The First Ministers and their political supporters (including the leaders of the two national opposition parties) are rushing to change our Constitution in ways that are either dishonestly meaningless or alarmingly substantial.

From one point of view, the accord is wordy, symbolic puffery, unworthy of the dignity of constitutional language. From another, it is a formula for a new Canada in which the range of opportunities and possibilities for the future will be tragically reduced.[37]

Yet that was only the beginning of Bliss's manifesto against an accord that he believed would see the federal government's role as a unifying body undermined, a dangerous proposal in a country where provinces have been able to accomplish little that binds them together into a unified state. He listed five areas of deep concern: Meech's changes to the federal spending power, the distinct-society clause for Quebec, directed immigration, senate and Supreme Court reform, and constitutionalized conferencing for first ministers on the economy. Of these conferences, he poignantly noted they 'will either become ritual griping meetings or they will evolve into major priority and policy-making sessions. In the former case, the country will have a ridiculous new institution, worse even than the Senate. In the latter, the provinces will have taken over responsibilities now handled by federal MPs. Ottawa will indeed be castrated.'[38] Bliss's indignation is unmistakable, yet it is leavened with reason and dressed with enough facts to ensure its palatability to readers who would have to think hard if they wanted to persuade themselves that Meech was a good idea. He struck his most compelling tones, however, when he pointed to the disastrous consequences Meech could have on Canadian democracy, particularly the proposal to give each province a veto over changes to Canada's political institutions:

The implications of the universal veto are mind-boggling. Anyone passingly familiar with Canadian history knows that modern Canada could never have been created under the proposed amending formula. There would not have been a Confederation in 1867, for the provinces would never have agreed on a Senate. Ontario would have vetoed Manitoba's entry into Confederation in 1870; Quebec or Manitoba would have blocked the creation of Alberta and Saskatchewan as new provinces in

1905; Quebec would have kept Newfoundland out of Confederation in 1949 unless it was given Labrador. For that matter, had other provisions of Meech ... been in force in the past, Canada would not have had the present schemes of unemployment insurance, old age pensions, health insurance or any other national social program.

Meech ... jeopardizes the aspirations of the people of the Yukon and Northwest Territories, most of them aboriginal Canadians, in the most cynical possible way. It also creates the possibility that the will of the 130,000 people of Prince Edward Island can stand in the way of the aspirations of 26 million Canadians. The notion of provincial 'equality' is being extended to smother basic and elementary principles of political democracy.[39]

Here was a call to democrats and those who supported aboriginals to oppose the deal, casting such opposition, just as he framed support for free trade, as a progressive position. It was, like so many of Bliss's opinion pieces, a brilliant mix of past and present, of optimism about the essential soundness of the country and its people, combined with a certain pessimism about the politicians' construction of and catering to special interests.

Perhaps the greatest testament to Bliss's influence in the country's constitutional debates of our times is suggested in what happened in the lead-up to the efforts by Brian Mulroney's Conservative government to revive Meech a year after its collapse in 1990. When governments went back to the negotiating table for a second time, few believed they could bring the outcome to pass without first consulting the Canadian people. Indeed, several provinces had passed legislation ensuring a referendum would be held if any such deal was proposed again. Backroom deals foisted on an unsuspecting public by politicians and their hangers-on had become non-starters. Bliss, during the Meech debates, was right when he argued the imposition of the deal was out of step with the democratic temperament of the times. In August 1992 the federal government concluded another constitutional deal, the Charlottetown Accord, which retained many of the same principles that were laid down in the Meech Lake Accord. The three main parties in Parliament supported it – the Conservatives, the Liberals, and the NDP – and an expensive and sophisticated campaign was devised to sell the deal to Canadians, who would be asked to vote on it in a referendum on 26 October 1992. The first stage leading to the 1992 deal began the year before when the basic elements of the constitutional proposal were first assembled and an effort was made to bring influential politicians and academics on side.

Most received a phone call from Ron Watts, Ottawa's top constitutional adviser. Only Michael Bliss received a personal call from Joe Clark, the government's point man on the Charlottetown Accord.[40] It made little difference. Bliss opposed Charlottetown, as did former prime minister Pierre Trudeau and, as it turned out on 26 October, a majority of Canadians as well.

From Michael Bliss's journalism on constitutional matters and the merits of free trade one can discern how he came to see Canada's evolution: what worked to unify the country – a strong central government – and what brought prosperity – free-market capitalism – as well as what held growth back, trade barriers. Yet his most compelling columns to reach print dealt with a far different dilemma, political corruption. Natasha Hassan, who was Bliss's editor at the *National Post* for several years, recalls most clearly the strong moral compass he brought to the paper's comment pages.[41] Integrity matters to Bliss and he thinks it should matter to Canadians as well. He eschews in his journalism those who write off pork-barrelling and unethical behaviour as the price of brokerage politics. Consider the following example from June 2002:

> Prime Minister Jean Chrétien is right in believing that the current ethics scandals in Ottawa fundamentally revolve around our expectations of Members of Parliament. He believes their job is to get out there and fight for their constituencies – fight for federal grants and federal projects. If fighting on behalf of constituents is seen to be unethical, then, the Prime Minister believes, MPs become eunuchs, castrated, unable to perform.
>
> Thus his particularly vigorous defence of Solicitor-General Lawrence MacAulay, who, in the Prime Minister's and his own mind, was only doing his job in lobbying the RCMP to give a grant to a community college in his riding. The fact that MacAulay's brother is president of Holland College is deemed insignificant because it's a public institution; the president would not derive direct personal gain from the grant.
>
> As the Prime Minister predicted, P.E.I.'s Conservative Premier, Pat Binns, and other Island politicians have risen to MacAulay's defence. He's just doing his job. As an editorial in P.E.I.'s, The Guardian, puts it: 'On Prince Edward Island, and in Canada generally, part of a politician's track record is the assessment of their success in bringing government spending to their home constituency.'
>
> This is the pork barrel defence. MPs are expected to help their constituents get government money, the more the better. This, of course, was also the Prime Minister's Shawinigate defence, and it was the government's

HRDC defence. Bringing home the bacon. Every student of Canadian history knows that our elected legislators have always scrambled to do this.

So where's the scandal?

Here it is: As we broaden our understanding of the concept of fairness in public life, we are beginning to expect politicians not to interfere with the disposition of public money. Millions of Canadians assume that access to government programs must be open equally, normally through open competitions judged by impartial arbiters. In such competitions, there is no room for meddling or lobbying or representations by Members of Parliament, any more than there is in, say, the hiring of civil servants.

Forget about Lawrence MacAulay's brother. The RCMP is perfectly competent to decide for professional reasons which programs it wishes to fund. No Member of Parliament, let alone the minister in charge of the agency, should have any business trying to influence its decisions to favour one group of Canadians over another group. MacAulay's intervention with the RCMP (and, now we learn, with the Correctional Service of Canada) should be seen as inappropriate as, say, a phone call to a judge on behalf of a constituent.[42]

This is the kind of insight editors are willing to pay for and that does not come out of journalism schools. It sells newspapers and educates the public by clearly outlining an issue and showing in this case how the prime minister, MPs, and even the press can be blinded to unethical behaviour and attempt to explain it away as part of the political process. The message Bliss sends to the reader is, Don't let prime ministers, ministers, or those who excuse them in the press dupe you into thinking that what is being done here, pork-barrelling, is acceptable. The average Canadian who is disgusted by such conduct learns from Bliss that they have every right to be, regardless of what politicians want them to think. This is an education, but it is also a confirmation: a validation of common sense and everyday morality.

Representing the interests of ordinary Canadians is the common thread in Bliss's writing on political corruption, but his indignation is not simply that of a populist. It comes from a principled understanding of how important honesty is to ensuring that the machinery of government, like that of business, operates effectively. When well-educated elites disregard the importance of honesty, Bliss sees it as an insult to those they represent and to the integrity of the entire political process. When the auditor general, Sheila Fraser, released her report on Adscam on 10 February 2004, Bliss's commentary on it appeared on the front of the *National Post* the next day, indicating not only the importance of the story but the fact that people would buy the paper to read what Bliss had to say about political corruption in Ottawa. He did not disappoint:

> The rot in Ottawa also has a class dimension. The other shoe is the way that our most wealthy and most powerful politicians, the Cabinet ministers of Canada, bypassed procedures to buy themselves brand new Challenger jet planes, while requiring the ordinary men and women of the Canada Forces to make do with vehicles of doubtful reliability. This is the mentality, not of English or French, but of the rich and privileged who take privilege and luxury as their due. One of the mentality's other characteristics is an inability to understand why citizens should make fusses about such useful facts of life as tax havens and flags of convenience.
>
> When the lid comes off, you deny knowledge, deny responsibility, and blame the underlings, exactly as prominent Liberals are doing today. There is a certain validity here: We ought to be very worried about incompetence or corruption in the civil service of Canada, the people who gave us the absurdity of the national gun registry, the people who under-estimated by ten thousand per cent the amount of business Canada does with Canada Steamship Lines, the bullies who tried to destroy the former president of the Canadian Business Development Bank for standing up to the former prime minister.[43]

To understand the appeal of Bliss's journalism (and this is something that many in the academy who think Bliss is a neo-conservative cannot allow themselves to grasp), it is essential to keep in focus his defence of principles that are in place to protect ordinary Canadians from greed and corruption. Taking seriously his duty as an educator, he teaches through his writing the importance of ethics and integrity and makes clear how they safeguard ordinary Canadians from exploitation by the country's elites.

Just as Bliss has used his journalism to give Canadians reason to reflect on their leaders and the political system that governs the country, he has also asked Canadians in his columns to reconsider the comforting myths that they wrap Canada in. This is particularly true regarding health care, where Bliss has long been a critic of the notion that medicare defines Canadians and that allowing private care is something akin to treason. In a column written for the *Toronto Star* in 1995, Bliss put the lie to those arguing socialized medicare was bred in the bone of Canadians:

Nor is socialist health care integral to the Canadian identity. For a century after Confederation we built a prosperous, free, humane and well-governed society and did our share in the wars of this century, all without universal health insurance.

Medicare came to Canada in 1968. Not long afterward we began systematically undermining our financial future – just ask our creditors – as we struggled to maintain a system that is no more Canadian than kippered herring or borscht.

Our pioneering ancestors understood that two-tier access to everything is the way of the world. Responsible people learn to save and provide for themselves in time of sickness. They pay for insurance policies to protect against calamity. Humanely they pay taxes to government to give the genuinely needy access to a basic standard of living, including health care.[44]

Bliss's op-eds on health care gave readers reason to ask who really benefits from the government's monopoly on health services and raised the question of individual rights. In an important piece written for the *New York Times* and republished in Canada by the *National Post*, Bliss summarized succinctly the problem with socialized medicine:

No sooner had governments implemented universal health insurance than they became horrified by its steadily rising costs. Under Canadian medicare, by the 1970s the single greatest policy problem was not to provide services to the people, but to find ways to limit expenditures. Not surprisingly, a generation of bureaucrats and civil servants grew up preaching the socialized-medicine dogma that costs could be contained if (a) providers, i.e., doctors, nurses and hospitals, were more closely controlled in their tendencies to do too much; (b) patients were controlled in their tendency to want too much. The way to stop provider and patient resistance to government health-care squeezes was to use the power of law to outlaw alternatives. The key legislation, the Canada Health Act of 1984, has made the provision of private medical and hospital services effectively illegal. Tommy Douglas never did that in Saskatchewan. Unlike today's socialists, he was committed to physician and patient freedom.

Since the early 1980s, we Canadians have had no choice but to accept the health care given us by our political masters. Claiming they know what's best for us, governments have conspired to cut our access to doctors, nurses, hospital and diagnostic facilities. Now the governments of Ontario and Canada want to limit our freedom as patients by forcing us to be 'rostered' with family practitioners who will effectively become salaried civil servants. It's a frying-pan to the fire solution that would create a truly horrendous mess, but is utterly characteristic of the naive socialist faith that a little more control, a few more limits on human freedom, are all you need to change human nature.[45]

Unlike the issues of free trade and dangerous constitutional proposals, Bliss cannot claim to be on the winning side of the health care debate. Canadians may be raising questions about their health care system, but they still cling to the belief that socialized medicine is progressive and the best system for them. What Bliss has done through his columns on health care is join a growing chorus that has made talk of private care respectable. In the end, as more and more individuals head to the Supreme Court of Canada to challenge restrictions on private health care that keep them languishing in long line-ups for treatment as a violation of their rights under the Charter of Rights and Freedoms, well, perhaps Michael Bliss will be proved correct once again.

Whether or not Michael Bliss was on the right or wrong side of the issues he took up in his journalism is, here, a moot point. What is evident is that he emerged as a national media personality and generated a following among the public and influential circles in the 1980s and 1990s, when Canada's political values were changing, a context that spurred editors and producers to look to experts, including historians, in our universities for comment giving context and guidance that audiences could use to make decisions about what direction the country ought to take. It's easy to label Bliss a neo-conservative and write off his contribution as a public intellectual as part of a broader right-wing agenda, but to do so would both misrepresent the media that turned Bliss into a media personality and Bliss himself.[46] Left-leaning publications, such as the *Toronto Star*, and broadcasters, the CBC in particular, sought out Michael Bliss, as did centrist magazines such as *Maclean's* as well as the conservative, libertarian-orientated *National Post*. His appeal runs across the political spectrum, and in that appeal rests new ways of understanding Bliss's contribution to our national debates and how the media shaped those debates by bringing him onto centre stage.

Michael Bliss offered intelligent and persuasive commentary on the merits of free-market capitalism and free trade as Canadians debated opening up the border to trade with the United States. When Canada was struggling with how to bring Quebec into the constitutional fold he advocated the importance of a strong central government in a fragmented country and highlighted the folly of a political elite tampering with political institutions that bind the nation. His writing on political corruption reminded Canadians to be vigilant and to hold their political leaders to account, while at the same time admonishing the press and politicians who tried to explain away ethical lapses as part of the political process in Canada. As his scholarly work turned towards medical history Bliss also gave context and insight on the burning political issue of the late 1990s and the early years of the new century. Bliss challenged the status quo in health care, arguing that medicare, like trade barriers, does not define the Canadian identity, and asked readers to consider whether individual rights should be suppressed, denying sick people access to timely treatment, in the name of socialized medicine. The media turned to Bliss because he had something interesting and insightful to say on questions Canadians struggled to answer. What he had to offer could not be generated in journalism schools, but was the product of a detail-oriented, scholarly mind that could frame issues inside Canada's national historical narrative, generating a large readership that could not be ignored by politicians who track the opinion of national audiences and develop public policy accordingly.

Michael Bliss's success depended on combining readability and expert knowledge with broader themes at a moment in Canada's history when the media craved expertise. At the same time, Bliss also felt as a teacher and a historian that it was his duty to enter these larger public debates. Media need and Bliss's sense of duty intersected at a critical moment in Canadian history, giving Bliss the opportunity to not just document history, but to become in his own way an actor in a larger historical process that brought important change to the country.

## NOTES

1 The Organization of American Historians held a seminar at its convention in April 2007 designed to improve understanding of the media. See http://www.oah.org/meetings/2007/ihrc.html.
2 Michael Bliss, 'Concentration Problem Found Not Worsening,' Letter to the Editor, *Financial Post*, 27 July 1985.
3 Examples of torqued headlines abound. One example that is worthy of note, however, is the *Toronto Star*'s 19 March 2006 front-page story 'Why Our Banks Have Abandoned the Poor.' The article alleged Canadian banks had abandoned the poor in Toronto's Regent Park, a community dominated by large public housing projects. But the story was bogus and

suggested the community had only one bank, when in fact it had two, giving the community more access to banking on a per capita basis than was
available in most other parts of Canada. The branch that was excluded was
600 metres from the front lawns of some Regent Park homes. John Turley-
Ewart, 'The Toronto Star's Smear on Banks,' *National Post*, 22 March 2006.

4  This is discussed in Neil Postman, *Amusing Ourselves to Death: Public
Discourse in the Age of Show Business* (New York: Penguin Books, 1984).

5  'National Amnesia,' editorial, *National Post*, 10 September 2001; *Saturday
Night*, Editorial, May 1997.

6  Afua Cooper, *The Hanging of Angelique: Canada, Slavery and the Burning of
Montreal* (Toronto: HarperCollins Canada, 2006).

7  A front-page article in the *Toronto Star* offers a fine example of this.
Cooper's work is dropped into the bottom of the copy, almost as an after-
thought, and the focus of the report is the Queen and the British prime
minister. Royson James, 'This Is a Disgrace,' *Toronto Star*, 28 March 2007.

8  http://www.histori.ca/minutes/minute.do?id=10166.

9  David Damrosch, 'Trading Up with Gilgamesh,' *Chronicle Review*, 9 March
2007.

10  Robert Fulford, *The Triumph of Narrative* (Toronto: Anansi, 1999).

11  Carol Goar, 'PM Sees Future in Canada's Past, *Toronto Star*, 24 November
2006. In this column Goar lauds Robert Bothwell's *Penguin History of
Canada*.

12  The importance of narrative storytelling is explored in the context of the
divide between narrative and analytical historians in Penny Clark, 'Engaging the Field: A Conversation with Mark Starowicz,' *Canadian Social Studies*
36, 2 (Winter 2002).

13  Charlotte Gray, 'History Wars,' *Saturday Night*, 7 October 2000.

14  Clark, 'Engaging the Field,' 00.

15  It is rare to see a professional columnist's work spiked, but it does happen
when a column is badly written or poorly argued and its publication would
serve the interests of neither the columnist nor the paper.

16  http://www.ryerson.ca/journalism/programs/#paper.

17  Robert Fulford, 'What Is the Point of J-School?' *National Post*, 31 July 2002.

18  Ibid.

19  Donna Logan, 'Educating Journalists in Today's World,' in *Journalism in the
New Millennium*, ed. D. Logan (Vancouver: UBC Press, 1998), 2.

20  Robert Marshall, 'A Shaken Nation Bares Its Anger,' *Maclean's*, 7 January 1991.

21  Neil Nevitte, *The Decline of Deference* (Peterborough: Broadview Press, 1996).

22  'The People Take Sides,' *Maclean's*, 1 August 1988.

23  Paul Kaihla, 'Truth and Consequences,' *Maclean's*, 23 March 1992.

24  Damrosch, 'Trading Up with Gilgamesh.'
25  Michael Bliss in conversation with the author.
26  Andrew Coyne in conversation with the author, 2006.
27  Christina McCall made these comments to Robert Fulford, who conveyed them to me in our conversations about journalism and Michael Bliss.
28  Michael Bliss, 'History on the Fly,' *Toronto Star*, 5 November 2002.
29  Ibid.
30  Universities that regularly contact me in my capacity as a comment-page editor using their public-relations departments to submit op-eds from faculty include the University of Toronto, University of Guelph, and Simon Fraser University. Often the departments that do submit on behalf of professors also edit the submission before it arrives, helping professors to bridge the gap between the writing styles in the academy and the media.
31  Michael Bliss, 'Academics: History Was Nothing but Relevance,' *Ottawa Citizen*, 28 December 1997.
32  Michael Bliss, address at 'Giving the Future a Past' conference, Association for Canadian Studies, Winnipeg, 20 October 2001, http://www.quasar.ualberta.ca/css/Css_36_2/ARteaching_canadian_national_history.htm.
33  Michael Bliss, 'Privatizing the Mind: The Sundering of Canadian History, the Sundering of Canada,' *Journal of Canadian Studies* 26, 4 (Winter 1991–2).
34  Robert Prichard in conversation with the author, 2006. When I was a TA for Bliss in his Canadian undergraduate class, it was obvious that he drew one of the most diverse groups of students to his undergraduate class of any Canadian historian and that many of them were there because they had read his work on newspapers or seen him on TV.
35  Michael Bliss, 'Tories Are Riding a Broad Social Trend,' *Toronto Star*, 16 October 1988.
36  A particularly striking example of Bliss drawing on his knowledge of business history to counter sentimentalist thinking is found in Michael Bliss, 'One Last Spike into a Canadian Myth,' *National Post*, 22 December 1999.
37  Michael Bliss, 'A Wild Constitutional Leap in the Dark,' *Toronto Star*, 30 June 1987.
38  Ibid.
39  Ibid.
40  Peter C. Newman, 'A Daring Strategy – and Bold Execution,' *Maclean's*, 7 October 1991.
41  Natasha Hassan, now deputy comment editor at the *Globe and Mail*, in conversation with the author, 2006.
42  Michael Bliss, 'Ottawa Needs More Whistle-Blowers,' *National Post*, 1 June 2002.
43  Michael Bliss, '"Angry All Over Again,"' *National Post*, 11 February 2004.

44 Michael Bliss, 'Two-Tiered Medicare Is No More Canadian Than It May Seem,' *Toronto Star*, 21 April 1995.
45 Michael Bliss, 'Health Care's Promised Land,' *National Post*, 2 February 2000.
46 A particularly egregious example of dismissing Bliss as a simple neo-con pundit and misrepresenting the media is Howard A. Doughty, 'Mark Kingwell: A Very Public Intellectual,' *College Quarterly* 8, 1 (Winter 2005).

# Politics and Business

# 4 Constructing Ignorance: Epistemic and Military Failures in Britain and Canada during the Seven Years War

E.A. HEAMAN

The press is generally touted as a good thing for public opinion and public life. But it can skew public debate in certain directions. Particularly in the heady early days of the development of the press, the more it was seen to play an important public role in the metropolis, the more its absence might be deprecated in provincial or colonial states. This essay investigates an early episode in the development of a public sphere. It provides an intellectual history of ignorance, so to speak, specifically the purported ignorance of the French Canadian population after the Conquest of 1760. That ignorance was one of the great 'truths' of post-Conquest British writing, developed and perpetuated by political correspondence, travellers' accounts, and the press. A variety of governors and pundits from the Conquest to the Quiet Revolution pronounced the *habitants* too ignorant for self-government and, consequently, susceptible to demagogues ranging from Louis-Joseph Papineau to Maurice Duplessis.[1] Lord Durham's report is perhaps the most famous example; perhaps the most telling is that of the Marquis de LaRochefoucault-Liancourt, who toured Canada in the 1790s. He was not allowed into Lower Canada, but was still able to say confidently that the French Canadians were ignorant.[2] Indeed, French Canadians could be found saying it of themselves in the early years of the British regime.[3] This paper explores what people meant when they spoke of ignorance. A close reading of the extraordinary efflorescence of pamphlets and journals during the Seven Years War reveals that the trope of French Canadian ignorance emerged very rapidly, within a particular intellectual and political context. There was always, implied or overt, a contrast with British public opinion, which was itself under serious political and philosophical scrutiny in the mid-eighteenth century. I analyse metropolitan arguments that British public opinion was not simply and unambigously knowledgeable and then provide local examples to show that Canadians were aware of the ambiguities.

The British themselves knew little and probably cared less about French Canadian cultural traits before the Seven Years War (1756–63), which the British avowedly entered in order to 'secure' North America for its colonists, who were being penned in geographically and harassed with bloody raids by the French and their aboriginal allies. With the war under way, the French Canadians became interesting to the British public, first as enemies, then as subjects. Only then, as the sketches of them multiplied, could the trope of ignorance become commonplace. But ignorance was not the first image of the French Canadians to circulate in Britain. Not until the 1760s did the trope of ignorance become dominant, and it reflected British ambivalence towards enlightenment and empire.

The British enlightenment and British imperialism of the mid-eighteenth century have received considerable attention from scholars in recent years, and no wonder. In their respective manners, British soldiers and British philosophers were conquering the world, and the British public followed their exploits in a public press that was noisy, opinionated, exuberant, and expanding almost day by day.[4] Britain was fast becoming a modern imperial power with the requisite 'far-flung' colonies, including most of North America. Whereas its North American possessions had hitherto been, for the most part, reassuringly British and concentrated along the eastern seaboard, during the Seven Years War Britain acquired the vast inland territory of New France, with its 80,000 or so (they reckoned) French-speaking, Catholic subjects.

The Conquest of 1760 raised problems regarding knowledge. It posed the question, Just what did one have to know in order to be British? French Canadians were offspring of the most 'civilized' nation in the world, so there was no question of their ultimate *capacity* for participation in the British polity.[5] That they had the rights of all British subjects was speedily recognized by the government. The minister responsible for colonies, the Earl of Egremont, observed that the French Canadians, 'being now equally his Majesty's subjects are consequently equally entitled to his protection' and must be allowed to 'enjoy the full benefits of that indulgent and benign government which constitutes the peculiar happiness of all who are subjects of the British empire.'[6] And yet in practical terms their distance from Britain and British language, history, and religion, as well as their lack of a public sphere, even of a printing press, meant that they lacked at least some of the prerequisites. The problem of French Canada highlighted the cultural density of Britishness.

The cultural density of Britishness is a hotly debated topic. Historians have pointed to the development of a British identity in or by the eighteenth century, but they disagree as to whether it was distinct from Englishness, and whether it was a civic or a cultural form of identity. The debate has largely focused on the Western Isles and the American colonies (which were largely peopled by kinfolk), with scant attention paid to the wider empire.[7] A richer sense of cultural diversity may shed more light on the question. For example, Jorge Canizares-Esguerra argues:

> It is very telling that the bulk of the scholarship critically addressing the epistemological and methodological proposals of the Enlightenment did not come from the British American colonies but from Mexico. Thomas Jefferson, Alexander Hamilton, and Benjamin Franklin did not offer any comprehensive methodological response to the negative views of America proposed by authors such as Buffon, de Pauw, Raynal and Robertson.[8]

Looking at Quebec can broaden the conceptual framework. Peter Marshall observes that 'no precedent existed for the effective imperial absorption of a non-British population.'[9] This question of absorption was debated by British politicians and parliamentarians during the 1750s, 1760s, and 1770s – they recalled their own conquest seven hundred years earlier in philosophical histories and they argued about their rights as conquerors in North America.

Rights mattered because the British exercise of power was not naked aggression and exploitation; it was cloaked in legitimacy. Antonio Gramsci is only one of many theorists to insist that hegemony is an important aspect of political consent and that it cloaks the naked use of force, which is illegitimate in the modern state. For Gramsci, hegemony is political consent exercised through culture – through such cultural organizations as political parties.[10]

In retrospect, there is clearly a problem. Cultural consent could exist in the Western Isles, where overlapping histories created a good degree of commonality in language, history, religion, laws. But British structures of hegemony couldn't obviously hold sway in a colony so far away as Canada, in the absence of any shared laws, customs, or institutions. Citizenship in Canada was far more problematic than citizenship in other British colonies in the 1750s, whether Ireland or Scotland or the United-States-to-be.

The cultural basis of consent was being theorized and articulated at precisely this moment by the leading figures of the British Enlightenment. Men of letters published sophisticated arguments about the ways in which culture and coercion intertwined. Hegemony was a hot topic in the 1750s. Something resembling a modern theory of hegemony was articulated by David Hume, who argued in 1742 that, because all rulers were vastly outnumbered by the ruled, they could not rule by coercion but only by opinion, even if only among the soldiers who enforced it. The worst dictator 'might drive his harmless subjects, like brute beasts, against their sentiments and inclination: But he must, at least, have led his mamalukes, or praetorian bands, like men, by their opinion.'[11] Similarly, Adam Smith, in his *Theory of Moral Sentiments* (published in 1759), argued that people were not simply chessmen to be moved around according to the whim of their leaders, but that 'in the great chess-board of human society, every single piece has a principle of motion of its own, altogether different from that which the legislature might chuse to impress upon it,' that the legislator resisted at his peril.

William Pitt's accession to power during the Seven Years War exemplified the point. Although the king disliked him personally and the reigning Whigs distrusted him, Pitt was too eloquent an opponent and too personally popular with the British public, and above all the London interests, to be left in the political wilderness, especially as military losses piled up during the early years of war. The howl of outrage and the cries of incompetence following the fall of Minorca in 1756 could only be assuaged by the execution of Admiral Byng and the appointment of Pitt as southern secretary (responsible for colonies) and the architect of the war effort. Pitt owed his advancement to public opinion, and in particular to his arguments for an aggressive war to take complete control of North America. Aggressive imperialism propelled him to power, but, as Marie Peters observes, public opinion was even more bellicose and imperialistic than Pitt himself, and it pushed him towards a stronger stand. The Canadian victories added considerably to his popularity and were celebrated with great pomp. The story of Pitt, the Great Commoner, reveals the growing importance and legitimacy of public opinion in mid-eighteenth-century Britain.[12]

Consent was an intriguing new problem in Britain, but it was all the more intriguing when the colonies entered the equation. Britons typically celebrated their own liberal political regime as more consensual than the more 'despotic' Bourbon regime in France. But the contrast failed to explain the success of the French in North America. Bafflingly, they seemed to have some 'secret' for 'conciliating the affections' of 'Indians' and thereby gaining their loyalty. Aboriginal traders would bypass Albany, and buy the same British goods at higher prices in Montreal and Fort Frontenac (Kingston), solely because they preferred to deal with the French.[13] It was this 'secret' affinity with the aboriginal population that made the French so dangerous in North America.

Naked force simply wouldn't work in Canada. By 1760, the British government had already spent, by popular agreement, too much money capturing a cold and poor country that the French had, more wisely perhaps, expended far less defending. It could not afford to garrison the place. It could hope that veterans would settle down on the land offered them, and many did, but the tide of immigrating Britons that Benjamin Franklin predicted would drown out the French settlers never materialized.[14]

Nor was deportation an option. The treatment of the Acadians was a case study in how not to govern. There was no appeal to Acadian culture, manners, or opinion, only a stipulation that the Acadians make a formal declaration of loyalty. When they didn't, and when the war broke out, colonial officials in Nova Scotia and in New York deported them to less strategically important locations elsewhere in North America.[15] The British did use a wholly coercive approach to the Acadian 'problem,' moving them around like men on a chessboard, treating them as beasts rather than men, objects rather than subjects. But that approach wouldn't work in New France. One the one hand, deportation would be strategically useless. Even if all the potentially hostile French Canadians (ten times more numerous than the Acadians) could be deported, the land would remain populated by potentially hostile aboriginal peoples.

On the other hand, this inhumane policy would have to run the gauntlet of British public opinion. It would be considerably more difficult to advocate wholesale subversion of the liberties of British subjects during a parliamentary debate, under the scrutiny of a partisan press, than outside parliament in the secret wartime councils of colonial governors. Indeed, the expulsion of the Acadians soon attracted condemnation. In 1758 the author of *An Address to the Great Man: With Advice to the Public*, observed: 'The Power of a Governor of a single Province, supported by the Opinion of a Council of War of Land and Sea-Officers, dealt them out in Parcels of four or five Hundred to every other English Government in America; where they mostly perished, through the Fatigue of long voyages, the Change of Climates, the bad Reception they as Catholics met with, and their own sullen Obstinacy.' With heavy irony he concluded: 'may this Business never appear to disinterested Nations in the Light of an unnecessary, impolitic, and perhaps cruel Extirpation.'[16]

In fact, this author believed that North American continental war was unnecessary: if the trade routes of the French Canadians could be cut off, then they would have to trade with 'their English Neighbours: and they would thence-forward cease to be our Enemies, soon commence profitable Allies, would establish an useful Barrier between us and the Indians, and in length of time possibly become our Subjects.' Wise government, which the pamphleteer expected of Pitt, would use interest rather than fear to turn bellicose and sullen colonials into peaceful and prospering allies and subjects. The same was true for their aboriginal allies: 'For the *Indians*, like the rest of the world, will bring their skins to the best market.'[17] Once the French state had been ejected from the New World, its subjects and allies could be won over to fidelity.[18]

According to this line of argument, if the British couldn't rule the Canadians – French and Aboriginal – by opinion, they couldn't rule them at all. But this did not seem to pose a great problem. On the whole, pundits were extraordinarily optimistic about the prospect of absorbing and conciliating the French Canadians. Some took a Rumsfeldian view, arguing that the Canadians would welcome the British as liberators.

When *Canada* and *Mississippi* were taken, our troops might march back to our own colonies, save only ten or twelve of the independent companies, and a few of the ships, to guard the country. But there need not be many left, because when once the *French* governors, their regular troops, and their priests are driven away, the poor planters would be glad to live there peaceably under his Majesty's mild government, especially as they are now kept most miserably poor under those bigots and tyrants, who oppress them to the last degree, because they were protestants when first sent there by *Lewis* XIII. after the siege of *Rochelle*, and continue so still, as far as they dare.[19]

Others argued that religious toleration, as guaranteed by the peace settlement, would suffice.[20]

But there remained a difficulty, if one continued to follow Hume, in making appeals to loyalty. They were always appeals to reason, and reason could never be a stable foundation for politics any more than it could be for the self. This point reverberates through all of Hume's writings, but it was made most explicitly in a new essay published (tellingly) in 1759.

Reason is so uncertain a guide that it will always be exposed to doubt and controversy: Could it ever render itself prevalent over the people, men had always retained it as their sole rule of conduct: They had still continued in the primitive, unconnected state of nature, without submitting to political government, whose sole basis is, not pure reason, but authority and precedent. Dissolve these ties, you break all the bonds of civil society, and leave every man at liberty to consult his private interest, by those expedients, which his appetite, disguised under the appearance of reason, shall dictate to him. The spirit of innovation is in itself pernicious, however favourable its particular object may sometimes appear.[21]

So, while Hume vested legitimacy in opinion, he vested opinion in 'authority and precedent.' This was the lesson of his *History of England*, published during the 1750s, which sought to rehabilitate the Stuart monarchs at the expense of the Tudors. Henry VIII had managed, Hume explained, to aggrandize royal authority and Protestantize the country, 'by insensible acquisitions, which escaped the apprehension of the people' and so were not rejected as usurpation. Hume showed that the exercise of authority rested on precedent, which is to say culture and history, and that these should be altered only gradually. By following that formula, one might indeed Protestantize a nation or a colony. Hume's work constituted a 'how-to' primer for the ambitious prince in the new age of public opinion.[22]

But how could a conqueror exercise legitimate authority over a distinct people? British customs, religion, and law might be a conservative force in Britain, but to impose them in a conquered country would be to impose precisely the sort of innovation that Hume warned against. It took very little experience of Quebec to see that the thin version of civic identity rested on the thicker version of culture. Every time the British government tried to cement the relationship between itself and its new citizens by extending civil liberties, it seemed to confirm their cultural distinctness. It could not grant them justice – the right to appear before the courts and participate in juries – without officially tolerating Catholicism and the French language, extending privileges not permitted in Britain. Moreover, because, as J.G.A. Pocock observes, property was the foundation of personality in Britain,[23] the British state had to confirm their possessions under French law because the alternative was to abolish all existing titles. As a result, these new British subjects were not wooed to British property laws or British justice, thought to be the best in the world, and these benefits were also denied to British immigrants to Quebec.

The problem was a practical one and it was also a theoretical and moral one. If the imposition of British institutions would eradicate existing property laws – laws that determined relations between parents and children, husband and wife – did the right of conquest include the right to private property? That sort of expansionist and assimilationist project on the part of the conquering Normans of 1066 was denounced as 'superfluous tyranny' by the conservative historians of the 1750s – David Hume and Edmund Burke.[24] The rights of the conquered were similarly upheld by the conservative Rockingham ministry in April 1766:

> To change at once the Laws and manners of a settled Country must be attended with hardship and Violence; and therefore wise Conquerors having provided for the security of their Dominion, proceed gently and indulge their Conquered subjects in all local Customs which are in their own nature indifferent, and which have been received as rules of property or have obtained the force of Laws, It is the more material that this policy be pursued in *Canada*; because it is a great and antient Colony long settled and much Cultivated, by French Subjects, who now inhabit it to the number of Eighty or one hundred thousand.

But when the Whigs tried to enact this policy in Parliament in 1774, they were criticized by conservative MPs, including Burke himself, who did an apparent turnaround to insist that the French Canadians should be forcibly anglicized: 'With a French basis, there is not one good thing that you can introduce. With an English basis, there is not one bad thing that you can introduce.' And many agreed with Burke's appraisal, albeit not enough to carry the vote.[25]

In short, the British agonized over the problem of legitimacy – political and cultural – in the new colony of Quebec. The British have not often paid much attention to Canada, but in the years around the Seven Years War, they wrote reams about it. They had to confront the problem of cultural difference and the fact that being British required cultural coinage. This was never described as culture, but rather as custom, which is to say history. The most common way of talking about the problem in the 1750s and 1760s was to talk of history and of knowledge. Participation in British laws and institutions required knowledge of history, British history, and that was something the French Canadians didn't have. From there, it was a short leap to say that these people were ignorant, too ignorant to be full citizens in the British polity; they must be half-citizens (deprived of self-government) until educated up to full citizenry. And this was precisely what happened, beginning almost immediately after the Conquest. But before the Conquest, the British press did not seem to consider the *habitants* particularly ignorant and was, indeed, more struck by the knowledge that they possessed, knowledge that seemed conspicuously lacking in Britons and British colonists.

The early observations came during the early years of the war, when Britain seemed to be losing it. There were terrible defeats in 1755 and 1756, including the defeat and death of General Braddock and the fall of Minorca. The losses led to much soul-searching and the debate between commerce and virtue flared anew.[26] Did a commercialized Britain still possess sufficient virtue to sustain martial values, such as a citizen militia, or should it rely on hired German mercenaries and control of trade to sustain its international position? In these debates, the contrast was always drawn between the peaceable British and the martial French. The French Canadians were understood to be, if anything, even more martial than the French themselves.

Because New France was commercially unprofitable, especially for farmers, its inhabitants lacked the commercial vices of British subjects. Though politically subservient, they had more manly military virtues than their British counterparts and might even be considered models to be emulated. When Braddock fell, the author of *Three Letters to the People of England* observed that 'a militia of French peasants which is to say slaves is doing better than our freemen, who aren't properly allowed to defend their country.' Even Indian chiefs, it was reported, noticed that 'the *French* behave like men, the *English* like women.'[27] A *Constitutional Querist* signalled the colonists' public spiritedness and energy, observing: 'It is this spirit in the French colonists that made them so powerful in Canada; it is this made us, at the beginning of the war, when our counsels were unprosperous, almost tremble for the fate of some of our colonies; and this it was that made the conquest of a province, in itself inconsiderable, be deemed a mighty acquisition.'[28] Another writer argued that Britain must fight the war in America by river and lake, not by land, because American farmers lacked the military prowess of the French settlers; yet another described the colony as a 'seminary for the soldiery that *France* must have in America'[29] The *London Magazine* observed that, barring a few priests, the settlers 'may be accounted so many soldiers, who are better for the service of that country than their best veteran troops, and even the Indians themselves' by reason of their fighting skill and their knowledge of the country.[30] Likewise, *An Address to a Great Man* observed that the Acadians 'missed few opportunities of promoting the French interest' and that 'it were devoutly to be wished' that British subjects copy them in this 'fault.'[31]

Some pamphleteers took the argument directly to the common people of England, who seemed all too reluctant to join a militia. 'A Plain Address to the Farmers, Labourers, and Commonality of the County of Norfolk' warned that, without a militia, the French might inflict on England the deprecations that the French colonials were inflicting on English colonials:

> The case is this, the *French* even in time of peace kept up the use of arms, and a good militia amongst their people; whilst ours neglected it, so that they were intirely unprepared for defence or resistance; and, (in which I am afraid we too much resemble them,) when the danger became imminent, and the *French* had even begun hostilities, instead of uniting closely, and pursuing vigorous and spirited measures, they were all divided, quarrelling among themselves, trying to shift off any little burthen and charge upon one another, and cavilling at, and opposing, every thing that was proposed for the public, service; and in this manner wasting their time, till destruction fell upon them; and now they severely feel the ill effects of their negligence.[32]

The debate about the militia bears remarking because it tempers the image of an educated English public and an ignorant French one. The English were *ignorant* of military knowledge: they had forgotten the arts that their forebears, skilled in the longbow, had possessed.[33] The French, by contrast, were *schooled* in military science. The leading jeremiad of the day, John Brown's *An Essay on Manners*, observed that 'their youth are trained up for all public offices in civil, naval, and military schools, at the national expence, and have NO MEANS to rise in *station* but by rising in *knowledge* and *ability.*'[34] This was a matter of political culture: whereas every French colonial was a soldier, disciplined to follow in unison the will of a unified executive, the British squabbled among themselves, the victims of their much-vaunted freedom of opinion.

The French knew warfare, the British knew peacefare, and the two seemed to be incompatible. British enlightenment – meaning both its knowledge and its liberties – counted for nothing if, in the end, the nation could not defend itself against its enemies. The French Canadians knew what one had to know in order to get ahead in the New World. British enlightenment, by contrast, seemed so much ignorance and blindness, with the only question left for debate whether the governing or the popular classes were the more to blame. And there were arguments for both sides. Some blamed irrational and unformed public opinion, insisting that tyranny, oppression, corruption, and folly must follow when 'the Minds of the People are not subservient to the Methods used for their Welfare and Security, but will indulge their own weak Opinions, in Opposition to their Superiors.'[35]

But other pamphleteers flattered their popular audiences and blamed the leadership. One exclaimed: 'I do not know any set of men, more likely to yield to reason, when it is honestly laid before them, than the farmers of *England.*'[36] Another, that 'the middle and lower class of people in *England*, are vastly altered and changed from what they were half a century ago, they will now see for themselves, they will now reason for themselves, they will no longer be amused and governed like fools and asses, as they have formerly been by their civil and ecclesiastical leaders, with foolish party-names and notions.'[37] These opposition pamphlets and papers blamed bad leadership for the military defeats. There wasn't much new in that: the opposition press had been denouncing the leadership so long as there had been an opposition press. The Machiavellian theme of a good people misled by corrupt rulers was freely articulated.

Historians have had a lot to say about the importance of morality and corruption to eighteenth-century political rhetoric, but they have had less to say about the concept and the practical workings of knowledge. The Seven Years War reveals that epistemology was as central to the political problem of the day as morality. The war proved the necessity for genuine, true knowledge of the world and ignorance at the highest levels was an obvious culprit. A prominent Tory, John Shebbeare, advanced the proposition at length. 'No man, I believe, will presume to deny, that a true Intelligence of what employs our Enemies, is necessary to all Ministers who would successfully oppose their Machinations.'[38] Natural justice was at work here: it was the 'settled Rule of Providence, that the best Understandings shall always prevail at last' – like the house in a Pharo game, they might lose a trick or two, but in the end they must win. But this knowledge of the enemy 'must be confessed to have been totally neglected' by the ministry, not from ill will but from incapacity, which was worse than ill will.

> Weakness and incapacity are even more fatal and destructive than a wicked Heart joined to superior Intellects in a M—r: This last, thro' pure Understanding, will exert every Faculty; conceiving his own and his Country's Interest inseparably united, his Judgment will correct his Mistakes, and re-instate what may have been originally wrong. But want of Intellect is irremediable; no human Power can correct that Error … It is the most incurable of all Diseases of the Mind.

Another pamphleteer observed that Britain would be better led by a Machiavelli or even a Count Richelieu, than by a Don Quixote, that paragon of stupid virtue.[39]

The fall of Minorca served to make ignorance a more prominent criticism than corruption. It was hard to see how the ruling Whigs benefited from the loss of the island, so corruption alone could no longer explain the government's failings. In the debate over that defeat, Byng's competence was set against that of the government, which had ignored French naval preparations at Toulon and sent Admiral Boscawen in the wrong direction. It proved as deaf to obvious warnings as were the antediluvians to the voice of Noah.[40] One cartoon showed the ministry plotting to disguise its neglectful ignorance of the real theatre of the war – as represented by a cobwebbed map of North America – by publicly smearing Byng and deceiving the public, which was so erroneously baying for Byng's blood. Henry Fox's co-conspirator, Lord Anson, the First Lord of the Admiralty (shown with a broken anchor), was depicted as a gambler, that is, as both corrupt and ignorant.[41] At a time when the ministry seemed hopelessly ill informed, it was one of Pitt's great appeals that he was always extremely well informed, thanks to an extensive network of American correspondents. Pitt gave the ministry the air of informed competence and helped to popularize that standard.

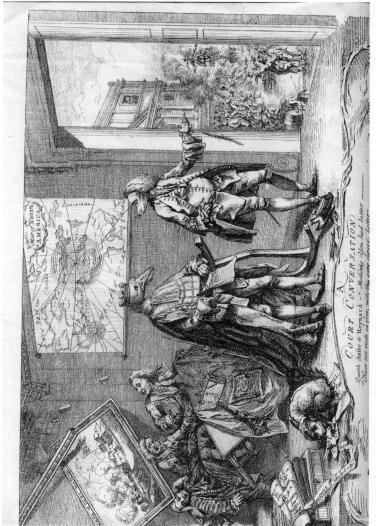

'Knowledge in disarray' (Courtesy of the British Library)

The British press trumpeted its role in spreading true and valuable knowledge. Journals were full of maps and verbose histories of North America and other theatres of war. They portrayed themselves as confronting head-on the corruption, ignorance, and dissimulations of the governing Whigs. John Wilkes launched his *North Briton* in 1762 with a bold panegyric to publicity and the press: 'A wicked and corrupt administration must naturally dread this appeal to the world, and will be for keeping all the means of information equally from the prince, parliament, and people.'[42] His was only the most vehement of the numerous calls for a public debate of the peace treaty.[43]

By 1762 the depiction of the 'enemy' had changed. France had lost the war and lost Canada to the decadent, corrupt British nation. The abashed, confused tone of pamphleteers quickly became triumphal. A British empire based on trade and on opinion – consensual and informed self interest – rather than on military domination and 'slavery' was vindicated. Knowledge of how to fight was not, it seemed, so valuable after all. The tactical advantages of the French were useless against the greater strategic knowledge of the English. Gramsci's metaphor of a war of position (in the trenches) versus a war of movement (the big battalions behind the trenches) seems appropriate, especially because the big battalions represented for him a dense civil society propped up by schools, associations, clubs, and political parties, things that hardly existed in French Canada.

Immediately, the trope of French Canadian ignorance began to emerge. The king's new subjects had virtues, but education wasn't one of them. Early in 1761 papers like the *London Magazine* and the *Annual Register* reprinted the Jesuit Pierre-François-Xavier de Charlevoix's description of the *Canadiens* as skilled marksmen and good subjects but probably 'unfit for the sciences.'[44] James Murray, the first civil governor, took a similar line, describing them as 'perhaps the best and the bravest race upon the Globe,' and, if their Catholicism were indulged, likely to become 'the most faithful and most usefull, set of men in the American Empire.' But even his earliest reports to the Board of Trade (which managed the colonies) observed: 'The Canadians are very ignorant and extremely tenacious of their Religion.'[45] The attachment to a superstitious religion was parasitical upon their ignorance, which had been carefully nurtured by jealous civil and religious leaders who 'practised upon their credulity.' Religious and political ignorance and servitude went hand in hand. As the Halifax *Gazette* observed in 1755: 'With very few Exceptions it may be said, that *Papists* are the most ignorant slavish herd of Bigots and understand no more of Religion than those Tyrants over their Faith, the Priests please to tell them.' Specific examples in the British press included Governor Vaudreuil's manipulation of French Canadian public opinion with false reports of success, even as the English were closing in and Wolfe's deprecation of the militia in favour of a trained soldiery.[46]

The Bible was only one branch of their purported ignorance; agriculture was another. Murray's report took pains to describe converted Huron as skilled farmers, implying a comparison unfavourable to the French Canadians, but also implying that the necessary skills could be taught. Likewise, one periodical in 1762 predicted that the French Canadians would become important consumers of British manufactures once, 'under the benignity of his majesty's reign, commercial ideas have spread among them, and they have been taught, by the wisdom of the *British* government, to make the most beneficial uses of their land.'[47] Being Catholic would, it was thought, slow the process down, as it had in Ireland, but the proximity of good examples by new settlers would help.

French Canadians were deemed ignorant of 'the inglorious arts of peace,'[48] arts that the British prided themselves they had developed to the highest degree. Britishness, to no small degree, consisted in one's relationship to trade and trading values. Commerce was an alchemy, turning private into public good, just the sort of alchemy that had to be enacted on the French Canadians to make them British. They had been public-spirited under France, now they had to learn private-spiritedness. In teaching them, the British would be assimilating them to British institutions as a whole. Murray recommended hemp: if the French Canadians raised it, they could become commercial farmers and supply the British navy. The hemp project initiated a sustained effort to reconstruct the French Canadian self through agricultural societies.

The problem with the agricultural societies was that they relied on the workings of that same ignorant *habitant* opinion that they were supposed to be reconstructing. And this paradox marked British efforts in Quebec from the start. Even as Murray denigrated French Canadian public opinion, he courted it. As the senior officer on the battlefield, and in charge of the garrison over the winter, he offered unusually generous terms to the inhabitants and local population, because his forces were too scanty to do otherwise.[49] As civil governor he continued to appeal to French Canadian opinion and loyalty. An early example is provided by the 'unhappy incident' of the grand jury presentment in the autumn of 1764. Grand juries played an important role in conveying local knowledge and opinion to the executive. In the absence of a legislature, they were an important source of political information and legitimacy.[50] The grand jury of 1764 (which included French Canadian jurymen) was specially charged with cultivating French Canadian public opinion:

> As we are but an Infant colony, I would beg leave to recommend it to your consideration by every means in your power to discourage any Advances towards disturbing the Public, or Individuals, either by personal invective or general calumny, either reduced to writing or verbal, as the promotion of such things serves for no other purpose than to weaken the community and to render us contemptible in the eyes of our so lately acquired Fellow Subjects.[51]

Murray's attempts to mediate between British merchants and French Canadian inhabitants failed. The grand jury demanded that Catholics be excluded from jury service, notwithstanding the presence of French Canadian Catholics on that very jury. Murray blamed political and linguistic ignorance that, he argued, left the French Canadians as vulnerable to manipulation by Britons as they had once been by the French. Likewise, commenting on an anti-French-Canadian memorial signed by some francophone Montrealers, Murray reflected (in a letter to military governor Colonel Ralph Burton) that

> Great pains, much art, and of course many misrepresentations, have been made use of to mislead the poor French people who have signed that memorial; indeed the memorial of itself sufficiently shews the truth of that Information. I have only to observe, that in my Opinion, the French will be good subjects, if properly managed, but if they are allowed to be led by Ignorant, licentious factious men, I foresee every bad consequence to the King's service, and to themselves.[52]

Here, Murray castigated both French and English as ignorant, not even exempting Whitehall in other letters. But the British did not much worry about British ignorance in the colony. By contrast, French Canadian ignorance was a political problem – and, of course, a political solution at the same time. Long after a legislature was created in 1791, the image of ignorance and manipulation was used to justify a great deal of illiberalism in the governance of the colony.

But another view was possible. Certainly British North American papers could just as easily fill columns deprecating the intelligence of the English peasants: the Halifax *Gazette*, for example, described the persecution of witches in Suffolk in 1753 as evidence that 'the Country People' there were 'full of Ignorance and Superstition.'[53] Murray's accusations of ignorance were not restricted to French Canadians, nor were those of Guy Carleton, who succeeded Murray as governor of Quebec in 1765. According to Carleton, French Canadians were ignorant in the way most people were ignorant: a few knew political principles and the rest merely clung to the laws they had grown up with.[54] By this standard, to complain of popular ignorance was to display one's own. That had been the lesson of the political philosophers. When Hume or Smith defended popular custom, they defended popular error. Governors who tried to govern against opinion might be correct in their ideas, but that didn't matter: any attempt to generalize them (any hasty attempt in Hume's formulation) would be wrongheaded. Truth existed under a regime: good truth supported the existing regime and bad truth destabilized it. Hume's sceptical philosophy led him to conclude that reason rested on both custom and an unfounded belief that future events would replicate past ones. There was no point in trying to debunk it. For Hume, the way in which beliefs were held – moderately or zealously – was far more important than the content of those beliefs: moderate views were good for political stability and zeal threatened it.[55]

Edmund Burke seconded the argument. His early essay *A Vindication of Natural Society* (1756) attacked the deism of Bolingbroke and Rousseau by extending their critique of 'artificial' religion to political society which, he showed, had caused incessant bloodshed and oppression throughout history. Political society and artificial religion were both products of artificial reason and amounted to the abdication of natural reason. People in political society were unable or unwilling to know truth or happiness: 'The Poor by their excessive Labour, and the Rich by their enormous Luxury, are set upon a Level, and rendered equally ignorant of any Knowledge which might conduce to their Happiness.'[56] And yet his scathing indictment of political history was a defence of that same political history. Political society was a Bedlam and a Newgate, to be condemned by natural or vulgar (speculative) reason, but it was necessary.

The fact that the essay uses politics to make an argument about religion requires the reader to look beyond the debates over deism to the political context of the 1750s. The newfound legitimacy of public opinion, the outbreak of a major war, and the prospect of conquering and being conquered, combined during this extraordinary decade. They pointed simultaneously to the promise and perils of knowledge in public life, the power and the fallacy of reason, the attractions and the dangers of relativism. Among his historical examples, Burke recapitulated the story of Athenian decay, whereby the people, unrestrained, became 'forgetful of all Virtue and publick Spirit, and intoxicated with the Flatteries of their Orators' and 'Truth became offensive to those Lords the People, and most highly dangerous to the Speaker.'[57] There were lessons to be learned here, but they were not lessons that could be easily conveyed by an appeal to popular reason. Burke's dark tract, which has 'baffled commentators over two centuries,'[58] was not written for a popular audience. Beneath the indictment of politics lay the foundation for Burke's defence of history as the source of morality and politics. History could not teach the reasoning mind which oppressive political system to prefer in the abstract, but it could and should teach citizens to prefer their system to others. Popular knowledge, which was really ignorance, and philosophical knowledge shared the same destination: a kind of patriotic acquiescence.

Hume and Burke were agnostics about knowledge. If public opinion was going to govern politics, it should not be like scientific opinion, zealously devoted to truth-seeking, but more like Livy's history, which entwined charming myth and empirical fact. Hume and Burke issued a clear warning against founding legitimacy on reason and knowledge. But their warning wasn't heeded. Knowledge seemed too powerful a legitimating grounds for governance and empire, especially in the new age of public opinion. During the Seven Years War, knowledge trumped virtue as the royal road to secure power in a threatening world. Apologists for imperialism insisted that they were not imposing one political culture atop another but were disseminating facts and the power to reason about them. The construction of French Canadian ignorance is part of this story.[59]

Hume was right of course. The appeal to public reason was always an appeal to an independent reason that might turn against the government. If the British governed by the power and the right of knowledge, then, if they could be shown to lack knowledge and local knowledge be shown to be autonomous, British laws were illegitimate. This would indeed become a powerful argument among the colonial reformers of the 1830s, voiced by Joseph Howe, the Patriotes, and even

Lord Durham.[60] But it didn't take that long for the conquered population to work out the argument, and a rebuttal was voiced almost immediately upon the establishment, in June 1764, of a local newspaper, the *Quebec Gazette*. In 1765–6, a series of letters to the *Gazette* used the idiom of ignorance to advance a serious critique of British governance. While the letters seem to develop and perpetuate the trope of French Canadian ignorance, read ironically they insist on local knowledge and metropolitan ignorance. The tone is oblique but this was, after all, a newly conquered country and some delicacy was required.

The point of departure was a letter by a French Canadian, Civis Canadiensis, which appeared in September 1765, observing that the *Gazette* had been full of alarums and complaints about attacks on British liberties in the form of the stamp duty, the cramping of trade, and the lodging of military men on the civilian population. Civis asked:

> Are they founded or are they not? You should not be surprised at my Ignorance. What can I, a new Subject of Great-Britain, know of the constitutional Rights of Individuals. Having however a Right, as a British Subject, to partake of those same Rights, Privileges and Liberties, I should be desirous of knowing what they consist in; but as no Body informs me what they are, all I can do is form Conjectures.

He continued: as part of the community, he would expect that his liberties should tend to the public good, but he had no way of knowing what that good was, and yet if he tried to express his ideas, 'if I, simple Individual as I am, should, under Pretext of Liberty, form Ideas, dive into Matters, and determine, by my private Opinion, in what the General Good of the Community consists, while there are others appointed for that Purpose, it will immediately be thrown in my Face, that it is easy to see, that I still favour of that Despotism under which I was formed.'[61] Civis closes repeating his plea for enlightenment, but not before voicing a statement which reveals that he did not believe himself quite so ignorant after all. A French Canadian had been heard lampooning friends and relations, and claiming that this sort of thing was done in England. Civis commented that, had this man 'been made acquainted with the Analysis of those English Liberties, which he gloried in the Enjoyment of, he would not have fallen into so gross an Error.' Clearly, Civis thought that he could distinguish between error and true liberty.

Civis's letter provoked a reply, again by a French Canadian, who defended his right to voice lampoons and then gave an orthodox description of British liberties as rooted in the control of selfish passions.[62] To my mind, this is beside the point: Civis was more interested in the political than the moral questions relating to British liberties.

The debate halted abruptly as the paper stopped publishing, due to the *Stamp Act*, but seven months later it was active again and a new series of letters appeared – under a different signature but written in the same tone, albeit less oblique. The purpose was an attack on metropolitan taxation policies. This time it took the form of a series of letters from a man in Quebec to his friend in Montreal. The author, signed 'Your real friend,' now openly accused the British of governing Canada ignorantly: 'I have never seen what you call the Mother Country, and consequently do not know whether her sight is so impaired as to oblige her to use Spectacles,' but, he insisted, 'the Mother Country is misinformed.' Britain clearly lacked 'Knowledge of a Memorial' that Canadians had signed and sent to the Board of Trade, which proved that Canada's productions did not pay for its imports.[63] The argument was, once again, hedged with protestations of the author's ignorance about British liberties. What information he could find about taxation was not fact but disputed opinion: 'After hearing so many different Opinions; I can form no judgment, and can only tell you with Certainty, that the Colony is not able to bear an Impost of any Kind.' Voluminous trade statistics cemented the argument.

The protestations of ignorance and pleas for enlightenment continued apace. One letter began: 'Sir, the astonishment with which you seem to have received the Information, *that no Body had as yet been able to inform me of the Privileges of your Nation*, has occasioned me to seek, with unparalleled Diligence, for that great Charter Magna Charta, to which you refer me for Information. I have found it, and now want nothing to satisfy myself but Interpreters.' The letter-writer found the language too archaic to be useful, and the comprehensible parts seemed to show rights granted only to the clergy and nobility, not to king or people.[64] The next letter had moved on (on advice) to Coke's interpretations, but several days' study convinced the author that taxes required 'the approbation and consent' of freemen and citizens.[65] The argument was, by now, explicit: no one seemed to know the constitutionality of taxes, and it was better to reason from the facts anyways. 'It is not my Business to examine whether His Majesty can order those Duties to be levyed, this I am ignorant of, here let us therefore leave Prerogatives, and bend our Thoughts to consider whether the imposing such Duties may not be productive of some Consequences prejudicial to Trade, the Colony, and the Mother Country.'

The Canadian author's protestations of ignorance are profoundly ironic. The letters overflow with statistics and the testimony of such authorities as Pitt and Franklin. He possesses decisive knowledge, and wields it like an axe to chop down the arguments from prerogative and constitutional history. Indeed, the author seems to advance some of the most modern political arguments available to him. His summary dismissal of the main tenets of Whig constitutional history sounds positively Humean. He also sounds modern in arguing from commercial facts to political ones, unlike his correspondent, who seems to argue from politics to economics, from the right to control trade to the power to control trade. And the anonymous author also shows that he clearly understands the British point of view, that a proper understanding of one's economic self-interest must simultaneously coincide with the proper economic interests of the metropolis.

But it goes further. That first letter, effectively a warning salvo shot across the bow, amounts to a defence of private judgment. The author is told that it is illegitimate for him to reason from his private judgment, but then he does exactly that. As Hume predicted, he can do no other than use his reason, and his reason leads him to disagree with his imperial masters. His request to be instructed in first political principles amounts to a dare that they try to tell him how he must think. The British may want deny him political representation so that they might train him up to genuine, informed, political agency – and indeed he begs them to do just that – but in point of fact he is already fully master of his reason and his economic self-interest, that is to say, fully politicized. The cultural project of discrediting French Canadian political and economic knowledge was always already intellectually bankrupt and was known to be such in both Britain and in Canada from the outset, because modern governance projects had to appeal to reason and opinion, no matter how dismissive of that reason they might be.

NOTES

1 See Gerald M. Craig, *Early Travellers in the Canadas, 1791–1867* (Toronto: Macmillan, 1955) and Adam Shortt and Arthur G. Doughty, eds, *Documents Relating to the Constitutional History of Canada, 1759–1835* (Ottawa: King's Printer, 1907–35); also Herbert F. Quinn, *The Union Nationale: A Study of Quebec Nationalism* (Toronto: University of Toronto Press, 1963).
2 Lord Durham observed: 'It is impossible to exaggerate the want of education among the habitans,' *Report on the Affairs of British North America*,

ed. Sir C.P. Lucas (Oxford: Oxford University Press, 1912); Le Duc de La Rochefoucauld Liancourt, *Travels through the United States of North America, the Country of the Iroquois, and Upper Canada in the Years 1795, 1796, & 1797; with an authentic account of Lower Canada* (London, 1799), 1: 314–20.

3 José Igartua, 'A Change in Climate: The Conquest and the *Marchands* of Montreal,' Canadian Historical Association *Historical Papers* 9 (1974): 115–34.

4 Linda Colley, *Britons: Forging the Nation, 1707–1837* (New Haven: Yale University Press, 1992), Kathleen Wilson, *The Sense of the People: Politics, Culture, and Imperialism in England, 1715–1785* (Cambridge: Cambridge University Press, 1995). On Canada, see Philip Lawson, *The Imperial Challenge: Quebec and Britain in the Age of the American Revolution* (Montreal: McGill-Queen's University Press, 1989); Vincent Harlow, *The Founding of the Second British Empire, 1763–1793* (London: Longman's, 1952–64); P.J. Marshall, 'A Nation Defined by Empire, 1755–1776,' in Alexander Grant and Keith J. Stringer, eds, *Uniting the Kingdom? The Making of British History* (London: Routledge, 1995), 208–22; Phillip A. Buckner, 'Was there a "British" Empire? The Oxford History of the British Empire from a Canadian Perspective,' *Acadiensis* 32 (2002): 110–28.

5 As compared to Native peoples of North America: see Joyce Chaplin, *Subject Matter: Technology, the Body, and Science on the Anglo-American Frontier, 1500–1676* (Cambridge, MA: Harvard University Press, 2001).

6 Egremont to General Amherst, 12 December 1761, quoted in Peter Marshall, 'A Nation Defined by Empire,' 213.

7 A recent survey of the scholarship is Krishan Kumar, *The Making of English National Identity* (Cambridge: Cambridge University Press, 2003).

8 Jorge Canizares-Esguarra, *How to Write the History of the New World: Histories, Epistemologies, and Identities in the Eighteenth-Century Atlantic World* (Stanford: Standford University Press, 2001), 210.

9 Peter Marshall, 'British North America, 1760–1815,' in P. Marshall, ed., *The Oxford History of the British Empire* (Oxford: Oxford University Press, 1999), 372.

10 Quinton Hoare and Geoffrey Nowell-Smith, eds, *Selections from the Prison Notebooks of Antonio Gramsci* (New York: International Publishers, 1971).

11 David Hume, 'Of the First Principles of Government,' in *Essays Moral, Political, and Literary,* ed. Eugene F. Miller (Indianapolis: Liberty Fund, 1985), 32; the observation's significance is discussed in Anthony Pagden, *Peoples and Empires* (London: Weidenfeld and Nicolson, 2001).

12 Marie Peters, *Pitt and Popularity: The Patriot Minister and London Opinion during the Seven Years War* (Oxford: Oxford University Press, 1980) and

Nicholas Rogers, *Popular Politics in the Age of Walpole and Pitt* (Oxford: Oxford University Press, 1989). On Pitt and the rise of the press during the war, see Paul Langford, *Public Life and the Propertied Englishman, 1689–1798* (Oxford: Oxford University Press, 1991); John Brewer, *Party Ideology and Popular Politics at the Accession of George III* (Cambridge: Cambridge University Press, 1976), H.T. Dickinson, *The Politics of the People in Eighteenth-Century Britain* (London: St Martin's Press, 1995); Bob Harris, *Politics and the Nation: Britain in the Mid-Eighteenth Century* (Oxford: Oxford University Press, 2002). See also David A. Copeland, 'Fighting for a Continent: Newspaper Coverage of the English and French War for Control of North America, 1754–1760,' *Early America Review* 1, 4 (Spring 1997): http://earlyamerica. com/review/index.html.

13  *London Magazine* 28 (1759): 25; 29 (1760): 543–5.
14  [Benjamin Franklin], *The Interest of Great Britain considered with regard to her colonies and the Acquisitions of Canada and Guadeloupe* (London and Boston, 1760), 47–8.
15  There is a voluminous literature on the subject. See, in particular, Naomi Griffiths, *The Acadian Deportation: Deliberate Perfidy or Cruel Necessity?* (Toronto: Copp Clark, 1969); Geoffrey Plank, *An Unsettled Conquest: The British Campaign against the Peoples of Acadia* (Philadelphia: University of Pennsylvania Press, 2002); John Mack Faragher, *A Great and Noble Scheme: The Tragic Story of the Expulsion of the French Acadians from Their American Homeland* (New York: W.W. Norton, 2005).
16  *An Address to the Great Man: With Advice to the Public* (London, 1758), 28.
17  *Gentleman's Magazine* 24 (1754): 504.
18  For example, *London Magazine* 29 (1760): 291.
19  *Gentleman's Magazine* 25 (1755): 391.
20  Once again, this was also true of Indians, *Gentleman's Magazine* 30 (1760): 351.
21  Hume, 'Of the Coalition of Parties,' in *Essays*, 495–6.
22  On Hume and the Enlightenment, see Philip Hicks, *Neo-classical History and English Culture from Clarendon to Hume* (New York: St Martin's Press, 1996); Mark Phillips, *Society and Sentiment: Genres of Historical Writing in Britain, 1740–1820* (Princeton: Princeton University Press, 2000); Roy Porter, *The Creation of the Modern World: The Untold Story of the British Enlightenment* (New York: W.W. Norton, 2000).
23  J.G.A. Pocock, *The Machiavellian Moment: Florentine Political Thought and the Atlantic Republican Tradition* (Princeton: Princeton University Press, 1975).
24  Edmund Burke, 'Abridgment of English History,' in T.O. McLoughlin and James T. Boulton, eds, *The Writings and Speeches of Edmund Burke* (Oxford:

Oxford University Press, 1997), 1: 472. Hume's criticism of the Norman understanding of the rights of conquest as 'very extensive in the eyes of avarice and ambition, however narrow in the eyes of reason,' was reprinted and discussed in the popular press: see *London Magazine* 31 (1762): 6–7.

25 *Debates of the House of Commons, in the year 1774, on the Bill for making more effectual Provision for the Government of the Province of Quebec* (London, 1839).

26 The classic statement is Pocock, *The Machiavellian Moment*.

27 *Three Letters to the People of England* (London, 1756).

28 *The Constitutional Querist* (London, 1762), 21.

29 *Gentleman's Magazine* 26 (1756): 211–13; 30 (1760): 551.

30 *London Magazine* 24 (1756): 286–7.

31 *An Address to a Great Man*, 26.

32 *Gentleman's Magazine* 27 (November 1757): 510–11.

33 Ibid.

34 *An Estimate of the Manners and Principles of the Times* (London, 1757), reviewed in *Gentleman's Magazine* 27 (1757): 171.

35 *A Political Treatise on National Humour* (London, 1756), 11–12.

36 *Gentleman's Magazine* 27 (September 1757): 407.

37 *A Letter to the Right Honorable William Pitt* (London, 1760), 13–14.

38 *Three Letters to the People of England* (London, 1756). Likewise, a Tory paper with which Shebbeare was involved, *The Monitor*, complained of the government's corruption in 1755, and of its corruption and ignorance in 1756. See also *London Magazine* 24 (1756): 403.

39 *Reasons for keeping Guadeloupe at a Peace* (London, 1761), 25.

40 *An Account of the Facts Which appeared on the late Enquiry into the Loss of Minorca* (2nd ed., London, 1757), 161–2.

41 *A Letter to a Member of Parliament in the Country, from His Friend in London, Relative to the Case of Admiral Byng* (London, 1756), frontispiece. See also the discussion in M. John Cardwell, *Arts and Arms: Literature, Politics and Patriotism during the Seven Years War* (Manchester: Manchester University Press, 2004), 87, 91.

42 Quoted in James Van Horn Melton, *The Rise of the Public in Enlightenment Europe* (Cambridge: Cambridge University Press, 2001), 36. Wilkes's campaign led to the end of parliamentary secrecy by 1771.

43 *Reasons Why the Approaching Treaty of Peace should be Debated in Parliament* (London, 1760).

44 *Annual Register* (1761), 'Characters,' 10; *London Magazine* 30 (1761): 25–7.

45 'General Murray's Report of the State of the Government of Quebec in Canada, June 5th 1762,' in Adam Shortt and Arthur G. Doughty, eds, *Documents Relating to the Constitutional History of Canada, 1759–1791* (Ottawa:

King's Printer, 1918), 47–81. See, by way of contrast, distrust of the French Canadians in the Upper Great Lakes: Kerry A. Trask, 'A Loose and Disorderly People: British Views of the French Canadians of the Upper Great lakes, 1760–1774,' *Voyageur Magazine, The Historical Review of Brown County and Northeast Wisconsin* 5 (1988–9) (also online at: http://www.uwgb.edu .wisfrench/library/articles/trask/trask.htm).

46 Halifax, *Gazette*, 15 February 1855 (citing a New York paper); *Annual Register* 3 (1760): 57.

47 *Gentleman's Magazine* 32 (1762): 532.

48 E.A. Heaman, *The Inglorious Arts of Peace: Exhibitions in Canadian Society during the Nineteenth Century* (Toronto: University of Toronto Press, 1999).

49 Fred Anderson, *Crucible of War: The Seven Years War and the Fate of Empire in British North America, 1754–1766* (New York: Alfred A. Knopf, 2000), 365.

50 Donald Fyson, 'Jurys, participation civique et représentation au Québec et au Bas-Canada: Les grands jurys du district de Montréal (1764–1832),' *Revue d'histoire de l'Amérique française* 55 (2001): 85–120

51 Library and Archives Canada (LAC), CO 42/2, p. 24, report by Murray to the Board of Trade. See Hilda Neatby, *Quebec: The Revolutionary Age 1760–1791* (Toronto: McClelland and Stewart, 1966), 37.

52 LAC, CO 42/1, Murray to Burton, 11 April 1764, p. 188.

53 Halifax, *Gazette*, 13 January 1753.

54 Shortt and Doughty, *Documents*, 295. See also J.A. Bourinot, *The Intellectual Development of the Canadian People* (Toronto: Hunter, Rose, 1881), 26.

55 Duncan Forbes, *Hume's Philosophical Politics* (Cambridge: Cambridge University Press, 1975).

56 'Vindication of Natural Society,' in Edmund Burke, *Pre-Revolutionary Writings* (Cambridge: Cambridge University Press, 1993), 53–4. The introduction by Ian Harris provides the deist context.

57 Ibid., 38.

58 Harris, in Burke, *Pre-Revolutionary Writings*, 4. Isaac Kramnick shows that the criticisms of contemporary society cannot be dismissed as merely satiric: see *The Rage of Edmund Burke: Portrait of an Ambivalent Conservative* (New York: Basic Books, 1977), 88–93.

59 Arguments for virtue would still be aired, but as an epistemological problem as well as a moral one, rooted in difficulties of communication and knowledge. Adam Ferguson, writing one of the last great British tracts in favour of public virtue in 1767, reflects the change with his wistful observation: 'If virtue be the supreme good, its best and most signal effect is, to communicate and diffuse itself.' Adam Ferguson, *Essay on the History of Civil Society* (5th ed., London, 1782), 1: 64. Available online at http://all.libertyfund.org.

60 In Yvan Lamonde, *Histoire sociale des idées au Québec 1760–1896* (Quebec: Fides, 2000), 223. Joseph Howe to Lord John Russell, 18 September 1839, in *The Speeches and Public Letters of Joseph Howe* (Halifax, 1909), 1: 235–6, 241–2, 252–3. Lord Durham: 'The colonists may not always know what laws are best for them, or which of their countrymen are the fittest for conducting their affairs; but, at least, they have a greater interest in coming to a right judgment on these points, and will take greater pains to do so than those whose welfare is very remotely and slightly affected by the good or bad legislation of these portions of the Empire.' *Report on the Affairs of British North America*, 282–3. See Philip A. Buckner, *The Transition to Responsible Government: British Policy in British North America, 1815–1850* (Westport, CT: Greenwood Press, 1985).

61 The French original invokes *knowledge* of the general good; this is an English translation that appeared soon after the French. Quebec, *Gazette*, 26 September 1765; English version, 3 October 1765.

62 Quebec, *Gazette*, 10 October 1765.

63 Ibid., 11 August 1766.

64 Ibid., 25 August 1766.

65 Ibid., 1 September 1766.

# 5 Common Knowledge: Theory, Concept, and the Prosaic in Making the Tariff of 1859

BEN FORSTER

The idea of a tripartite national policy exercises a continuing fascination; it is well ensconced as part of the intellectual feedstock of the Canadian educational system. Certainly, it seems to have broad explanatory power, as it appears to expose the internal logic of transcontinental expansion and industrialization within the nation state. After all, the trinity of immigration and western settlement, railway construction, and tariff protection appeared to intermesh to aid in the creation of a staple-producing, export-oriented western hinterland that at the same time provided a market for the manufactures of Ontario and Quebec. Here was the recipe for a balanced and dynamic national economy, replete with its own internal tensions, both regional and class. Sceptics may suggest, of course, that much of the fascination of the national policy lies in its potential for nationalist or regional myth-making, but there are other levels to its appeal. It is useful for didactic purposes, as a simplified (and thus by necessity partly misleading) means of comprehending the direction of Canadian development in the sixty years after Confederation. From another perspective, it functions as an interpretation, an abstract structure, formulated by historians to provide a model or explanation of Canadian economic growth. More emphatically, historians have implied or asserted that the tripartite national policy was a developmental policy consciously framed and applied by Canadian politicians and businessmen. These four levels at which the tripartite policy can be perceived are not readily disentangled of course, and are commonly concatenated.[1] After all, the deconstruction of the tripartite national policy as a historical reality or an effective interpretation leads the historian to view it as a form of mythology and to doubt its usefulness as a didactic device.

This paper will undertake to disentangle some of these elements in the context of the tariff of 1859. In doing so it will argue that the historical projection of a tripartite policy to this early date is incorrect. It will reject the notion that the chief architect of the tariff, Alexander Tilloch Galt, introduced radical and little-understood concepts of his own in the tariff, with primary and powerful protectionist intent. Instead, Galt implemented concepts well understood by the business community, and intended to maximize revenue for a government in desperate need. The tariff of that year was a revenue-maximizing concoction within which protectionist structural elements were given notable play. Moreover, Galt later drew away from the protectionism he accepted in 1859. In peeling back the conceptual and ideological layers relating to the making of tariffs in this period, the paper emphasizes the fiscal and political complexity of tariff-making, and asserts that political and pragmatic intentions were paramount.

Certainly before 1896, the national policy did not represent a realized economic reality. The concept does not adequately explain the dynamics of Canadian economic life, for the economy grew considerably between 1867 and 1896, a growth predicated on the expansion of industrial central Canada, not of a staple-exporting western agricultural hinterland. The success of Quebec and Ontario in industrial terms does not seem to have been crucially dependent on the prairie west, even after 1896, as Ian Drummond has forcefully demonstrated.[2]

Yet if the national policy is of doubtful value as a historical understanding of Canada's economic development in the last half of the nineteenth century, it still might be the way that many or at least key Canadians projected the development of the country. There can be little doubt that westward expansion was a vital concern to articulate observers in central Canada beginning in the 1850s, as Doug Owram has shown.[3] Even in the late 1840s, the prairie west controlled by the Hudson's Bay Company began to be seen as a new agricultural frontier by Ontario farmers, Montreal grain dealers and transportation men, pamphlet writers posing as national prognosticators, and a variety of politicians. By the late 1850s, Thomas D'Arcy McGee, Alexander Tilloch Galt, and other leading men perceived the west as a means of breaking out of the depression that had begun in 1857 and, at the same time, a means of transcending the stultifying political framework of the Union of the Canadas. Obtaining the Hudson's Bay lands in 1869–70 was crucial to the making of Confederation; thereafter, the construction of a transcontinental railway was important not only for fending off imagined or real American expansion in the Canadian west, but also as a means of inducing British Columbia to enter the union. The next fifteen years were explosive with the politics of transcontinental railways. Intimately associated with the taking of the west and its opening by railway was the need for population growth in the region. While some Ontario farmers functioned under politician-fostered misapprehensions that the west should be saved as a reserve for their excess progeny, the importance of immigration to the opening of an agricultural west was widely accepted. The evident success (1870–3, 1880–3, and after 1896) or lack of it (1874–80, 1884–96) in obtaining people for the west encouraged lengthy debate in the House of Commons, and the matter had been of great concern during the Confederation debates of 1865. Immigration and westward railway construction have an undoubted intimate link. Thus, if a tripartite national policy is to be seen as being fully articulated and consciously applied by businessmen and politicians, the proof revolves around the protective tariff policy – the 'National Policy' capitalized.[4]

A reductionist assertion would make the tripartite national policy the economic essence of Canadian nationality. Donald Creighton, who can usefully function as our straw man here (though a careful reading of some of his work shows how constrained he could be in his claims), saw the national policy both as an interpretation of the period and as a consciously constructed architecture of development. However, Creighton, who was fully acquainted with the Confederation debates, found no evidence in the mid-1860s of linkages between tariff protection and the strongly stated Confederation aim of westward expansion. Consequently, in his view, the tripartite policy had to wait until the 1870s, particularly the later 1870s, to be both fully articulated and implemented: 'The Fathers of Confederation and their successors were sure from the beginning about some features of their programme; but about others they were hesitant and divided. It took them some time to decide on certain parts of their plan; and it was not until 1878 that the last great decision in policy, the protective tariff, was taken.'[5] Creighton modulates the tripartite approach to present three separate national policies: immigration and western settlement, railway construction, and tariff protection, linked together as part of an overarching plan.[6]

Creighton's chronology, though not his underlying interpretation, has been disputed, and it has been argued that the elements of the tripartite policy were fully linked and articulated in the later 1850s. Thus, Alexander Tilloch Galt as inspector general and then finance minister

(Galt changed the name) was the first politician to link westward expansion and the tariff in an overall strategy of development for a prospective transcontinental Canada. In this interpretation the tariff of 1859 was emphatically and primarily protectionist in character. It was intended to foster the creation of a nation state though the development, in careful states, of primary, secondary, and tertiary industry. This case rests on a parsing of Galt's speech in introducing his Confederation resolutions in the provincial assembly, and on an examination of the 1859 tariff he introduced. Galt is thus portrayed as a protean figure, dynamic and original in his conception of nationality and the policy directions necessary to bring a new nationality into existence.[7]

But was Galt the decisive intellectual architect of protection in 1859, and was the tariff of that year a decisively protectionist device? Certainly, there seems to be no dearth of evidence to show that the tariff was protectionist. D.F. Barnett's close analysis shows that its structural characteristics were rooted in a sophisticated approach intended to foster industry through what is now called 'effective protection.' The tariff of 1859 was built in three ranges of tariff rates, each higher level reflecting an additional level of value-adding labour and capital. Thus, in simple terms, raw materials were to have the lowest possible rates of duty, at zero per cent, those same raw materials partially manufactured had intermediate rates of duty (10%), and finished products made of those raw materials had the highest rates of duty (generally at 20% in the 1859 tariff). In addition, the tariff was based on an understanding of how value added in the processing of input goods significantly increased the level of protection provided.[8] This structure and its underlying 'effective protection' basis is deftly drawn out of the 1859 tariff by Barnett, who assumes that it was really Galt's conceptual device. And certainly Galt was fully aware of how a carefully designed tariff could foster productive capacity in Canada, particularly in terms of value-added labour. In rough notes, probably for a speech to be given in early 1859, Galt noted three conceptual areas in which protection might be usefully provided in manufacturing:

> Those articles of which the raw materials exist in the country are proper subjects for protection.
> Those which requiring the smallest ... value of capital in fixed machinery, in proportion to the value produced.
> Those in which unskilled labor can be employed most fully, as thereby reaching the greatest class whose labor it is desired to raise in value.[9]

Throughout this note, Galt displays an obsessive concern with the development of low-level, labour-intensive manufacturing, and thus with labour-value-added protection. Yet Galt was not a significantly original thinker in terms of the tariff's structural qualities. Indeed, the massive incoming correspondence to Galt and his immediate predecessor Cayley from businessmen suggests that the business community was substantially aware of theoretical – to them very practical – considerations in the making of tariffs. On a pragmatic front, businessmen explored aspects of economic theory far beyond the limits of Galt's brief note quoted above, though of course the quote by no means expresses the limits of Galt's economic thinking.

Thus, for example, a number of manufacturers effectively pressed the infant-industry argument for protection on Galt. Framed in theoretical terms in the 1830s by John Rae while that economist was a teacher in Upper Canada,[10] the argument posited that those who first started manufacturing in a specific industry faced particular risks and burdens, and until well established, incurred costs that made these first movers especially vulnerable to competition. So those who initiated industries in a country justifiably needed protection against external competition until their manufactures were fully established. Thomas Ferguson Miller of Montreal undertook this argument at length with John Rose and A.T. Galt[11] when he asserted that his undertaking to establish a scrap-iron remanufacturing plant had special one-time capital costs and required the importation of skilled labour, and thus in this instance it was proper, 'in consideration of said proposed branch of industry being new and not without hazard, of the great economic utility and importance of the undertaking in a public point of view, of its first introduction being necessarily attended with uncommon expense and difficulty, the result uncertain and success problematical,' that the duty on producer-goods machinery be reduced or removed. D. Crawford, in writing to Galt on 7 March 1859, also placed his perspective within an implicit infant-industry framework. 'Several years ago since a differential duty was placed on roasted over green Coffee, prior to the imposition of that duty, not a single coffee mill could sustain itself in the Province, but since then ten establishments have opened and continued in operation Viz. One in Quebec, three in Montreal, two in Kinston [sic], three in Toronto, and one in Hamilton. If the differential duty is done away the practical result will be, that in a short time the establishments will again be closed.'[12] Numerous others implicitly or explicitly used this argument, without any reference to

Rae; the theoretical origins of the infant-industry notion were of no concern to businessmen lobbying Galt for protection. Yet they had the conceptual apparatus to hand, and Galt, who knew it as well, did not apparently dispute it.

No one, of course, has asserted that the infant-industry argument was Galt's idea. Galt's real apparent genius lay in building the tariff in such a way as to provide encouragement for value-adding labour and capital in the province. The three-tiered structure of the tariff, corresponding with raw materials, partially manufactured goods, and finished products, was the common stuff of lobbying by businessmen seeking tariff changes. An examination of the correspondence held in the Department of Revenue Records from 1856 to 1860 shows that this way of modulating tariffs was widely understood among those businessmen who wrote to Galt, to his predecessor William Cayley, and to their higher-level officials in the Departments of Revenue and Finance. Manufacturers intent on improving the competitive position of their factories frequently argued that producer goods (machinery and the like) intended for their plants should be allowed in duty-free. Eliminating taxes on expensive producer goods reduced input costs, and thereby conformed to the tiered structure of the tariff targeting domestic production and import substitution. Thus, a wallpaper manufacturer making inquiry as to whether he should move his operations from New York to the Canadas wanted to know if 'the Government will allow us to bring in our patterns, Models and Designs, and tools etc. such as *are only used in the manufacture of the Goods. I mention the above as they are for use and not for sale.*'[13] Rather later, the Montreal capitalist and banker George Stephen conceived of the trick of having woollens-manufacturing machinery held in bond in the factory. The machinery was conceptually still in the customs port-of-entry bonded warehouse as a result, so duties did not have to be paid on it, it never having been officially imported![14]

But producer goods were only part of the equation. That a tiered structure was the best form to provide protective levels for value-added manufacture was fully evident to manufacturers. The tariff propounded by the Association for the Promotion of Canadian Industry in April 1858, intended to push the then inspector general William Cayley along a protectionist path, was three-tiered. It reflected the interests of the association's membership, industrial and commercial, and was not a governmental policy model.[15] A massive memorial to Galt, dated 11 March 1859, from Frothingham & Workman and nearly forty manufacturers and importers of Montreal, displayed considerable sophistication on this front. They urged that protection should be reflected in low rates of duty on input items: 'Due regard will be given to the acknowledged principle of encouraging industry of the Province by admitting at the lowest possible rate of duty all articles that are considered raw material & which are not produced in the Country,' that manufactured goods produced in the country should be well protected, and that partly manufactured goods like iron and copper wire, bars of metal, or sheets thereof should not pay a low rate of duty.[16] William Hibbard of Montreal, a leather manufacturer, displayed a complete confidence in his understanding of the process. It was a principle that was already embedded in previous tariffs, and he knew that Galt was well aware of it:

> May I take the liberty of directing your attention to an omission of some importance in the last tariff, which possibly may not have come under your observation.
> Viz: – Leather, previously paying a duty of 15% was advanced to 20% without any distinction between 'Finished' and 'Unfinished' or 'In the rough' as it is technically termed. The latter is employed for the manufacture of 'Leather Belting' and Patent Leather, requiring large expenditure of labour which ought to be retained in the Province.[17]

Joseph Rogers, a hat manufacturer of Toronto, had made the same point to a customs official two years earlier, sending along as evidence of the necessary additional labour involved in manufacturing a finished felt hat from an unfinished felt-hat body, samples of each. The felt-hat body should be charged what at that time was 2.5 per cent rather than 15 per cent, he thought, and the finished product 15 per cent. That he was more concerned with cheap imports than manufacturing is not the issue here; he fully understood the principle.[18] Fish-oil manufacturers also had an excellent grip on the concept, as their memorial of 17 March 1858 to the then inspector general, William Cayley, clearly indicated:

> We beg respectfully to call your attention to the interpretation of the Reciprocity Treaty with the United Stated acted upon by the Customs Department with reference to the Article of Oil. The Treaty provides for the free admission of Fish, Fish oil, the product of fish, and all other creatures living in the water, from which we infer that *crude fish oils in their natural state*

is intended, but a different construction of the act is carried out by the Department, in the admission free of duty, of all *manufactured fish oils*, which go through an elaborate process of pressing & bleaching to extract the drug and refine them [*sic*], such as Winter pressed Elephant, whale & Sperm oils, to the great injury of our own fisheries, whose crude oils have to compete with their manufactured article, and also to an important and very extensive branch of industry carried on by ourselves, and others through the Province.[19]

That Galt was attempting to construct the tariff of 1859 on these well-understood lines, and on a consistent basis, was evident in the memorial from the premier metals importers in the Canadas of 29 November 1858, in which they asked for the importation of smelted copper at the low rate of 5 per cent, 'which would simply be carrying out the spirit of the present Customs Tariff.'[20] In proposing specific duties on cigars, R. Thompson of Hamilton, a cigar manufacturer, particularly wanted protection against cheap German cigars, and noted that if the protection were not provided, 'we will have to become dealers in German cigars and send the money out of the country that would otherwise be used in giving employment to our own people ... There will not be any more cigars used and the amount of Revenue you will derive from this source will be more than lost by the number of persons now engaged in making cigars and who will be obliged to leave the country in consequence of the alteration.'[21] Here the sharp end of the labour-value-added perspective becomes clear – if labour was not employed in adding value as a result of protection, a loss of labour population would result.

The notion that high-value components of finished goods should receive low rates of duty was also understood: 'Your Memorialists conceive that Vaneers [*sic*] ought to be considered as *Sawed Lumber* and should be included in the list of raw materials and admitted as heretofore *free of duty.*'[22] Veneers greatly enhanced the value of furniture and pianos as finished products. But while a year later the matter of veneers had been resolved to the satisfaction of the manufacturers, piano manufacturers had found other inconsistencies based on the same principles. Here the subtleties of value added escaped some of the lobbyists. That a higher rate of duty might be charged on component parts necessary for manufacturing an item than on the finished product, as long as the component part did not form a large part of the finished product's value, was not clearly understood. Thomas Flood, a piano manufacturer of Montreal, complained to John Rose that with the exception of veneer, the raw products for piano-making paid 15 per cent duty, and that finished pianos imported from the United States only paid 7.5 per cent – while his exports to the United States had to pay 25 per cent. He rather ambitiously calculated his total costs at 40 per cent when exporting there. That certainly made the contrast with the 7.5 per cent paid by the American imports into Canada startling, though it misconceived the value added perspective.[23] It was, of course, nearly impossible to actually calculate rates of effective protection because there existed no immediately useful mode of measuring value added in manufacturing in 1858–9. Galt, Cayley, and their correspondents depended on the tariff-rate spread between input and output items to estimate protection.

Similar misconceptions informed the perspectives of Greene and Sons, one of the most active lobbyists during the making of the 1859 tariff. Greene and Sons, who were able to present a wide array of sophisticated arguments relating to tariff matters, nonetheless saw it as 'suicidal' to place the tariff on headgear at the same rate as the goods necessary to its manufacture – hat plush and dressed skins. The duties being the same, they were convinced, would result in the 'prostrating [of] the industrial trade.'[24] Clearly the writers, no slouches at self-interest, wanted a return to the former duty on hat plush of 5 per cent. The notion that the value added in the manufacturing process had a direct impact on the level of protection was not addressed in their submission.

But others, in a practical way, understood this theoretical conception, at least when it accrued to the benefit of those doing the lobbying. A sole-leather manufacturer decried the placement of his product at an intermediate level of duty in Cayley's 1858 tariff because 'it takes *more* fixed capital to establish a Sole leather factory in proportion to the business done than either [cotton or woollens or] Boots & Shoes, [for which] a building can be hired, [and] a few hundred dollars will supply the fixed tools of the craft.'[25] The farmers of Dundee and surrounding townships requested the use of American fulling and carding mills just across the border. They wanted to send their raw wool across to the United States and have it manufactured, but they did not want to pay duty on the material when it was brought back, only on the value added to the wool through the carding and fulling process. Thus, they wanted relief granted 'by paying duty upon the actual labour done to the articles in the States, and not upon its value as Cloth.'[26] While some misconceived elements of the value-added protectionist ladder, at least when their ox was gored, others played the theory to their advantage.

Protection was clearly an issue of importance in the tariff of 1859, and of the tariff that preceded it. Historians who have viewed that tariff as an essentially or exclusively protectionist device can certainly be forgiven their perspective given the mass of evidence that suggests that conclusion. This mis-perception is all the more understandable given that the Association for the Promotion of Canadian Industry, a lobby group formed in 1858 in order to foster a protectionist tariff, obtained a great deal of contemporary and subsequent attention.[27] The association did much to trumpet its own self-importance. Its intent was to 'co-operate with the government in the work of tariff reform, without regard to political affinities.' The 'national policy for Canada must prevail, and ... its triumph is but a matter of time,' a pro-protectionist newspaper frankly stated.[28] But even in this context, where there existed an overwhelming protectionist bias, non-protectionist functions for the tariff could not be entirely ignored.

To better grasp these it is useful to explain briefly the functional characteristics of customs duties. Tariffs are schedules of customs duties that are paid on goods imported into a country. Duties are paid by the importer and their cost is generally passed on to the consumers of the goods. The duties can take two forms, one a specific duty (a set sum on a particular good), the other an *ad valorem* duty (a percentage of the value or cost of the good). The monies are collected at ports of entry into the country, and once collected become part of governmental revenue. Customs duties are, in administrative terms, easy to collect, given relatively modest overhead costs and their imposition at a limited number of locations. Their protective function derives from the impact they have on prices. They increase the cost of imported goods, and thus encourage import substitution in the country of importation, thereby fostering domestic capital formation and jobs. At the same time, they can increase the cost of living, as they function as regressive taxes on consumption. As taxes, they provide government with income. From Confederation until well into the twentieth century, the tariff generated 60 per cent or more of the central government's revenue. In the Union period, from 1841 to 1866, the tariff generated some three-quarters of all revenue. On some key goods (such as alcoholic products) customs duties could be balanced on the domestic side with excise taxes, so if applied with care in these contexts, customs duties did not encourage smuggling in an untoward fashion.[29] The tariff was in end effect a regressive consumption tax. That the tariffs as taxes were regressive and increased the cost of living did cause some concern. There was considerable opposition to heavily taxing 'necessities' such as tea, sugar, and foodstuffs.[30]

So the tariff had the chief and largely unquestioned role as the major generator of government income, before the era of the income tax. Its chief flaw as a revenue generator lay in its great sensitivity to trade cycles – a commercial depression could have powerful, negative impacts on governments as imports and revenue both would fall sharply. As expenditures could not easily be brought into conformity with such a fall in revenue, a government could be placed in especially tight spots. In an expansive economy, when growth is driven by a government incurring heavy debt loads, such a commercial downturn and associated sharp decline in government revenue would be particularly dangerous.

This is what indeed happened in the Canadas in the late 1850s. Michael Piva's thorough and conclusive exploration of government finance during the Union period examines the impact of these converging forces on the efforts of the government of the Canadas to remain afloat fiscally.[31] There was a commercial collapse in 1857, at the tail end of a period of particularly expansive growth, a portion of which was directly related to railway construction. Imports declined sharply, and so did government income. The railway construction that had taken place was underwritten by a variety of guarantee and bond mechanisms proffered by the government of the Canadas. These came emphatically into play beginning in 1856 as the railways, particularly the Grand Trunk, failed to generate the income expected.[32] So the governmental financial pressures that began to grow in 1856 became intense by 1858 and 1859. Galt fully knew that the financial position of the Province of Canada was precarious after becoming inspector general in 1858, if he had not been aware of its full extent before.[33] To some men of financial acumen it seemed that the province was staggering towards bankruptcy, especially as the commercial depression triggered in 1857 showed no signs of lifting. A bloated and unprofitable Grand Trunk Railway soaked up government money and bond guarantees; the Great Western Railway, though not as troubled, sought government manna with almost equal avidity. The provincial credit was directly tied to the fortunes of these ventures, and the London money market judged provincial bond issues accordingly.[34]

Though Galt's predecessor as inspector general, William Cayley, tried to paint a bright financial picture, those behind the scenes were gloomy. In June of 1858, the auditor general, John Langton, told Cayley with appalling frankness that things were much worse than Cayley thought; that an annual ongoing deficit of £600,000 (equal to about half the province's budget) could be expected in future years, and that no amount of cutbacks in expenditure or increase in customs duties would suffice: the province might well be driven to direct taxation of some form.[35] In fact, Cayley had undertaken to increase the revenues as early as 1856, and had at that time indicated that the pressures generated by the railways could only be dealt with by further government borrowing, direct taxation, or through the increase of customs duties, the last of which was the only real choice in his mind. His intention generated considerable opposition as well as protectionist opportunism.[36] By 1858 his efforts to increase revenue through tariff increases had grown more desperate; this, and the tenuous hold on political power by the government of which Cayley was a member, made him amenable to the tide of protectionist pressure generated by the economic downturn. Even so, Cayley had not grappled fully with the revenue needs of the province, as Galt recognized when he replaced the politically shattered Cayley after the infamous Double Shuffle. The dubious financial position of the Canadas remained, as Galt acknowledged. The large deficit that had been run in 1857 was coupled by another serious one in 1858, and the Grand Trunk difficulties did not go away, even after the imposition of higher tariffs in 1859. 'The truth is that my difficulties, financially, which have been sufficiently great arising out of the position of the Province, when I assumed office, are augmented every day by the necessity of supporting interests [e.g., the Grand Trunk] which it would be most disastrous to allow to succumb.' So wrote Galt to Thomas Baring, one of the British bankers dealing with Canadian-related debt issues in the London market.[37]

In late 1858 and 1859, as Galt formulated his budget plans, he initially looked to reducing the expenditures of the province as a mechanism to meet at least in part the difficulties it faced. His emphasis on retrenchment was not a mere pose, struck for the benefit of British banking houses and British bond purchasers, and thus possibly meant to disguise pure protectionist intent. Galt, as his confidant and fellow minister of the Crown John Rose indicated to a key British correspondent, planned to rid the exchequer of 'local bloodsucking if we live.' The province had to 'prune down gradually the Grants to institutions etc enter on no more Public works that do not offer a reasonable prospect of being remunerative ... Galt & I have determined to devote ourselves seriously to the task of making both ends meet.'[38] Galt made strenuous efforts to reduce government expenditures, but here his hands were tied by the need to maintain political power and the irreducible quality of basic expenditures, as well as the potential and real liabilities the railways imposed. The efforts to 'retrench' could only do so much, and as events proved, the savings were much less than Galt had estimated. Even as he planned his budget, Galt recognized that greater tax revenues were necessary.

As Rose acknowledged, 'our Tariff must be kept for some years to come up to the highest revenue pitch.'[39] The business community recognized the importance of revenue needs as well. William Cayley had been informed in mid-1858 that imported iron could readily withstand a *'Revenue* duty' and that many importers agreed with the letter writer.[40] Even vigorously protectionist sources acknowledged this as a matter of some importance, indicating that government revenues clearly had to improve.[41] Of course, manufacturers sought to find shelter for protectionist ends under the revenue umbrella. The manufacturers of tobacco pulled out the argument that American manufacturers had the advantage of slave labour, and that the Canadian 'Coloured population of this province, most of whom are acquainted with the manufacture of this article,' would find work if an appropriate differential duty on the manufactured product were imposed. Besides, an increased duty *'would yield a larger amount of revenue* than what is now derived from that source.'[42]

The same attitudes were evident after Galt took over. When he modified and then shepherded the Cayley tariff through to law in 1858, Galt noted: 'The cheerfulness with which under very severe mercantile distress our community have submitted to increased taxation ought to give our British creditors, increased confidence in our securities.'[43] When the Montreal Board of Trade provided its perspectives on possible tariff changes, they were cautious not to provide specific suggestions, 'as they do not know the amount of Revenue that has to be collected.' The Quebec Board of Trade urged that 'whenever the state of the Revenue would permit the Duties on Sugar and Molasses be reduced.'[44]

Galt undertook to calculate how the revenue could be maximized given governmental needs. He was quite willing to acknowledge publicly that he hoped to raise as much revenue as possible in the dire circumstances the government faced. As he told protectionist deputations that opportuned him, 'Revenue must be had, duty [would be] increased where [an] article could bear it; duty [would be] reduced where it could not to increase importation and thus revenue.' Here too lies an explanation of Galt's occasional raising of duties on raw or semi-processed goods. While it might be reasonable to try to create protectionist support for an intermediate product, it might also be possible to generate more revenue through input items required by industries that had moved beyond the infant-industry stage, despite their protests. The conceptual apparatus he could bring to bear was sophisticated, but in functional terms could not be precise. Clearly enough, if a duty on an item was at zero, no revenue could be raised. As well, an exceedingly high customs duty would be prohibitory of imports, and thus could not generate income for the government. So, as rates moved up a sliding scale, steadily higher revenues could be obtained, though the rate of increase in the revenues would slow as the imported goods become increasingly expensive, import substitution took place, and fewer consumers purchased imported goods. A maximum point of revenue could thus be reached, for if the tariff rates continue to rise indefinitely, imports begin to fall off sharply through the combined pressures of import substitution, increasingly high consumer prices on the imported goods, and smuggling, all tendencies well understood in the business community of the late 1850s: '... *High duties* on light articles generally such as dry goods ... are in some measure a premium for smuggling, over an extensive and open frontier like ours and must therefore operate prejudicially to the interests of the Revenue,' the Toronto Board of Trade noted.[45] So high rates of duty undercut revenue not only because of import substitution but because they encouraged the development of an underground economy – smuggling in some instances and the deliberate undervaluation of goods in others.[46]

Revenues derived from customs duties thus follow a curve that first rises then falls, as the rate of customs duties steadily rises. Observers will immediately recognize this as a Laffer curve (see fig. 5.1), named after the supply-side economist Arthur Laffer.[47] There is considerable dispute as to how well the Laffer curve, as an element of supply-side economics, models reality, but in its usage here it is emphatically a model of revenue maximization, and should not be deemed to carry supply-side baggage. It is a model of the way in which Galt understood how revenue could be obtained for customs duties. The point t* is what Galt had in mind: for there the maximum revenue could be obtained, and he believed he had approximated that level or lay below

Figure 5.1    The Laffer Curve

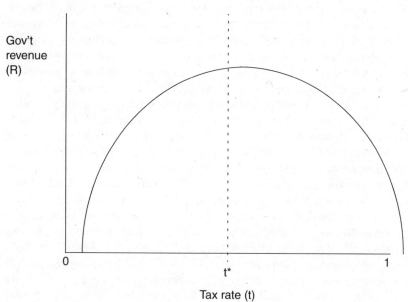

it in the tariff of 1859.[48] As he later articulated his revenue intentions, 'The point to be desired is evidently to fix such a rate of duty as will not by a diminution of consumption, defeat the object of obtaining revenue and the undersigned contends that this point has not been exceeded in the 20% duties.'[49]

Galt's contemporaries understood the concept. Those concerned with the customs duties on sugar played the revenue issues with considerable intensity. Importers, who naturally wanted duties as low as possible on sugar, made the argument that excessively high duties on the manufactured item would 'materially reduce the demand for sugar in the country and thereby adversely effect the revenue.'[50] A moderate view came from the Montreal Board of Trade, which felt it necessary to strike a balance between importers and manufacturers, and so urged on Galt 'the propriety of reducing the duty on refined Sugars ... to 30% instead of 40% as we conceive the 30% on the enhanced value of refined, over Raw Sugar, is a sufficient protection to native industry, and will not prevent the importation of such goods. While at the rate of 40% no Revenue of moment will be derived.' The board of trade exhibited not only a clear understanding of how higher tariffs might lead to lower revenue, but also an awareness of how labour value added functioned within the tariff structure.[51] Peter Redpath, who manufactured sugar in Montreal, carefully suggested a three-tiered structure for sugar duties, arguing that they should vary according to the value added – raw molasses at the lowest rate and white sugar at the highest, with other grades in between.[52] He understood the subtleties of the tariff mechanism.

So businessmen readily grasped that protection was to be provided within the framework of revenue needs. Years later, in 1871, Sir Francis Hincks, as finance minister of Canada, suggested that a purely revenue tariff was at the 10 per cent level.[53] Galt, in 1859, set the tariff level for goods not otherwise specified at 20 per cent, which he felt approached the point of maximizing revenue for many goods. Under that umbrella, a considerable amount of industrial protection could exist in the tariff, particularly given the three-tiered structure that Galt, as well as many members of the business community, found attractive. As one correspondent from the Quebec Board of Trade noted, when 'forming a Tariff for Revenue purposes special care should be taken that while giving moderate protection to the manufacturer the rates of Duty should so moderate as not to interfere too much with the regular import nor to encourage contraband Trade.'[54] This is what Galt called 'incidental protection,' a phrase that goes back to the late 1840s. *Incidental* protection was not *accidental*,[55] but was a planned secondary phenomenon – secondary to the needs of maximizing revenue. Given this principle, Galt's intention to maximize revenue provided headroom for protectionism. As the Montreal Board of Trade articulated this principle, 'Sound policy requires that raw materials shall be admitted free, or at a nominal duty; and that in framing a Tariff for Revenue purposes, founded on just principles of taxation, regard should be had to the encouragement of such branches of Manufacturing as can be advantageously prosecuted in this Country.'[56]

Indeed, if one examines the rate levels in the tariff of 1859 as revenue generators, the tiered structure that to this point has appeared so forcefully as a protectionist framework becomes ambiguous, shot through with revenue imperatives. While protectionist manufacturers sought, in their tiered-tariff proposal of 1858, to have the highest level at 25 per cent, and the intermediate level at 15 per cent, Galt resisted their imperatives, and created levels of 20 and 10 per cent. Given that Galt asserted that his rates would 'not by a diminution of consumption, defeat the object of obtaining revenue,' the refusal to raise the rates to levels that manufacturers desired was an assertion of the primacy of revenue. And while Galt may have structured the tariff to encourage industries not yet in existence by placing finished products not yet made in Canada at the highest tariff levels – such as Sheffield-equivalent cutlery – it was perhaps more reasonable to assume that such goods were placed at the 20 per cent level in order to generate the maximum revenue. The likelihood of a high-quality batch-steel manufacturing industry in Canada was remote at that time. It is true that the manufacturers' suggested tariff urged the placement of many intermediate products at a 25 per cent level out of pure self-interest, and that Galt lowered many of those to 10 per cent. But that too could be seen as a mechanism intended to generate a higher level of income for the government. The 10 per cent level, by allowing for greater levels of importation of intermediate goods, could produce more revenue than 25 per cent. Galt's frank statement – 'Revenue must be had, duty [would be] increased where [an] article could bear it; duty [would be] reduced where it could not to increase importation and thus revenue' – is thus revealed in his implemented tariff as counterpoised to the manufacturers' demands. The tariff structure was in large part a creature of revenue needs, not merely of protectionist intent.

Those historians who assert that Galt was trying to implement a scheme of national integration involving a tripartite national policy perhaps necessarily assert that his tariff policy was essentially or only protectionist. It was not. However, a planned protectionist policy, even if it were secondary to the tariff's revenue function, might still stand as a kind of marker towards the larger goal, if there were evidence that the protectionist policy was being consistently and persistently pursued. Galt certainly had the opportunity to assert protectionism as a long-term goal, given that he was in office from 1858 to 1862, again from 1864 to 1866, and again in 1867. An examination of his record over this period, however, provides much evidence to show that Galt was not a protectionist by nationalist or ideological conviction, and did not see tariff protection as a necessary element in Canadian transcontinental expansion.

Galt's commitment to tariff protection can be examined in terms of his policy inclinations in the period after 1859. Some of the evidence is equivocal, particularly that relating to the tariff changes he brought into place in 1866. At that time, Galt as finance minister reduced the general tariff rate to 15 per cent from 20 per cent. This large reduction in customs duties might be and was viewed as a move towards free trade. In 1866 it was certainly politically convenient to reduce the tariff, given that lower tariffs were deemed necessary to persuade the Maritimes to enter Confederation. Some hard-hearted central Canadian protectionists believed that the concession was nothing but a temporary ploy. As the cotton manufacturer Donald McInnes wrote to his Hamilton confrere, the merchant and protectionist nationalist Isaac Buchanan, 'I look upon Confederation as a great gain to Canada & the Maritime Provinces we all know are very jealous as to any increase in the way of customs[. P]erhaps the wisest course would be to leave it in abeyance till that is accomplished. Protection for our growing manufactures we *want* & *shall have*. We cannot be anything without them.'[57] As well, an examination of the 1866 tariff indicates that significant industrial protective elements were left largely intact, with some important revenue-producing elements suffering major rate cuts. For all the kow-towing to Maritimes interests, moreover, one should note that an element of agricultural protection was included to attract Ontario farmers. So Galt, if he held protectionist views as strong as those of McInnes and Buchanan, might well have disguised his longer-term intentions by lowering some tariff rates at that time as a matter of political convenience. One view held of his operations at the time was nonetheless that he announced for free trade, and then was forced back to a more protectionist stance by lobbying and political pressures.[58] Thus, his stance in 1866 is ambiguous.

However, Galt's perspectives and actions at times when he was less constrained by circumstance strongly suggest that he was not ideologically attached to protectionism. For example, in proposing an unimplemented 1862 budget, he declared that the model for trade systems he had in mind was the European, not the American, system. The American system was unquestionably that of protection – the Americans had sharply increased their tariff in 1860. The European system to which Galt referred was the interlocking system of trade treaties that the British, French, Germans, Austrians, and others were in the process of establishing in order to remove barriers to the movement of goods. The Cobden Treaty of 1862–3 between the British and French was the system's crowning jewel.[59] Galt's 1862 tariff wasn't implemented because of the political turmoil of the era, but Galt certainly declared for a free-trade direction. His actions in 1862 followed on a position he took in early 1861 in a memorandum approved by the cabinet and intended for the British government's consumption. In this instance, Galt was in pursuit of a customs union of the British North American colonies. 'Free Trade,' Galt wrote, requires the removal of all artificial burthens upon Trade ... the unrestricted interchange of the labor, skill and capital of mankind. The circumstances of the world and the jealousies of nations will probably forever prevent its universal adoption, but an approximation should be sought wherever practicable ... This is precisely the object sought by the Canadian Government, they desire to bring the North American Provinces under one system ... My Lords must surely admit that the proposition of Canada, is one that tends to remove existing restrictions upon trade ...[60]

Of course, the options available for 'European'-style trade agreements for the Canadas were limited. They consisted of, first, the British North American colonies, second, of the British empire, and third, arrangements with the United States. The first was under way through the movement towards confederation. The third was quite pressing. The Americans passed notice of abrogation of the 1854 Treaty of Reciprocity in March 1865. The venerable treaty was thus to come to an end a year later. So if existing trade relations were not to be disturbed, something had to be done quickly. The various British North American provinces actually undertook to provide a framework for further negotiation with the United States through the 1865 British-government-sanctioned Confederate Council on Commercial Treaties, which met in Quebec in August of that year. Yet in November Galt deliberately ignored the directives of the council, and undertook personal negotiations in Washington without authorization. His actions indicate how desperately he sought a continuation and extension of the treaty. In terms of trade goods, the arrangements of 1854 had included essentially only raw materials. As reported by the railwayman C.J. Brydges, who obtained his information in lengthy conversation with the most impeccable source of all, Galt himself, Galt's proposal to the Americans included that 'the area of the interchange of commodities should be largely increased, extending to manufactures as well as to natural productions – that the list should include agricultural implements – all kinds of tools, boots & shoes, iron & hardware, cotton & woollen goods, and a large variety of articles, the duty on these, if any, to be equal to their internal taxes.'[61] Moreover, as Brydges recounted, Galt proposed to have the same rates levied on goods from all other nations, thus approximating a broad move towards free trade. It was this precipitate action by Galt that brought George Brown, himself an ardent free trader, to resign from the government.[62] In the process, Galt displayed a wanton disregard for the sacred principles of protection in the pursuit of extending free trade. If Galt desired to constrain and limit foreign industrial competition for the prospective Canadian nation and to bind together its internal markets, then surely he would not have displayed such a desperate eagerness. Though these actions by Galt did not bring about the trade agreement by mutual legislation he had in mind – the Reciprocity Treaty came to its predetermined end in March 1866 – they showed that Galt was a committed opportunist, and quite possibly a free trader.[63] The protectionist elements of the 1859 tariff were not deeply rooted in Galt.

Beginning in the late 1850s Galt was a key political actor in the attempts made to escape the economic instability and cultural and political conflict that plagued the province. As finance minister his own efforts were dual in character, reactive and defensive, on the one hand, and aggressively growth-oriented, on the other. Galt's acceptance of government office during the infamous Double Shuffle of 1858 (at one point during this crisis the governor general actually requested that Galt form a government, which would have made him prime minister; so his political importance was great)[64] was predicated on the government pursuing some scheme of colonial union. However, to think of Galt as a self-actuated man, an independent and original thinker who took the opportunity of office to insert views not fully comprehended by others into public policy, is not accurate. He was never free to forward ideas exclusively his own to begin with; he was constrained by the men about him, by his background connections with Montreal commercial and industrial communities, by the position in public life he had, by received ideas, and by the political, economic, and institutional framework in which he operated. In putting forward the 1859 tariff, he was acting within this context. Admittedly, the conceptual apparatus Galt brought to bear in making the tariff of 1859 was theoretically perceptive: a revenue-maximizing concoction into which was blended a limited labour-value-added model of effective protection. However, that apparatus was a distillation of ideas and perceptions in broad circulation among businessmen of his time. One should not attribute originality to him in this regard. He was, as with many politicians, deeply pragmatic in his outlook.

Thus, Galt's protectionism was not profound, or ideological, or tied directly to a conception of nationality. Revenue was his chief concern in 1859; protection, in his mind, was an important, though secondary, and most particularly a temporary, consideration. In the late 1850s his province was suffering in a profound commercial depression. It had just gone through an initial cycle of industrialization, of which Galt was intensely aware, if in no other way than through the vigorous lobbying he experienced. The protectionist elements of his 1859 tariff were intended to meet the needs of the time. In the early and mid-1860s, the Canadas were undergoing a cycle of prosperity more broadly based than that of a decade earlier, rooted much less in the frantic expansion of debt-laden infrastructure, and more solidly based in industrial expansion. The planned transcontinental state could then potentially exist without the artificial prop of protection, especially if access to American markets continued to grow. Galt's 1859 tariff was thus a heavily revenue-oriented instrument; the protectionist elements were confined by revenue needs; the intense need for revenue was a product of the harsh economic climate. By the early 1860s and beyond the climate had changed, and protection could be dispensed with, so at least Galt thought. The tripartite vision was no more, if ever it existed in Galt's mind.

The implications for an understanding of a tripartite national policy are considerable. That Galt had such a vision is unlikely, given his limited adherence to industrial protection. All we know is that he probably used the phrase 'national policy' in his budget speech, but reports of that speech do not provide any obvious context for its insertion. If he used it, it could well have been in reference simply to the tariff. It was a phrase in circulation in 1859, and the protectionist Isaac Buchanan had no qualms in claiming it for his own and for tariff protection alone. Notions of exploiting an agricultural west, which Galt certainly had, focused in immediate practical terms on the United States, where a staple-producing hinterland already existed, one that could feed the Canadian transportation network.[65] Linkages between western expansion and tariff protection had no apparent purchase on the mind of his contemporary Canadian expansionists, as is evident from Doug Owram's *Promise of Eden*. Thus, the burden of proof for a tripartite national policy, in any of its guises, as a basis of Canadian nationality, shifts back to an exploration of the 1870s and beyond.

NOTES

1 See, for example, Alvin Finkel and Margaret Conrad, *History of the Canadian Peoples*, vol. 2, *1867 to the Present* (Toronto: Copp Clark, 1998), 47–8, and R. Douglas Francis, Richard Jones, and Donald B. Smith, *Destinies: Canadian*

*History since Confederation* (Toronto: Harcourt Canada, 2000), 46, 51, 151. My views, very succinctly expressed, are to be found in Ben Forster, 'National Policy,' in *The Oxford Companion to Canadian History*, ed. Gerald Hallowell (Toronto: Oxford University Press, 2004). At greater length, see Ben Foster, *A Conjunction of Interests: Business, Politics and Tariffs, 1825–1879* (Toronto: University of Toronto Press, 1987).

2 In *Progress without Planning: The Economic History of Ontario from Confederation to the Second World War* (Toronto: University of Toronto Press, 1987) Drummond observes substantial economic growth largely unlinked to the west. See also E.J. Chambers and D.F. Gordon, 'Primary Products and Economic Growth: An Empirical Measurement,' *Journal of Political Economy* 74 (1966): 315–32, which offered a controversial counterfactual view of the western wheat economy's evident failure to contribute to industrial development.

3 D. Owram, *Promise of Eden: The Canadian Expansionist Movement and the Idea of the West, 1856–1900* (Toronto: University of Toronto Press, 1980).

4 John F. Dales utilized the distinction between a capitalized National Policy, to mean the tariff, and the uncapitalized, to mean the tripartite policy, in his critique of the economic implications of tariff protection. See his *The Protective Tariff in Canada's Development* (Toronto: University of Toronto Press, 1966).

5 Donald Creighton, *Canada's First Century, 1867–1967* (Toronto: Macmillan, 1970), 25.

6 Ibid., 23–40. Much earlier, Creighton firmly concluded a paper on the economic origins of Canada by stating that 'the Dominion of Canada completed its program of national unification with the National Policy of Protection.' See his 'Economic Nationalism and Confederation,' *Canadian Historical Association Report* 24 (1942): 44–51.

7 A.A. den Otter, 'Alexander Galt, the 1859 Tariff and Canadian Economic Nationalism,' *Canadian Historical Review* 63 (1982): 151–78. This perspective is partially derived from D.F. Barnett, 'The Galt Tariff: Incidental or Effective Protection?' *Canadian Journal of Economics* 9 (1976): 389–407. Barnett closely analyses the structure of the tariff, attempting to prove its protective character, and ascribing to Galt first-mover status in conceptualizing a sophisticated protectionist function, particularly in the notion of 'effective protection.' This view of the importance of the 1859 tariff as a protectionist device has deep roots. For a full early exploration that emphasizes the tariffs of 1858 and 1859 as protectionist, see Edward Porritt, *Sixty Years of Protection in Canada, 1846–1907: Where Industry Leans on the Politician* (London: Macmillan and Co., 1908), 130 7, 187–8, 218–42. Den Otter asserts that it was Galt who named the over-arching tripartite strategy the 'national policy.'

8  The amount of protection provided to a product is not measured by the spread between the customs duty imposed on a final product and on its chief input item. A hypothetical example might illustrate this. A simple spread calculation on wooden furniture might be that furniture gets 10% protection because raw or partially processed wood gets 10% and the nominal rate on wooden furniture is 20%. The effective rate of protection is rather higher. In the process of manufacture, a great deal of value is added to the wood. Assume the manufacturing process provides double the value of the furniture item over the wood input. The actual calculation would give an effective protection rate of 30% in this hypothetical instance. However, wooden furniture utilizes many additional input items: glue, nails, screws, stain, varnish, veneers, and at times upholstery, to name the most obvious. All of these might have different rates of duty, and would be calculated at varying costs as components of the final product. Because of consequent complexity in calculation, Galt and his contemporaries took comfort in constructing tariffs that had clear spreads between input and output, and Barnett takes similar comfort in doing the same in his analysis of the tariffs. It is important to note that rates of effective protection could vary considerably, even wildly, if the value added is not known. The conceptual apparatus associated with effective protection was first substantially delineated by Clarence Barber, 'Canadian Tariff Policy,' *Canadian Journal of Economics and Political Science* 21 (1955): 513–30. For exhaustive treatment by an economist, see W.M. Corden, *The Theory of Protection* (Oxford: Clarendon Press, 1971) and his *Trade Policy and Economic Welfare* (Oxford: Clarendon Press, 1974).

9  Library and Archives Canada (LAC), Department of Finance Records (DFR), vol. 3368, filed under January. This is undated and unsigned, but is clearly in Galt's handwriting. Internal evidence suggests 1859 as the date of authorship.

10  R. Warren James, *John Rae, Political Economist* (Toronto: University of Toronto Press, 1965).

11  LAC, Department of National Revenue Records (DNNR), vol. 204, 17 January 1859 petition; letters to Rose and Galt, 10 January and 20 June 1859, respectively.

12  LAC, DNNR, vol. 373. LAC, Buchanan Papers, vol. 58, 46645–50, Wm. Weir to I. Buchanan, 10 January 1860, addresses the infant-industry argument at some length, and as well refers to any resultant tariff policy as a national policy.

13  LAC, DNNR, vol. 373, Thomas Fuller to R.S.M. Bouchette, 28 April 1859.

14  LAC, DNNR, vol. 220, G. Stephen to A.T. Galt, 28 May 1866.

15 Isaac Buchanan, *The Relations of the Industry of Canada* (Montreal, 1864), 483–7, and W. Weir, *Sixty Years in Canada* (Montreal, 1903), 105–18. Barnett's dissection of this proposal in comparison to both the 1858 and 1859 tariffs elucidates some of the weaknesses in the thinking of manufacturers. See also LAC, DFR, vol. 3368, J.B. Forsyth on behalf of the Quebec Board of Trade, to A.T. Galt, 31 January 1859, which urges low duties on raw materials.

16 LAC, DFR, vol. 3368, 11 March 1859.

17 LAC, DFR, vol. 3368, Wm. H. Hibbard, Montreal, to A.T. Galt, 7 March 1959.

18 LAC, DNNR, vol. 370, Joseph Rogers to unknown recipient, 26 February 1857.

19 LAC, DNNR, vol. 203, John Mathewson & Sons to Wm. Cayley, 17 March 1858. This petition was victorious, as J. Hopkins to R.S.M. Buchette, 8 September 1858, DNNR, vol. 147, makes clear.

20 LAC, DNNR, vol. 203, Frothingham & Workman et al. to A.T. Galt.

21 LAC, DNNR, vol. 115, to A.T. Galt, 4 March 1858; and see also LAC, DFR, vol. 3368, George Peck & Co. to A.T. Galt, 7 March 1859.

22 LAC, DNNR, vol. 209, Petition from cabinet makers and piano manufacturers to A.T. Galt, 30 July 1861. LAC, Buchanan Papers, vol. 21, 18064–6, B. Clark to I. Buchanan 3 July 1858.

23 LAC, DNNR, vol. 203, to John Rose, 10 March 1858.

24 LAC, DNNR, vol. 204, Greene & Sons to John Rose, 10 March 1859.

25 LAC, Buchanan Papers, vol. 21, 18182–3.

26 LAC, DNNR, vol. 78, Petition to R.S.M. Bouchette, 14 September 1861.

27 For contemporary attention, see the Hamilton *Spectator*, 19 April 1858 and 9 September 1858, 2.

28 *Spectator*, 10 July 1858, 2. See also ibid., 8 July 1858, 2; 7 July 1858, 2; and Letter Canadaensis ([Isaac Buchanan], *Spectator*, 6 July 1858, 3.

29 LAC, Galt Papers, vol. 10, 107–11, Letterbook, A.T. Galt to G. Glyn, 7 February 1862. LAC, Buchanan Papers, vol. 50, 40248–50, J. Osborne to I. Buchanan, 16 March 1859.

30 LAC, Buchanan Papers, vol. 118, 76438, Wolfred Nelson et al., Petition for a Commercial Policy Favouring Canadian Industry, 22 February 1856. See also Buchanan's intended amendment to the tariff of 1859, in vol. 118, 76424. Also LAC, DFR, vol. 3368, Montreal Board of Trade, John G. Dinning Secy. to A.T. Galt, 19 January 1859; or LAC, Toronto Board of Trade Papers, vol. 2, Meeting of 5 July 1868, Council Minute Book, 30 April 1850–24 January 1871. Ben Forster, 'Customs Duties,' in *Oxford Companion to Canadian History*.

31  M. Piva, *The Borrowing Process: Public Finance in the Province of Canada, 1840–1867* (Ottawa: University of Ottawa Press, 1992). This book provides a compellingly clear picture of the nature of the revenue and expenditure problems the province faced.

32  William Cayley in bringing down supply. Debates of the Legistative Assembly, 11 April 1856. Reported in the Montreal *Gazette*, 15 April 1856, 2.

33  LAC, Galt Papers, vol. 1, 4–7, Galt to Thomas Baring, 16 August 1858.

34  LAC, Glyn, Mills Papers, G. Glyn to A.T. Galt, 23 November 1857, Letter-books, no. 4, 1857–59, p. 52, notes the desperate circumstances as they first emerged: 'No one is disposed to touch the [Grand Trunk] bonds at any price … It is in vain attempting to raise money for the Company under existing circumstances and I really must say that it appears to me that no other course was open than an appeal to the Government unless the engagements of the Company were to be unpaid'

35  LAC, DFR, vol. 3367, J. Langton to W. Cayley, 27 June 1858.

36  *Gazette*, Montreal, 15 April 1856, 2. LAC, Toronto Board of Trade Papers, vol. 2, Council Minute Book, 1860–71, 99–100, Meeting of Council, 21 April 1856. LAC, Buchanan Papers, vol. 118, 76438, Petition.

37  LAC, Baring Papers, A.T. Galt to Thomas Baring, 14 July 1859.

38  LAC, Ellice Family Papers, vol. 34, 11249–53, John Rose to E. Ellice, 3 January 1858 [*sic*].

39  Ibid.

40  LAC, DNNR, vol. 203, James Anderson, Board of Arts and Manufactures, Montreal, 26 June 1858.

41  Hamilton *Spectator*, 23 June 1858, 2.

42  LAC, DNNR, vol. 372, Geo. Peck & Co., Toronto, to R.S.M. Bouchette, 1 May 1858.

43  LAC, Galt Papers, vol. 1, 1 4–17, Galt to T. Baring, 16 August 1858.

44  LAC, DFR, vol. 3368, J.G. Dinning to A.T. Galt, 19 January 1859; see also LAC, Kingston Board of Trade, Edward Berry to A.T. Galt, 15 March 1859; J.B. Forsyth to A.T. Galt, 31 January 1859.

45  See LAC, DFR, vol. 3368, Toronto Board of Trade, C. Robertson to A.T. Galt, 3 February 1859.

46  LAC, DFR, vol. 3367, Thos. Murphy to Inspector General, 2 July 1858. LAC, DNNR, RG 16 A-1, vol. 202, John Smith Montreal to T. Bouthillier, 28 March 1857; and see vol. 115, P.J. Ware, Hamilton, to R.S.M. Bouchette, 19 March 1859; also vol. 203, Savage & Lyman to Wm. Cayley, Montreal, 27 May 1858.

47  In the form applied by supply-side economists, there is much concern about the impact of taxes on the propensity to work and thus on productivity and economic growth. Tax cuts are deemed to spur economic growth.

Arthur Laffer apparently sketched this out in November 1974, and more
fully expounded it in the company of other economists in 1982. He does not
claim absolute originality. Victor A. Canto, Douglas H. Joines, and Arthur
B. Laffer, eds, *Foundations of Supply-Side Economics – Theory and Evidence*
(New York: Academic Press, 1982).

48 Hamilton *Spectator*, 12 March 1859.

49 LAC, Province of Canada, Executive Council Office, State Minute Book, V,
38–47, 16 March 1860.

50 LAC, DNNR, vol. 204, J&J Mitchell, Montreal, to John Rose, 10 March 1859.

51 LAC, DNR, vol. 3368, J.G. Dinning, for the Montreal Board of Trade, to A.T.
Galt, 15 March 1859. And see ibid., Edward Berry, for the Kingston Board of
Trade, to A.T. Galt, 15 March 1859. LAC, Buchanan Papers, vol. 21, 18064–5,
Benjamin Clark to I. Buchanan, 3 July 1858. Ibid., vol. 50, 40257–8, John
Osborne, for the Hamilton Board of Trade, to Isaac Buchanan, 9 March 1859.

52 LAC, DFR, vol. 3368, P. Redpath to A.T. Galt, 6 January 1859.

53 LAC, Macdonald Papers, vol. 167, 68447–56, Sir F. Hincks to Sir J.A.
Macdonald, 15 February 1871.

54 LAC, DFR, vol. 3368, J.B. Forsyth, on behalf of the Quebec Board of Trade,
to A.T. Galt, 31 January 1859.

55 Barnett, 'The Galt Tariff,' falls into this error.

56 LAC, DFR, vol. 3368, J.G. Dinning to A.T. Galt, 19 January 1859.

57 LAC, Buchanan Papers, vol. 45, 36011–13, D. McInnes to I. Buchanan,
4 October 1866.

58 LAC, Baring Papers, vol. 4, 1925–9, John Rose to T. Baring, 26 July 1866.

59 S.B. Clough, *France: A History of National Economics, 1789–1939* (New York:
Scribner, 1939), 184–88.

60 LAC, Macdonald Papers, vol. 215, 92103–8. Memorandum by Galt
approved by the Committee of the Executive Council of the Canadas, 2 January 1861, ibid., 92096.

61 LAC, Watkin Papers, item 83, C.J. Brydges to Sir E. Watkin, 11 December
1865.

62 See J.M.S. Careless, *Brown of* The Globe: *Statesman of Confederation, 1860–
1880* (Toronto: Dundurn Press, 1989), 211–17.

63 Of course, it might be countered that Conservative protectionists in later
years were always ready to negotiate reciprocity with the United
States. Macdonald tried to do so in the meetings that led to the Treaty of
Washington in 1871; there was a clause in the National Policy Tariff of 1879
providing for reciprocity with the United States; Sir Charles Tupper
engaged in some preliminary negotiations in 1887. But there is a crucial
difference between these later Conservative efforts and that of Galt. After

Confederation, the Conservatives, while being willing to undertake trade negotiations, limited their shopping list to the raw products of mines, forests and the sea – never manufactures.

64 LAC, Galt Papers, vol. 1, 3, Lord Mock to A.T. Galt, 4 August 1858.

65 LAC, Galt Papers, vol. 1, 28–31, A.T. Galt to Brassey, 13 February 1859, makes it clear that the trade of the west necessary to make the Grand Trunk and the Canadian canal system going concerns was the trade of the American west. LAC, Baring Papers has two letters confirming Galt's perspective that the increase in traffic was an *immediate* necessity to provide support for the Grand Trunk, and that could only mean traffic from the American side of the border. A.T. Galt to T. Baring, 13 October and 12 November 1859. This paper has passed by the importance of commercial protection in the tariff of 1859. One of Galt's chief aims in the tariff was to force as much traffic as possible through the railways and canals of the Canadas, so as to make them less a drain on the finances of the province.

# 6 Business, Culture, and the History of News, 1870–1930: A Case Study of the 'Political/Commercial' Dichotomy

GENE ALLEN

The past fifteen years have seen a proliferation of thought-provoking work on the history of journalism. With the cultural turn in historical studies, the newspaper and other news media have appeared as subjects meriting closer and more imaginative exploration; and the importation of concepts and methods from cultural studies, the history of the book, and other disciplines has provided an array of new and revealing approaches to what was once a narrowly institutional and biographical field.[1] Though his work predates the recent crop of material by more than twenty years, Jürgen Habermas's influential notion of the newspaper as central to the emergence of the public sphere, and indeed to the historical emergence of such a thing as 'the public,' has emphasized the centrality of news to modern Western societies generally; and Benedict Anderson's equally influential idea that modern nations are imagined communities gives newspapers an equally central role in the formation of modern social consciousness.[2] In this recent scholarship, the news media are seen less as mere chroniclers, sources for studies of other, more important subjects, and more as significant historical phenomena in their own right.

In dealing with one central question, though, some of the recent journalism history loses its sophistication. While there are many noteworthy exceptions, a questionable but persistent thread of interpretation concerning a crucial period in this history – the emergence of the mass press between about 1880 and 1920 – has firmly woven itself into the literature. In this view, the transformation of the newspaper from an explicitly partisan organ, receiving much of its revenue from party funds and explicitly playing the role of partisan cheerleader, into a big business seeking the largest possible circulation, relying on advertising

revenue and conventions of 'objectivity' (so as to offend as few potential readers as possible), is a profound diminution of its role in creating
and sustaining a meaningful public sphere. Once addressed as citizens,
readers became mere consumers. The mass press may have reached a
larger public, but it was a very different, politically impoverished, kind
of public.[3] This distinction between a pre-1880 or pre-1890 'partisan'
press and an increasingly 'commercial' press after that date has
become an accepted shorthand for describing a broad and highly significant process of change.[4]

The partisan/commercial dichotomy does capture many important
aspects of the transformation of the press in the years around 1900, but it
is inadequate and in some respects misleading as an overall account of
what happened. An emphasis on the change from partisan to commercial orientation oversimplifies at both ends of the period, losing sight of
the commercial orientation of many newspapers before 1880 and the
continuing partisan affiliation of most well into the twentieth century. It
relies on a romanticized account of the focus on partisan politics that did
indeed characterize most newspapers before about 1880: the public
sphere defined by the press before 1880 was no broader, and was in
several respects narrower, than that of newspapers after the turn of the
century. Most important, the partisan/commercial dichotomy imposes a
much too restrictive reading on twentieth-century newspapers, one that
focuses on their divergence from a pre-defined ideal of citizenship as
coterminous with engagement in (or at least exposure to) electoral politics. In fact, most twentieth-century newspapers did actively address
their readers as citizens, as long as citizenship is defined broadly
enough to include questions of class (however obliquely presented),
gender roles, ethnicity, religion, social morality, and attitudes toward
collective interests and individual rights, as well as the broader, ritual-
ized elements of group-identity affirmation through communication
that James Carey has so effectively described.[5]

Twentieth-century newspapers did this at the same time as they
addressed their readers as consumers, sought to entertain them, and
relied on a business model that was based on selling advertising,
attracting large numbers of readers, and using capital-intensive production methods. For example, the emergence of women's pages in
newspapers was clearly related to the necessity of attracting female
readers in order to appeal to advertisers of goods that women were
likely to buy. The content of these women's sections did much to promote the consumption of goods and, in a sense, taught their readers

how to be consumers. But the women's pages also cast women in new public roles, publicized the work of women's associations, and provided a new place where questions about women's position in society could emerge.[6]

As this example suggests, a deterministic view of the influence of business organization on newspaper content flattens the historical reality. A complex and changing interplay between the reader as citizen and as consumer, on one hand, and between the newspaper as public institution and as profit-seeking business, on the other, is reduced to a simple opposition in which triumphant business values largely eradicated whatever went before. There is little room in this analysis for the notion that readers exercised some degree of meaningful choice, and that the newspapers produced in increasing numbers succeeded because their content genuinely appealed to readers. One need not accept the traditional assertion of industry apologists – that newspapers simply and transparently give readers what they want – to reject the equally improbable view that readers are essentially automata who buy and read whatever is put in front of them so long as it includes sufficient quantities of entertainment, scandal, and celebrity. (Even these types of content may have more social meaning than is apparent at first glance: as one recent article suggests, sensationalism need not be seen merely as empty entertainment, but carries important messages about morality and order.)[7]

In short, the 'commercial' model of the post-1880 press focuses almost entirely on the supply of news, while paying very little attention to questions of demand, of why readers in large numbers bought certain kinds of newspapers and not others. Twenty-five years ago, Michael Schudson insisted that literacy and technology by themselves could not explain the emergence of the penny press in the 1830s and 1840s: the questions of why literacy was worth acquiring and why some technologies were valued essentially require cultural and social answers.[8] In the later period as well, business and cultural history must be closely integrated in order to provide an adequate account of the evolution of news.

One scholar who has explicitly examined the evolution of newspaper content during the 'partisan' period from a broadly cultural perspective is Richard Kaplan.[9] Like Schudson, he criticizes analyses of the transition to mass-audience journalism that see it as 'a quasi-biological process of natural evolution, or ascribed to one or two inevitable forces such as increasing modernization or commercialization of the media.' In Kaplan's view, these accounts ignore the cultural shaping of news – the interplay between the expectations and desires of readers, journalists' assessments of what these expectations and desires were, and their own predispositions to consider some subjects legitimate and newsworthy, and others not.[10] He explicitly rejects the idea of an obvious and automatic link between business considerations and content: 'Profit orientation is only secondarily concerned with the message of the news.' The attempt to attract more readers (and hence more advertising) 'may entail stories of celebrities and scandals, and even a fictionalization of the news, but not necessarily. *Depending* upon the cultural expectations of readers and the structure of the market, the news may or may not respond to democracy's need for diverse, critical perspectives and reliable information.'

This study examines the validity of the partisan/commercial dichotomy by focusing in detail on specific editions of two Toronto newspapers in 1870, when the 'partisan' model is assumed to have still held sway, and again in 1930, when the 'commercial' press had established its dominance. The two newspapers are *The Daily Telegraph* and its later incarnation, *The Evening Telegram*; and *The Globe*. These two were chosen, first, because they both had clear partisan affiliations; and, second, because they addressed different audiences and exemplified different styles, the *Telegraph/Telegram* being a populist evening paper, and the *Globe* being a more serious morning paper aimed at a business and professional readership.[11]

A brief examination of both newspapers' histories illustrates that 'partisan' is a notably imprecise term as a blanket description for nineteenth-century newspapers. Is a partisan paper one financed and controlled by a political party? One that receives financial support but is influenced rather than controlled directly? One that is financially independent but generally supports a particular party in its columns? These newspapers were indeed both partisan, but in different ways, and in ways that changed over time. The *Telegraph* was established in 1866 and went through six years of on-again, off-again support of the Conservative party, with on-again, off-again party financial backing, before going out of business. It was re-established in 1876 as the *Telegram*, and from then on followed a course of independent and sometimes eccentric Conservatism.[12] The *Globe* was, of course, Canada's pre-eminent Liberal newspaper in 1870 and continued to play this role. But though it had relied on party funds in its early years and continued to receive preferment whenever Liberal governments were in office,[13] by 1870 the *Globe* was a power in its own right, seen as dictating party policy more than carrying out orders from party chiefs in Ottawa. (It may be more realistic to see 'partisan' publishers or editors such as George Brown – or, by the 1920s, Joseph Atkinson of the *Toronto Star* – as semi-independent satraps representing particular strands of party opinion, rather than as party functionaries.)

As Paul Rutherford notes, party-affiliated papers were not necessarily slavish exponents of whatever their political allies or financial backers wanted.[14] This may have been because, as Thomas Walkom's valuable calculations show, federal patronage between 1874 and 1906 never constituted more than 3 per cent of the total revenue of any Toronto daily.[15] Explicit partisan affiliation declined rapidly after 1914 in keeping with an overall reduction in the availability of discretionary political spending – but even after this, many newspapers continued informally to support one party rather than another.[16]

Nor was partisan affiliation inconsistent with a strongly commercial orientation. George Brown's *Globe* began as a vehicle for a Canadian faction of the Presbyterian Church, and soon after became an organ of the Reform party. But well before the purported 1880 watershed it had also become an intensely commercial venture, buying expensive new presses, providing costly telegraphic news, and aggressively pursuing an ever-larger circulation. These very things helped make it a particularly valuable Liberal ally.[17] After 1880, commercially-oriented publishers recognized that partisanship helped attract readers in competitive markets, as Walkom and Kaplan have both shown in their detailed studies of newspapers in Toronto and Detroit, respectively.[18]

Nonetheless, proponents of the 'partisan' characterization accurately point out that virtually all newspapers before 1880 were devoted to covering partisan politics – which, in the Canadian case, meant the proceedings of parliament in Ottawa. It is said that newspapers do not so much tell their readers what to think as what to think *about*; and an examination of the *Telegraph* and *Globe* editions of 10 March 1870, clearly indicates that readers were expected to think a great deal about federal politics. (See table 6.1.)

Thus, in a four-page paper of thirty-six columns, the *Globe* devoted 1.5 columns to a summary of the previous day's events in parliament, four columns more to a detailed account of parliamentary proceedings (something like a combination of an official journal and Hansard) that duplicated and expanded on most of the items discussed in the summary, and another full column of other parliamentary stories. On top

Table 6.1
Toronto *Globe* and *Daily Telegraph*, 10 March 1870: breakdown of contents

|  | Globe | Telegraph |
|---|---|---|
| Advertising (columns) | 12.75 | 15.5 |
| Editorial (columns) | 23.25 | 20.5 |
| News (columns) | 18.7 | 12.7 |
| Advertising as % of total space* | 35 | 43 |
| Editorial as % of total space | 65 | 57 |
| News as % of total space | 52 | 35 |
| Editorial content (major categories) |  |  |
| News as % of all editorial content | 70 | 62 |
| Editorials, commentary (% of all editorial content) | 6 | 10 |
| Business (% of all editorial content) | 11 | 19 |
| Literary (% of all editorial content) | 5 | 6 |
| News content (major categories) |  |  |
| Ottawa politics and government (as % of all news) | 61/42** | 60 |

* Percentages have been rounded off to the nearest whole number. In cases where the figures do not total 100 per cent, uncategorized, miscellaneous content makes up the difference.
** The first figure shows the result if the Red River correspondence is classified as parliamentary coverage; the second, if it is not.

of this, the *Globe* printed more than three columns of correspondence released in Ottawa about the situation at Red River (disclosing the fact that the recently appointed governor of the territory had made a serious error in judgment by asserting Canadian sovereignty prematurely). In all (if the Red River correspondence is included), about three-fifths of the *Globe*'s news space that day was dedicated to parliamentary news; even if one leaves out the Red River material, the proportion of parliamentary news was more than 40 per cent. The *Telegraph*'s devotion to parliamentary coverage was similarly single-minded: a half-column summary of the day's parliamentary news, fully 5.5 columns of detailed proceedings (as with the *Globe*, repeating and expanding on most of the points referred to in the summary), and 1.75 columns of other parliamentary stories, constituting 60 per cent of its entire news content.

What kind of political engagement on the part of readers might this extensive parliamentary coverage have entailed? Most assessments of the partisan/commercial dichotomy in newspaper history assume that the partisan press did a particularly good, or at least a better, job of serving readers' democratic or societal interests than the mass-audience press. But as Schudson has asked, was this really the case?[19]

Certainly the lengthy and detailed reports of parliamentary proceedings in the two newspapers were hardly the kind of thing to set partisan blood boiling, with their deliberate itemization of every stage of that day's legislative process: petitions, committee reports, introduction of bills, motions, second reading of legislation, and so on. The discussion that ensued on each of these points was reported at length, though not verbatim; the Liberal *Globe* was more likely to include telling points made by opposition MPs or embarrassing admissions by ministers, while the Conservative *Telegraph* made its selections in a similar vein of pronounced but hardly virulent partisanship. The publication of these proceedings was intended, probably, less to convince – the *Globe* or *Telegraph* reader already knew which side he or she was on – than to inform the faithful of the party's position on whatever issues were current, from the minutiae of parliamentary procedure (whether the proper steps had been followed in introducing a bill that amended another bill already before a legislative committee, for example) to more weighty and controversial questions such as a fisheries dispute with the United States or the abolition of dual representation. All were reported, one after another, in the order they had been raised and in the same decorous, if sometimes pointed, tone of parliamentary debate.[20]

While the Ottawa reports covered the full range of parliamentary proceedings, the public sphere that the newspapers defined did not extend much beyond this. Daniel Hallin has presented a simple but useful way of analysing the range of journalistic coverage that is useful here.[21] Hallin distinguishes three spheres: the sphere of consensus, covering those topics on which virtually everyone is assumed to be in agreement (such as, in twentieth-century North America, the appropriateness of nations as forms of political organization, or of private property and wage labour as bases of the economic system); the sphere of deviance, which includes topics or viewpoints universally considered beyond the pale and not meriting serious discussion (say, a subject like homosexual marriage in the 1950s); and the sphere of legitimate controversy, where opposing points of view are regularly presented in the mass media (such as the question, after 1968, of whether continuing military involvement in Vietnam served the United States' best interests). In the 1960s, Hallin points out, the sphere of legitimate controversy in the United States was roughly defined by the differences between the two main political parties, or between competing factions in the bureaucracy.

If one applies this analysis to the pre-1880 press, the differences between 'partisan' and 'commercial' publishers seem less striking. When publishers wore partisan affiliation on their sleeves, the zone of public debate was circumscribed primarily by the differences between the major political parties – much as Hallin found it to be in the 1960s. Minority viewpoints on fundamental economic and social issues (the sanctity of the family, the racial superiority of whites, property rights, or the predominance of the Christian religion, for example) were no more likely to get a respectful hearing before 1880 than afterward.[22]

In fact, Walkom and David Paul Nord have shown that, in Toronto and Chicago, the market-driven search for larger audiences brought an increase in labour-oriented, radical, and Progressive journalism for at least thirty years after 1880 – the beginning of the 'commercial' press period, according to proponents of this view.[23] Walkom, who studied the evolution of the mass-audience press from 1871 to 1911, concludes that newspapers deliberately began to address 'issues of power, privilege, wealth and class' as an essential element of their commercially-motivated efforts to expand their circulation to different social strata, especially the working class.[24] Nord analysed three Chicago newspapers of markedly different political and market orientations between 1870 and 1900 and concluded that all were 'early proponents of progressive-era business values, notably a commitment to public interest consumerism, an obsession with commercial order and social control, and a growing faith in organizational/bureaucratic modes of conflict resolution.'[25] For the period up until the First World War, then, the evidence suggests that a more commercial, market-driven press went along with a socially and ideologically broader, rather than narrower, view of the public interest.

Some scholars have suggested that the public sphere of the partisan era might be considered healthier in that newspaper readers were regularly addressed as engaged partisans, as citizens actively involved in politics. But a key method of such journalism was the routine distortion of coverage for partisan advantage and the exclusion of the opinions and arguments of political opponents. As Gerald Baldasty, whose analysis of the commercialization of American newspapers is reflected – sometimes in an oversimplified form – by proponents of the 'partisan/commercial' dichotomy, notes, partisan editors in the United States did not set out to increase public understanding of issues, but to gain political advantage. 'There's no evidence that these editors engaged in debate because they idealized the *process* of debate … Certainly [patronage] limited press content. Party editors did not detail their opponents' views in any evenhanded way. They skirted discussions that would undermine the power of their political parties.'[26] Moreover, as Schudson has observed, nineteenth-century mass politics was 'politics of affiliation, not politics of assent'; the voter's identification with his party was communal and ritualistic, rather than the outcome of a process of disinterested evaluation of the issues that led to an independent choice.[27] Both by the slanting of coverage and by the nature of voters' involvement, the Habermasian public sphere of rational-critical debate was correspondingly limited; this reduced the possibility of genuinely comparing alternative views that is often considered to be at the centre of democratic politics. Under the later practice of 'objectivity,' with all its limitations,[28] readers were more rather than less likely to see different partisan viewpoints presented in a relatively even-handed way. In short, readers of partisan papers might have been engaged, addressed as active participants in politics, but were not necessarily particularly well informed or open to genuine debate. Moreover, beyond the 'sphere of legitimate controversy' that partisan politics represented, minority or radical perspectives received less exposure in the partisan era than they did later on.

How did the content of these two newspapers change by 1930? Editions of the *Globe* and the *Telegraph*'s successor, the *Evening Telegram*, of 13 March 1930 bear out many of the commonly accepted generalizations about what had changed since 1870. Most obviously, both were much larger than in 1870: the *Globe* had gone from four to twenty pages, and the *Telegram* from four to forty-four.[29] Interestingly (see table 6.2), the ratio of advertising to editorial content in the *Globe* was the same as in 1870. The *Telegram* corresponded more closely to the general view of an increase in advertising space that was both absolute and relative. Advertising now accounted for about three-fifths of its total space – a substantial increase from the 43 per cent found in the 1870 edition.

Measured in absolute terms, the amount of editorial and news content in both papers was also substantially greater than it had been earlier. The *Globe* published 223 per cent more editorial content than in 1870, and 59 per cent more news. The populist *Telegram* published

Table 6.2
Toronto *Globe* and *Evening Telegram*, 13 March 1930:
advertising, editorial, and news content

|  | Globe | Telegram |
|---|---|---|
| Total space (columns) | 160 | 352 |
| Advertising columns | 55.7 | 219 |
| Editorial columns | 104.3 | 133 |
| News columns | 41.3 | 61.25 |
| Advertising as % of total space | 35 | 62 |
| Editorial as % of total space | 65 | 38 |
| News as % of total space | 26 | 22 |

367 per cent more editorial content than in 1870, and 247 per cent more news. Proportionally, though, there had been a reduction in the share of the newspapers' total space dedicated to news. In the *Globe*, editorial content accounted for the same proportion of the whole newspaper as in 1870, but news coverage only accounted for half as much as it had earlier – 26 per cent as opposed to 52 per cent. In the *Telegram*, editorial space (38 per cent as opposed to 57 per cent) and news content (22 per cent versus 35 per cent) both accounted for around one-third less of the newspaper's total space than in 1870. For both papers, then, general news made up both a smaller proportion of overall content and a much larger absolute amount than in 1870.

Editorials and commentary also declined as a proportion of content, markedly so in the *Telegram*. These changes were offset by a variety of new types of content: notably sports,[30] women's pages, and, to a lesser extent, entertainment coverage (mainly radio listings and program notes), comic strips, and games. (See table 6.3.) By contrast with these new types of content, business coverage remained the largest non-news editorial section, just as it had been in 1870.

The sharp decline in parliamentary coverage from Ottawa as a proportion of all news was striking. From being by far the largest category of coverage in 1870, Ottawa political coverage had declined in the *Globe* to the point that it occupied only one-third as much space as news about Toronto, and was merely one of five categories that each accounted for around 10 per cent of overall news coverage. In the *Telegram*, the decline of parliamentary news was dizzying: from 60 per cent of all news content in 1870 to merely 3 per cent in 1930.

Table 6.3
Toronto *Globe* and *Evening Telegram*, 13 March 1930: breakdown of editorial content

|  | Globe | Telegram |
|---|---|---|
| News (as % of total space) | 26 | 22 |
| News (as % of all editorial content) | 40 | 46 |
| Editorials + opinion columns (% of all editorial) | 4 | 2 |
| Business (% of all editorial) | 19 | 14 |
| Literary (% of all editorial) | – | 1 |
| Entertainment (% of all editorial) | 5 | 4 |
| Comics, games (% of all editorial) | 2 | 5 |
| Humour, children's (% of all editorial) | – | 1 |
| Sports | 16 | 12 |
| Women's (non-news)* | 8 | 8 |
| Farm news and prices | 4 | – |
| | | |
| Breakdown of news content (on main news pages) | | |
| | | |
| Ottawa politics and government (as % of all news) | 11 | 3 |
| Other Canadian news | 1 | – |
| Ontario politics and government | 10 | 5 |
| Other Ontario news | – | 11 |
|   Civic life, associations | | 7 |
| Toronto: | 32 | 26 |
|   Politics and government | 10 | 10 |
|   Civic life, associations | 13 | 9 |
|   Accidents, fires etc. | | 4 |
|   Miscellaneous | 9 | 3 |
| Foreign | 11 | 10 |
| Courts and crime | 11 | 16 |
| Accidents, disasters | 10 | 15 |
| Economy/business | 5 | 3 |
| Oddities | 1 | 1 |
| Other | 8 | 10** |

\* Some women's page stories are classified as news.
\*\* Includes feature stories, oddities, obituaries.

An increase in coverage of provincial and municipal politics and government made up for this to some extent. When these categories are included, political news accounted for more than 30 per cent of all news content in the *Globe* and 18 per cent in the *Telegram*. The increasing importance of local coverage in both newspapers underscores the mass-circulation newspaper's character as a particularly urban phenomenon. As many scholars have observed, a different kind of journalism, connecting people in new ways, had come into being as cities grew larger and more complicated.[31] The growing news focus on municipal democracy was part of this trend. It is not surprising that scholars such as Nord, whose early work focused on the urban reform movement of the late nineteenth and early twentieth century, have emphasized popular journalism's central role in the emergence of a municipal public sphere.[32]

While political coverage is particularly important for a newspaper's public character – especially national and local politics, where readers are potential voters – this was not the only kind of public sphere in which readers could be involved. For example, the 1930 *Globe* and *Telegram* both devoted around 10 per cent of their respective news space to foreign coverage, and much of this concerned major international topics such as European negotiations on mutual security and disarmament. No one would dispute that such stories did address readers as citizens, even though they may never have had an opportunity to vote directly on the immediate issues raised.

In local coverage, much non-political news fell into a category that might best be described as 'civic and associational life.' These were stories about such things as a planned public meeting on unemployment, a Masonic Lodge banquet, the dedication of a new church organ or opening of a factory, the election of a new president of a chapter of the Ladies' Liberal-Conservative Association, and so on. If this type of coverage, with its clear public-interest character, is included along with more explicitly political news, the 1930 *Telegram* devoted about one-third of the space on its main news pages to public life; for the *Globe*, the total was almost 45 per cent. In both cases, this was more in absolute terms than had appeared in 1870.

Other apparently non-political stories that appeared in the 1930 editions also addressed readers as citizens, but in new ways. Consider, for example, the extensive reports on the conclusion of a Toronto coroner's inquest that appeared in both newspapers. The case concerned a woman who had died while under anesthetic at the Toronto General Hospital, and the jury concluded that there had been no medical negligence – that her death was unavoidable. The story had news value because this had been the latest in a string of deaths of patients in Toronto operating rooms. This role of publicly scrutinizing the actions of large institutions was typical of twentieth-century journalism at a time when public and private bureaucracies affected growing areas of peoples' lives, and any individual's influence on them was correspondingly limited. This, surely, was part of the twentieth-century citizen's increasingly complicated world.

Other prominent stories from March 1930 illustrate that 'community' is a complex, multi-faceted concept, and that straightforward, univocal methods of classifying content often fail to capture the multiple meanings of events. The top story in both newspapers on 13 March was the death in a plane crash of Lt.-Col. William Barker, who had been Canada's number two fighter ace in the First World War. At first glance, this might be categorized as a story about an accident or disaster, evidence of a movement towards less serious, less meaningful news coverage. But when one reads such stories, it is clear that much of the event's impact involved the memory of Barker's glorious successes, which were related explicitly to the sacrifice of thousands of Canadian soldiers and airmen who had been engaged in the same heroic struggle. The Canadian Press article published in the *Globe* referred in the first paragraph to Barker's 'daring exploits,' describing him as 'the gallant aviator.' His wartime achievements, which included the documented shooting down of fifty-two enemy aircraft, were recounted extensively, and introduced as 'a romance which illumines a phase of Canada's accomplishments in the Great War with a glow that will remain long in the memory of this generation.' In a separate article, the provincial premier, Howard Ferguson, noted that the mission in which Barker won his Victoria Cross 'has stuck vividly in my mind, ever since the first meagre details of it were flashed back to us in Canada, nearly twelve years ago now. To me it represented then, as it does now, just about the finest example of courage that a man could aspire to.' Seeing these as mere reports of a fatal accident involving a prominent person fails to take account of their powerful and emotional evocation of Canada's participation in the war, which was explicitly seen as a noble collective enterprise.[33] These were exercises in the active construction of national memory and national purpose. James Carey's description of the ritual functions of communication – in which reading a newspaper is seen 'less as sending or gaining information and more as attending a mass, a situation in which nothing new is learned but in which a particular view of the world is portrayed and confirmed'[34] – captures much of what was involved here.

While coverage of an event like Barker's death sought to define a community of readers by inclusion, other articles focused on excluding those who did not belong, as the stories and commentary involving 'Reds' in both newspapers illustrate. For example, in their coverage of the law courts, both papers reported with obvious distaste the vagrancy case of Harvey Jackson. In the *Telegram*, the story appeared under an attention-grabbing headline: 'Unemployed "Outfit" Named Red Subsidiary.' According to a police inspector's testimony, Jackson had been 'spending time with Communists, stirring up trouble, getting recruits from among the foreigners at labour bureaux, at missions, at flop houses ...' The *Globe* made more of the angle that Jackson, although asserting that 'the Communists ... were the only ones trying to provide work for those in need,' had refused a police officer's offer to find him a job and had been arrested when he showed up at city hall as part of a delegation seeking relief payments for the unemployed. Again, these might be classified at first glance as crime or court stories, further examples of newspapers' moving towards sensational rather than public-spirited coverage. But they were also, particularly when taken together with the other dismissive references to 'Reds' in both newspapers, an exercise in defending the boundaries of Hallin's sphere of legitimate controversy. A heavily ironic suggestion on the *Globe*'s editorial page that unemployment could be alleviated 'by providing the Reds free transportation to the Soviet Elysium and seeing that it is used' made clear what was involved: this was an assertion of who was part of the community and who was not.[35]

Consider, too, the more obviously political stories that both newspapers carried about reactions to a parliamentary vote on whether a divorce court should be established in Ontario. The bill had been defeated by just one vote; Ontario MPs were divided fairly evenly, but MPs from Quebec, apparently motivated by religious objections to divorce, had voted unanimously against the bill. In the *Telegram*, delegates to a convention of the Orange Lodge were quoted as expressing 'amazement' that MPs affiliated with their organization had voted against the bill, 'a measure that very definitely upheld Ontario's rights as against Quebec domination.' In the *Globe*, the Orange Order's president described the vote on the divorce bill as 'an example of Papal domination unknown previously in Canada.' As Rutherford has noted, such Protestant-English intolerance had been a characteristic of Canada's English-language press since the 1870s; its persistence into the 1930s suggests continuity rather than a sharp break.[36] It also illustrates that the attempt to evoke a sense of community among newspaper readers was not necessarily the same as establishing a Habermasian public sphere of dialogue and rational-critical debate, characterized by open-minded consideration of opposing views.

Numerous other examples can be cited of coverage in areas that might initially seem to indicate a move away from public engagement. By 1930 both newspapers had substantial women's sections, whose appearance directly reflected the requirements of advertisers. Much of their content concerned domestic and personal matters – fashion, who's who in society, recipes, advice columns – rather than a public sphere broadly conceived as political. As Marjory Lang has pointed out, the women's section was a kind of ghetto, both for subjects related to women and for female journalists – a way of setting them apart from the broader sphere of public affairs.[37] But several of the women's section articles did have public significance, and this was something new. For example, both papers reported fairly prominently and straightforwardly the election of new leaders of the Toronto chapter of the Imperial Order Daughters of the Empire and the Ontario Girl Guides, the kinds of organizations in which women, increasingly, were able to play public roles. Other women's page articles discussed the need for special programs to keep the 'non-academic child' from drifting into criminality or the requirements of crippled children (with guest speaker Franklin D. Roosevelt). In coverage of these issues, one can see the beginnings of a broader, more socially oriented, public sphere. Moreover, both papers offered support to numerous women's organizations – Women's Institutes, chapters of the Women's Missionary Society and other church-affiliated groups, C.G.I.T. (Canadian Girls in Training) chapters, and so on – by publicizing and covering their meetings.[38]

The rise of separate sections such as women's news and sports, along with the greatly increased size of the newspaper, suggests another way in which the experience of reading was different in 1930 than it had been sixty years earlier. In a four-page newspaper, dominated by parliamentary coverage, one could reasonably assume that most readers looked at much of the same material; if one bought the newspaper at all, there was simply not much choice about what to read in it. In the larger, much more varied newspaper of 1930, the possibilities for fragmentation of the audience were much greater. Some might read the front page and the business section, others the women's section and entertainment, others sports and entertainment, others a bit of everything. Thus, the readers of the newspaper might best be understood as making up distinct, though overlapping and related, communities of readership. Offsetting this trend to some extent was the wider range of techniques available to editors to emphasize stories they considered especially newsworthy. The evolution of the front page as the newspaper's most important space and the use of multi-column display headlines and photographs helped ensure that the biggest stories of the day would register with more rather than fewer readers.[39] Stories that were prominently displayed for several days running would have had an even better chance of registering widely, and thus of providing shared points of reference for large numbers of readers.

Still, fragmentation meant less consensus about what was important; some readers may well have opted out of anything more collective than following the fortunes of a favourite sports team. But fragmentation is not the same thing as lack of interest in public affairs. Part of what was happening was that readers had more choice about which aspects of public life to be involved in, or about what merited consideration as 'public' at all.[40] In addition, each newspaper retained its own overall identity and style. Even a reader who picked up the *Telegram* strictly for its sports coverage could not have been ignorant of, or indifferent to, its anglophilia, its dismissive treatment of Roman Catholics and non-whites (whether the 'five Chinamen' facing trial for assault in a Page 1 story or 'Gandhi's Gang,' in the words of a headline about Gandhi's Salt March), or its devotion to crime as low comedy. To the extent that a newspaper implicitly divided the world into 'us' and 'them,' most of those who chose to read it would have seen themselves, if only approximately, as 'one of us.'

This question of a publication's personality reminds us that the newspaper is not just a collection of discrete stories: by juxtaposition, it presents many possible connections and associations. The sheer variety of coverage, and hence the possibility of drawing connections among the newspaper's various elements, was by 1930 almost overwhelming. The front page of the *Telegram*, for example, carried no fewer than twenty-seven separate items, and the inside pages were just as busy.

How might such associations have been drawn? One could suggest, for example, that some readers saw a connection among the following items: a short Page 1 'brightener' about the dilemma facing U.S. government agents who had to dispose of $30,000 worth of fine pre-war liquor; a Page 2 courts item headlined 'Strap Threat for Boozer' about an alcoholic given a stern judicial lecture for neglecting his family; and a Page 3 story about proposed new provincial rules requiring some buyers of alcohol to make purchases only at designated stores so their consumption could be controlled more closely. By one obvious classificatory scheme these would be an oddity story, a crime story, and a provincial government story, respectively; but it is perhaps more plausible to see them as threads in a single discussion about individual rights and the state's responsibility for moral order in the wake of Prohibition.

Or from the *Globe*, consider the connections that might be drawn among the following: a major Page 1 story about a sharp decline in the price of wheat; a shorter article about Australia's plans to introduce an unemployment insurance plan; a Page 2 story about a proposed Canadian trade agreement with New Zealand; an article about the fraud trial of two stockbrokers whose business went bankrupt, causing serious losses to many of their clients; a report about the problems of the livestock industry, in which it was noted that 'the apparent disregard of the middleman for the problems of the primary producer was the cause of considerable dissatisfaction'; a report of a vote by the Manitoba legislature asking that former soldiers be given more leeway to pay back loans for the purchase of farmland; the story of Harvey Jackson, the Communist arrested for vagrancy; and, on Page 13, news of the settlement of a garment workers' strike in Montreal. As Canada approached the first spring of what would later be known as the Great Depression, might not readers have seen these as threads in an emerging discussion about economic insecurity and the various possible responses to it, finding connections among apparently disparate articles that reflected their current concerns? One of the few scholars to study the form of news articles closely, Teun van Dijk, has stressed that they invariably presuppose an enormous amount of knowledge on the reader's part, without which they cannot be made sense of.[41] Similarly, when newspaper editors speak of 'timeliness,' one of the things they mean is how a given story will resonate with the things that are already on their readers' minds. While it is difficult (though not impossible)[42] to know for certain what might have been on readers' minds at a particular point in the past, content cannot properly be understood without considering the associations it evokes, and these associations often place small or apparently trivial stories into larger frameworks of public meaning.

None of this is to say that the newspapers of 1930 were on the whole more serious or high-minded that their 1870 counterparts. On a strictly quantitative basis, it is difficult to make a simple determination: should one emphasize the larger absolute quantity of serious material, or the smaller proportion of the whole it represented? Certainly the 1930 newspapers contained much more non-serious content than did their predecessors. Sports coverage, oddities, and trivialities abounded. Many crime stories were prominently reported simply for their shock value. The *Telegram*'s coverage of the law courts was written to be entertaining (but then, so had it been in 1870). National politics – a centrally important element of citizenship, though not the only one – was covered much less. Ethnic minorities, non-whites in particular, were treated no better (though not notably worse either).

But if we are seeking to understand the newspaper's social role at different times, such comparisons may not be very helpful.[43] Readers in 1930 did not compare their newspapers with what had appeared sixty years earlier. The newspapers they read included substantial amounts of material that put forward conceptions of common citizenship, as seen from a variety of angles. The range of subjects addressed in this way was much broader than in 1870. The absolute volume of such material was considerable, even if it made up a smaller proportion of the newspaper than previously, and much of it was prominently displayed on Page 1 or the main news pages inside.

Newspapers in 1930 did operate more like big businesses than they had done sixty years earlier. Capital requirements and barriers to entry were much higher. They paid less attention to formal politics, especially at the national level; they were more concerned with entertaining, as well as informing, their readers; they reinforced relentlessly the gospel of consumption. But the act of publishing news and delivering it to thousands of people still situated readers in an emphatically public sphere – it still addressed them, and in a sense constituted them, as a public.[44] Reading the same newspaper each day gave them a shared exposure to events outside their personal realms, shared points of reference, a sense not only of what they knew as individuals, but of what was socially known. Benedict Anderson's central insight remains extremely valuable: newspaper readers are aware of the presence of other readers and imagine the presence of many more. A major part of the reader's experience is coming to know what others know, being part of the community of readers. This public character, the awareness that the newspaper's content is inherently shared knowledge, gives the newspaper much of its weight and authority. Anderson's approach can be applied more broadly: the imagined community of readers need not only be a nation, but can include Toronto, the British Empire, or Protestantism; the community of non-Chinese, non-Catholics, non-boozers, and non-Reds; members of the Women's Institute, I.O.D.E., or Girl Guides; or the amalgam of all of these that made up the intended audience of the *Evening Telegram* or (somewhat more decorously) the *Globe* on any given day.

The community of readers can be conceived in another way too. When editors put together a newspaper each day, they make hundreds of choices about selection and emphasis. In the aggregate, these choices outline the shape of their intended audience – their imagined audience, if you will. No two readers are likely to respond to this presentation in the same way; there is a correspondence between editors' intentions and readers' reactions, but only a rough one.

Asserting the essentially public character of newspapers does not mean that they always carried out this role in the same way. The *kind* of public that newspapers addressed, and the ways in which it was addressed – who was presented as belonging and who was not, which kinds of events in the world were emphasized and which ignored, which sources of information were seen as credible, how the news was presented – these did change substantially, and with important effects, over time.[45] Indeed, one of the objections to the partisan/commercial dichotomy is precisely that it flattens out important differences in time and across space: political partisanship continues in newspapers to this day, but it had a different, specific form in 1930 than in 1950 (or in 1970 or 1990). The presence or absence of competition is particularly important when thinking about the newspaper's public role; in highly competitive markets like Toronto, readers had more choice (though never anything like a perfect choice) about which of the various 'us' groups being offered seemed to fit best.

The different groups of readers to which newspapers were addressed need not all be seen in a positive light. There is in much of the literature an implicit (sometimes explicit) criterion of judgment: whatever fosters community is good, and whatever does not is bad; since the evolution of newspapers has substituted consumption for community, things are worse than they used to be. But is every form of community sentiment desirable? In James Huffman's insightful study of the emergence of a mass press in Japan, he notes the contradictory forces at work. On one hand, a public community was created that for the first time recognized the common people as citizens, and saw them as having a role in government and politics; on the other, it was a public community united by extreme nationalism, militarism, and the cult of the emperor.[46] An examination of Toronto newspapers in 1930 makes it clear that community was defined by exclusion and intolerance as well as inclusion.

Could the public addressed by the *Telegram* or *Globe* in 1930 have been more inclusive, more authentic, more effectively mobilized to defend its best interests? Obviously, yes. But a convincing analysis of what the newspapers failed to do must begin with an adequate account of what they actually did. It is a difficult assignment merely to divine the shape of the public community that a newspaper proposed at a particular time. Coming to grips with the dizzying profusion of words and images in just one edition of one newspaper, without resorting to simplistic categorization, is challenging. When one adds the additional dimension of change over time, and attempts to weigh the often incommensurable claims of what has been gained against what has been lost, the task becomes harder still.

It is here that the inadequacy of the partisan/commercial dichotomy becomes most apparent. It captures some aspects of what changed, but obscures the new ways in which readers were addressed as a public. The changes in business structure and practices that newspapers embraced in the last decades of the nineteenth century and the early twentieth influenced and constrained, but did not determine, either the newspaper's content or its cultural role. Culture is not entirely autonomous either; only through the interplay of business and culture can the historical evolution of newspapers be understood.

Business history, in short, needs cultural history, and vice versa. This applies not only to newspapers – or, for that matter, to other cultural businesses like advertising, public relations, and marketing (which, in the twentieth century, came to involve the production of virtually all consumer products). Business historians have increasingly recognized the importance of considering culture in all areas of their work, including the internal organization of firms, attitudes towards hierarchy and authority, definitions of rationality, and the functioning of the market.[47] The influence on business of cultural products, such as the newspaper, deserves particular attention: how information is gathered, organized, and made available is increasingly seen as crucial to understanding the evolution of the environment in which business operates.[48]

The suggestion that business can only be understood in its social and cultural context would come as no surprise to Michael Bliss, to whom this volume is dedicated. His first book, *A Living Profit*, had a revealing subtitle: *Studies in the Social History of Canadian Business*.[49] It was about what businessmen thought (or 'thought they thought,' to use the words of Edward Kirkland, whose study of American business ideology inspired Bliss's work),[50] and one of its main conclusions was that they thought (and did) many different things.

Some men in business were extraordinarily money-hungry, others thought profit a by-product of excellence in business. Some beat and kicked their workers, others paid high wages and built baseball diamonds. Some corrupted legislatures, others worked for civil service reform and honest government. Some formed combines and gouged the public, others combined in the literal hope of making a living profit.[51]

The idea that all businessmen acted the same way – or worse, that they could all be assumed to act the same way – is not that different from the assertion that a uniform set of 'business values' systematically undermined the public role of newspapers after 1880.

As an empirically-grounded historian, Bliss is sceptical of models and explicit theory; the business historian builds up generalizations cautiously, dealing in specific, differentiated cases rather than seeking the law-like accounts of the economic historian.[52] In Bliss's business history, there are just a few great, continuing, and interconnected verities: the inevitability and value of competition, the importance of the entrepreneur, the value of open markets.[53] But even here, businessmen were not all in agreement. In *A Living Profit*, Bliss documents their deeply ambivalent attitudes toward competition, insisting on one hand that workers and the young, for example, must steel themselves to face the lash of competition while seeking regularly to avoid its harshest demands themselves. Similarly, *Northern Enterprise* is full of cautionary tales about businessmen who sought to circumvent competition through reliance on the state.

The newspaper industry embodied contradictions too. There was always a tension between newspapers' historic and inescapable public role and their character as profit-making private businesses. The nature of this tension changed over time. Newspapers were much bigger after 1880, more capital-intensive, more dependent on advertising and large circulation; and all these things drove them increasingly to entertain as well as to inform their readers. But it was a case of 'as well as,' not 'instead of'; the fact that readers were addressed as members of a public sphere, broadly conceived, was one of the main things newspapers had to sell.

NOTES

1 James Carey, 'The Problem of Journalism History,' in Eve Stryker Munson and Catherine A. Warren, eds, *James Carey: A Critical Reader* (Minneapolis: University of Minnesota Press, 1997), 86–94. There is a large volume of high-quality recent work about the history of journalism; in addition to

those mentioned elsewhere in this essay, a few examples are Jean K. Chalaby, *The Invention of Journalism* (Basingstoke, London, New York: Macmillan and St Martin's Press, 1998); Charles E. Clark, *The Public Prints: The Newspaper in Anglo-American Culture, 1665–1740* (New York: Oxford University Press, 1994); Robert Darnton, 'An Early Information Society: News and the Media in Eighteenth-Century Paris,' *American Historical Review*, 105, 1 (February 2000): 1–35; Dean de la Motte and Jaennene M. Przyblyski, eds, *Making the News: Modernity and the Mass Press in Nineteenth-Century France* (Amherst, MA: University of Massachusetts Press, 1999); Brendan Dooley, *The Social History of Skepticism: Experience and Doubt in Early Modern Culture* (Baltimore, London: Johns Hopkins University Press, 1999); Hanno Hardt and Bonnie Brennen, eds, *Newsworkers: Toward a History of the Rank and File* (Minneapolis: University of Minnesota Press, 1995); Jeffrey L. McNairn, *The Capacity to Judge: Public Opinion and Deliberative Democracy in Upper Canada, 1791–1854* (Toronto: University of Toronto Press, 2000); Joad Raymond, *The Invention of the Newspaper: English Newsbooks, 1641–1649* (Oxford: Clarendon Press, 1996); Elizabeth Sinn, 'Emerging Media: Hong Kong and the Early Evolution of the Chinese Press,' *Modern Asian Studies* 36, 2 (May 2002): 421–65; Mary Vipond, 'The Mass Media in Canadian History: The Empire Day Broadcast of 1939,' *Journal of the Canadian Historical Association*, new ser., 14 (2003): 1–21.

2 Jürgen Habermas, The *Structural Transformation of the Public Sphere: An Inquiry into a Category of Bourgeois Society*, trans. Thomas Burger (Cambridge, MA: MIT Press, 1989); Benedict Anderson, *Imagined Communities: Reflections on the Origin and Spread of Nationalism*, rev. ed. (New York and London: Verso, 1991).

3 For example, Minko Sotiron's *From Politics to Profit: The Commercialization of Canadian Daily Newspapers, 1890–1920* (Montreal, Kingston: McGill-Queen's University Press, 1997) is explicitly structured around the question of how Canadian newspapers reached the state of concentration of ownership decried by the Senate Special Committee on the Mass Media in 1970. According to Sotiron, 'The period from 1890 to 1920 … marked the transition from the politically oriented newspaper of the nineteenth century to the corporate entity of the twentieth' (10). Gerald Baldasty covers similar territory in relation to the U.S. newspaper industry in a more nuanced way, but his conclusions point in a similar direction: 'When commercial considerations dictate the general news process, the press will serve democracy only when such service is financially profitable.' Gerald Baldasty, *The Commercialization of News in the Nineteenth Century* (Madison: University of Wisconsin Press, 1992), 9, 144. In *The Form of News* (New York, London:

The Guilford Press, 2001), Kevin Barnhurst and John Nerone recognize that 'the newspaper will figure its reader as citizen on one level and as consumer on the other, as self-controlled rational investor on one level and as emotion-driver buyer or fan on another, and so on' (3). Even so, their overall view is that 'some things newspapers simply used to do better. They engaged readers better. They invited people (albeit especially white men) into politics better. They presented multiple voices better. They encouraged argument better' (25).

For a critical assessment of this view as 'almost pure functionalism, even economic determinism,' see David Paul Nord, 'The Business Values of American Newspapers: The Nineteenth Century Watershed,' in D.P. Nord, *Communities of Journalism: A History of American Newspapers and Their Readers* (Urbana, Chicago: University of Illinois Press, 2001), 134. Habermas has also rejected as 'too simplistic' his own earlier conclusion that increasing commercialization of journalism brought about a change from a 'culture-debating to a culture-consuming public'; see 'Further Reflections on the Public Sphere,' in Craig Calhoun, ed., *Habermas and the Public Sphere* (Cambridge, MA and London: MIT Press, 1992), 438–9.

4 See, for example, the recent survey by Paul Starr, *The Creation of the Media: Political Origins of Modern Communications* (New York: Basic Books, 2004), 146.

5 James Carey, 'A Cultural Approach to Communication,' in Carey, *Communication as Culture: Essays on Media and Society* (New York: Routledge, 1992, first pub. 1989).

6 Marjory Lang, *Women Who Made the News: Female Journalists in Canada, 1880–1945* (Montreal, Kingston: McGill-Queen's University Press, 1999), 1–11. See also Barbara Freeman, *The Satellite Sex: The Media and Women's Issues in English Canada, 1966–1971* (Waterloo, ON: Wilfrid Laurier University Press, 2001).

7 Joy Wiltenburg, 'True Crime: The Origins of Modern Sensationalism,' *American Historical Review* 109, 5 (December 2004): 1377–1404. See also Henrik Ornebring and Anna Maria Jonsson, 'Tabloid Journalism and the Public Sphere: A Historical Perspective on Tabloid Journalism,' *Journalism Studies* 5, 3 (2004): 283–95.

8 Michael Schudson, *Discovering the News: A Social History of American Newspapers* (New York: Basic Books, 1978), 31–43.

9 Richard L. Kaplan, *Politics and the American Press: The Rise of Objectivity, 1865–1920* (Cambridge, New York: Cambridge University Press, 2002).

10 As Kaplan puts it, accounts based on modernization or commercialization ignore 'the role of such social variables as power and culture in the consti-

tution of news … The variable ways in which the media enhance or inhibit democratic discussion are lost, and the actual social construction of the news is neglected.' Ibid., 6–7.

11 In *A Victorian Authority: The Daily Press in Late Nineteenth-Century Canada* (Toronto: University of Toronto Press, 1982), Paul Rutherford describes the *Telegraph* as one of the first 'people's papers' in Canada (53–4).

12 Ron Poulton, *The Paper Tyrant: John Ross Robertson of* The Toronto Telegram (Toronto, Vancouver: Clarke, Irwin & Co., 1971), 26–62; Minko Sotiron, 'John Ross Robertson,' *Dictionary of Canadian Biography* 14; Rutherford, *Victorian Authority*, 43; Thomas L. Walkom, 'The Daily Newspaper Industry in Ontario's Developing Capitalistic Economy: Toronto and Ottawa, 1871–1911,' PhD diss., University of Toronto, 1983, 31.

13 J.M.S. Careless, *Brown of* The Globe, vol. 1, *The Voice of Upper Canada* (Toronto: Macmillan of Canada, 1959), 77, 105, 121; Walkom, 'Daily Newspaper Industry,' 345.

14 Rutherford, *Victorian Authority*, 212. It is also relevant that the party system had a markedly different history in Canada than in the United States, which means that accounts of newspaper partisanship there will not necessarily apply here. For example, Jeffrey Pasley illustrates clearly that by the 1830s many American newspapers were integral elements of the emerging system of mass political mobilization; Jeffrey L. Pasley, *'The Tyranny of Printers': Newspaper Politics in the Early American Republic* (Charlottesville, London: University of Virginia Press, 2001). National politics in Canada did not even begin until forty years later, and the integration of national and provincial party machines before 1900 was much less extensive.

15 Walkom, 'Daily Newspaper Industry,' 346, and table VII-1, 375. Newspapers outside Toronto depended more heavily on patronage.

16 Brian P.N. Beaven, 'Partisanship, Patronage and the Press in Ontario, 1880–1914: Myths and Realities,' *Canadian Historical Review* 64, 3 (1983): 348–9.

17 Careless, *Brown of* The Globe, 1: 46–8, 64–5, 228, and *Brown of* The Globe, vol. 2, *Statesman of Confederation, 1860–1880* (Toronto: Macmillan of Canada, 1963), 5–6, 68, 268–70, 280, 340, 368–9; Walkom, 'Daily Newspaper Industry,' 35–6.

18 Walkom, 'Daily Newspaper Industry,' 53, 99–101, 348–9; Kaplan, *Politics and the American Press*, 9. It is also worth remembering that newspapers' commercial character and the treatment of news as a commodity were not innovations of the late nineteenth century. As Habermas observed, the very emergence of the public press in the seventeenth century was a response to the requirements of commerce and had essentially to do with news' character as a commercial commodity. Habermas, *Structural Transformation*, 21.

19 Michael Schudson, 'Was There Ever a Public Sphere?' in Schudson, *The Power of News* (Cambridge, MA, and London: Harvard University Press, 1995).

20 See also Walkom, 'Daily Newspaper Industry,' 194: 'Usually there was no need to bias, either overtly or covertly, the actual accounts, since readers of each paper knew what connections they were supposed to draw.'

21 Daniel C. Hallin, *The 'Uncensored War': The Media and Vietnam* (New York: University of California Press, 1989; first published 1986), 116–18.

22 Kaplan, *Politics and the American Press*, 189–90.

23 Sotiron recognizes this phenomenon as well, but dismisses it as participation in 'the elitist civic reformism and non-partisan movements of businessmen'; *From Politics to Profit*, 160.

24 Walkom, 'Daily Newspaper Industry,' 468.

25 Nord, 'Business Values,' 145.

26 Baldasty, *Commercialization of News*, 34; Kaplan, *Politics and the American Press*, 190.

27 Michael Schudson, *The Good Citizen: A History of American Civic Life* (New York: The Free Press, 1998), 6; Schudson, 'Public Sphere,' 199–200.

28 There is a voluminous literature on the development of objectivity. Besides Schudson, *Discovering the News*, and Kaplan, *Politics and the American Press*, see David T.Z. Mindich, *Just the Facts: How 'Objectivity' Came to Define American Journalism* (New York, London: New York University Press, 1998) and Chalaby, *Invention of Journalism*.

29 Because the standard page size was smaller in 1930, the available space was 220 per cent (*Globe*) and 604 per cent (*Telegram*) greater than it had been 60 years before.

30 One or two very short sports items had appeared in the 1870 editions, all related to horse racing, but there was nothing like a sports section.

31 Baldasty, *Commercialization of News*, 49–52, notes specifically that the new newspaper was essentially an urban phenomenon. See also Rutherford, *Victorian Authority*, 135–6.

32 One of Nord's first publications was *Newspapers and New Politics: Midwestern Municipal Reform, 1890–1900* (Ann Arbor: UMI Research Press, 1981). See also Nord, 'The Public Community: The Urbanization of Journalism in Chicago,' in *Communities of Journalism*, 108–32.

33 See Jonathan Vance, *Death So Noble: Memory, Meaning and the First World War* (Vancouver: UBC Press, 1997).

34 Carey, 'Cultural Approach to Communication,' 20.

35 For examples of the same approach to labour radicals in Chicago in the 1870s and 1880s, see Nord, 'Business Values,' 139, 141–2, 144.

36 Rutherford, *Victorian Authority*, 167–8.

37 Lang, *Women Who Made the News*, 6–9.

38 For the significance of coverage of such 'club women,' *Women Who Made the News*, see Lang, 216–47.

39 For the evolution of Page 1 from 1885 to 1985, see Barnhurst and Nerone, *The Form of News*, 181–218.

40 Schudson interprets this as part of a shift from an 'informed citizen' model to a 'monitorial' model of citizenship; *Good Citizen*, 309–12. The emergence of gender issues is a good example of a once-private matter becoming public and thereby political.

41 Teun A. van Dijk, *News as Discourse* (Hillsdale, NJ: Lawrence Erlbaum Associates, 1988), 29, 33–4, 36–7, 75.

42 For successful attempts to understand the reader's perspective, see Nord, 'Readership as Citizenship in Eighteenth-Century Philadelphia,' 'Reading the Newspaper: Strategies and Politics of Reader Response, Chicago, 1912–1917,' and other chapters in *Communities of Journalism*.

43 To quote Michael Schudson: 'The use of history should not be to condemn the present from some purportedly higher standard of the past, but to know where we stand in time.' *Good Citizen*, 9.

44 The analogy with language is instructive: just as language shapes the understood world for us, rather than merely describing it, so newspapers constitute their different publics, rather than merely selling a product to a public that already and independently exists. On the public role of newspapers, see also Nord, 'Business Values,' 145: though editors and publishers were devoted to ideas of private property and private enterprise, 'their product and the function of their product were inherently public … As urban newspapers began to expand their definition of news and to expand their circulations to broader audiences in the mid-nineteenth century, the realm of public life expanded for them as well. *Through the act of publication itself newspapers asserted that a particular issue was no longer a private matter'* (my emphasis).

45 Baldasty, *Commercialization of News*, 96–7, makes a convincing argument that the emergence of the beat system of reporting, with its reliance on official sources (police headquarters, city hall, etc.) reflects the large newspaper's demand for a regular, predictable supply of news that goes along with mass-production methods. Here there does seem to be a plausible link between organizational imperatives and a specific kind of content.

46 James Huffman, *Creating a Public: People and Press in Meiji Japan* (Honolulu: University of Hawai'i Press, 1997) 202–4, 210–13, 220–22, 338–41, 357.

47  Kenneth Lipartito, 'Culture and the Practice of Business History,' *Business and Economic History* 24, 2 (Winter 1995): 1–41. As Lipartito succinctly notes, 'All behavior, even supposedly easy responses to unambiguous market lessons, is filtered through cultural lenses by all actors all the time' (25). For a recent example of how cultural perspectives are being integrated into large-scale structural approaches to business history, see Naomi R. Lamoreaux, Daniel M.G. Raff, and Peter Temin, 'Beyond Markets and Hierarchies: Toward a New Synthesis of American Business History,' *American Historical Review* 108, 2 (April 2003): 404–33.

48  See, for example, the various essays in Alfred D. Chandler, Jr, and James W. Cortada, eds, *A Nation Transformed by Information: How Information Has Shaped the United States from Colonial Times to the Present* (New York: Oxford University Press, 2000); and Oliver Boyd-Barrett and Terhi Rantanen, 'The Globalization of News,' in Boyd-Barrett and Rantanen, eds, *The Globalization of News* (London: Sage Publications, 1998): 'We regard the development of the concept "news" as a process that lies at the heart of modern capitalism and which also illuminates process of globalization which modern capitalism has helped to generate … The links between modernity, capitalism, news, news agencies and globalization are an outstanding but neglected feature of the past 150 years' (2).

49  Michael Bliss, *A Living Profit: Studies in the Social History of Canadian Business*, 1883–1911 (Toronto: McClelland and Stewart, 1974) .

50  Edward C. Kirkland, *Dream and Thought in the Business Community, 1860–1900* (Ithaca, NY: Cornell University Press, 1956).

51  Bliss, *Living Profit*, 136–7. Throughout his career, Bliss has questioned the 'continuing belief held by liberal, "progressive" intellectuals that the values of liberal culture and high profits were necessarily opposed … Whatever these studies prove, they originated in the belief that neither the past nor the present is quite that simple.' Ibid., 13.

52  The biography form is particularly well suited to examining the varied ways that ideas and material circumstances influence one another, and in *A Canadian Millionaire* Bliss showed how Joseph Flavelle's innovative and paradigmatic business practices coexisted with his Methodism and ideas of public service; *A Canadian Millionaire: The Life and Business Times of Sir Joseph Flavelle, Bart., 1858–1939* (Toronto: Macmillan, 1978). Flavelle's somewhat quixotic experience with the *Toronto News* fits interestingly into the discussion here of how business values and newspapers went together (or not) in the early years of the twentieth century. Flavelle got into newspapers not for business reasons at all, but through motives of public service; he was concerned about the debasement of public taste which, he believed,

accompanied the increasing reliance of the press on advertising and a mass audience. He encouraged his editor to attack businessmen who, in Flavelle's view, violated accepted business standards, and eventually sold out after losing between $300,000 and $400,000 – an indication that even idealism had at some point to come to terms with commerce, or at least with the circulation department. The *News* illustrates that civic high-mindedness in journalism is not always the best way of attracting readers. Bliss, *Canadian Millionaire*, 149, 171–2, 182–3.

53 Bliss, *Northern Enterprise*, 579–84.

# Family and Religion

# 7 'I thank God ... that I am proud of my boy': Fatherhood and Religion in the Gordon Family

DAVID B. MARSHALL

In the early 1920s, when King Gordon was attending Oxford University, his father, Charles Gordon, wrote a letter to him reminiscing about their relationship.

> The thing that bored its way into my heart was this that the days of your boyhood were over and that henceforth your days at home would only be your holidays. I confess the thing quite appalls me. But I must meet this as part of life and find for it such help as I do for other things that constitute life's burden. We have had a great time together boy a great & good time – a very heart satisfying time ... this I want to say now King my boy that looking back over the twenty-two years I would not care to change one day of your conduct toward me. And what more could a father ask and why should I complain that we cannot have the great carefree fine days of comradeship together any longer. Not many fathers have the memory your father has – none that I have known. So we will look bravely as we can and without whining at the new conditions that life and duty impose upon us.[1]

This outpouring of intimacy and sentimentality marked just one occasion when Charles allowed his son a glimpse of the depth of his fondness and admiration. This letter was typical of many from Charles to his son especially in its candour about their relationship and his expectations. Charles recognized that a particularly intimate and intense period, in which he had a direct hand in nurturing and guiding his son, was nearing an end. King, now twenty-two years old, had grown out of boyhood and into manhood, and he no longer required the same amount of direction and mentoring as he had previously. Clearly, Charles was struck by the irony of fatherhood: by raising his son to be able to go his own way in the world he had fostered the self-reliance that would, in part, take his son away from him. Letters such as these reveal a man who was intimately involved in raising his children. Charles Gordon is a perfect example of what historians have called 'masculine domesticity,' best understood as a model of behaviour in which fathers take on significant responsibility for some of the day-to-day tasks of raising the children, particularly playing with them and teaching them about the world around them.[2]

We are more familiar with the public Charles Gordon, better known as the popular novelist 'Ralph Connor,' not the father in the letter above who was lamenting his son's growing independence and the decline of their daily intimate contact. 'Ralph Connor' was the author of numerous best-selling novels, including *Black Rock* (1898), *The Sky Pilot* (1899), and *The Man from Glengarry* (1900). By 1914 Connor had published nine best-selling novels. Each one had sold over one hundred thousand copies. The most popular was *The Sky Pilot*, with sales in excess of three hundred thousand copies. *The Man from Glengarry* had sold two hundred and fifty thousand copies and *The Doctor* had sold just over two hundred thousand copies by the beginning of the First World War. Publishers' reports indicate that the total sales of all Connor novels by 1914 had reached 1.6 million, with just over one million copies sold in the United States and over three hundred thousand copies in both the Canadian and British markets. The last best-selling Connor novels were the two wartime tales *The Major* (1917) and *The Sky Pilot in No Man's Land* (1919). Gordon continued to write Connor novels throughout the twenties and thirties, but sales had trailed off significantly. His early best-selling novels remained in print throughout the 1920s and 30s and frequently had annual sales of over a thousand copies.[3]

Connor fiction was formulaic and can be considered to be typical examples of the adventure tale set in the far reaches of the British Empire, specifically, the Canadian west. Connor heroes, often missionaries or North West Mounted Police, personified all the qualities of the cult of masculinity that emerged so powerfully in the popular culture of the late nineteenth century.[4] They were strong, aggressive, courageous, competitive, adventurous, passionate, loyal to their cause, and sometimes violent. In Connor novels, the heroes transformed their masculine energy, tough-mindedness, and determination into tools or weapons in the battle for moral order, religion, and civilization on the rugged frontier. They were muscular Christians. Indeed, President Theodore Roosevelt, who 'epitomized manly zest' and the quest to revitalize modern manhood,[5] was a fan of Ralph Connor novels and he corresponded with Gordon about their merits.[6] Gordon drew heavily on the dominant code of manliness, which extolled action, determination, duty, independence, and moral and physical courage in writing his Connor novels. This public Charles Gordon of the Ralph Connor novels is a perfect example of the cult of manhood and is best known to historians.[7]

Charles Gordon's notoriety, however, went far beyond his fame as a best-selling author. He was a leading proponent of the social gospel in the Presbyterian Church in Canada. Through his work for temperance in Manitoba, cleaning up various forms of vice in Winnipeg, crusading for the preservation of the Lord's day, and acting as a labour conciliator in protracted and bitter strikes in the coal fields of western Canada, Gordon was widely known as an activist minister who was in the forefront of many moral and social reform movements. He also spearheaded many programs that promoted muscular Christianity.[8] He was particularly concerned about the fate of young men, for he knew they did not attend church in the same numbers as women, and was most alarmed by the lack of suitable men for work in the church and especially in the mission fields. Only vigorous, robust men who possessed the qualities of courage, determination, a willingness to sacrifice material well-being, and an ability to endure hardship could meet the challenges of the mission field. Like many of his contemporaries, Gordon worried that these masculine virtues were lacking in young men raised in modern society. Gordon built much of his reputation in the Presbyterian church as a recruiter of young men to the cause of Christianity, and he was prominent in many crusades designed to save young men from the decadent influences of alcohol, the bar, gambling, and the billiard hall. St Stephen's Presbyterian Church in Winnipeg, where Gordon was the minister, was one of the first institutional churches on the Prairies. It boasted a gymnasium, games room, and meeting rooms where clubs and organizations for young men and businessmen could gather. To an extent, Gordon was instrumental in making St Stephen's a place that was a counter-attraction to the many baneful influences that were undermining the character, moral fibre, and health of young men. Ultimately, Gordon demonstrated his firm commitment to the principles of muscular

Christianity in a highly visible and public way. He volunteered for the chaplain's service and served overseas during the First World War.

How do we reconcile the public Gordon of the Ralph Connor novels and the dedication to the values of muscular Christianity with the private Gordon, the devoted, nurturing, and sometimes very sentimental father? On the surface these two models of masculinity seem to be irreconcilable. Indeed, adventure novels such as those by Ralph Connor are cited as examples of men's desire to flee, at the very least in their fantasy world, from the domestic sphere for a more exciting life on the imperial frontier, where they could exercise their manly attributes unencumbered by the confines of domesticity and the influence of women.[9] Moreover, muscular Christianity was designed to rescue imperilled manhood or redeem boys and young men from the overly feminine and domestic influences of modern society that were thought to have an enervating influence on the male character. These two models of masculinity are not mutually exclusive or necessarily contradictory, however. Perhaps it is best to suggest that men at the turn of the last century were constantly negotiating between the energetic and tough-minded adventure-seeking male and the sentimental, nurturing domestic male.[10] Put another way, men were constantly moving in and out across the threshold of the home.[11] Any concerns that men had about the continuation of masculine character in boys necessitated fathers becoming more involved in their sons' upbringing. To an extent, men's involvement in the domestic sphere and especially child-rearing was rooted in their concerns about the preservation of masculinity. To preserve the rugged, ambitious male they had to sacrifice some of their toughness and independent spirit and assume a greater nurturing role in the home and family circle.[12] As John Gillis explains: 'Fathers at the threshold ... defined the borders between home and the world. Threshold rites gave expression to male ambivalence, reflecting the tension between men's longing for home and their anxiety not to be too closely identified with the feminine domain.'[13]

Perhaps we get the best glimpse of Gordon the muscular Christian, determined to promote an adventurous, outdoor, even primitive masculinity, and the caring father when he was at the summer cottage he purchased at Lake of the Woods. He took two months off from his preaching and pastoral duties at St Stephen's church each summer so that he could spend as much time as possible with his family at a rugged wilderness retreat. The Gordon cottage was located on an island called Birkencraig, named for birch trees that grew from the island's

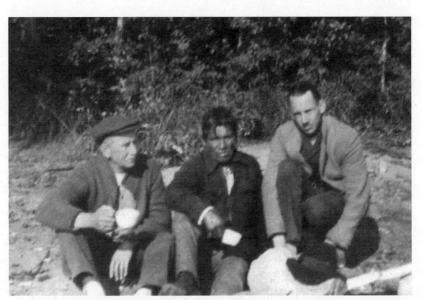

Charles and King Gordon, with an unidentified man in the middle, at Birken-craig, Lake of the Woods; date not known. (Photo reproduced with permission from the Department of Archives and Special Collections, The University of Manitoba, Photograph Collection 76-2-4)

lichen-covered crag. On Birkencraig, where the cottage was sur-rounded by primeval forest, Charles had the opportunity to teach King the pioneering skills of chopping wood, rock climbing, and canoeing, those very skills that were being lost in modern urban society to the detriment of the masculine character of young boys. This summer retreat in the wilderness was also where Gordon was fond of recount-ing romantic heroic tales of the *coureurs de bois*, 'when along these very waters, the fur fleets were wont to make their way, their gay chansons ringing in rhythm with the swing of their paddles ... [they] came to rest at this very spot.'[14]

A great deal of the literature on men and masculinity has been based on the prescriptive literature and images of males presented in popular culture. The construction of the 'cult of manliness' through schools, popular literature, boys' organizations and clubs, sporting activities, games, public celebrations, and the military has been emphasized. Drawing on public sources to understand the cult of masculinity and family life overlooks the fact that a great many masculine virtues were not solely passed on through public institutions, such as schools, advice manuals, magazines and periodicals, or popular boys stories.[15] The passing of masculine virtues and characteristics through advice and example within the domestic sphere and especially from father to son, was equally, if not more, important. As Anthony Rotundo has explained, there were many influences upon a boy as he learned the ideals of manhood: ministers, teachers, popular fiction and school-books, scouting, sports and games to name a few. But of all the influences on boys developing ideals and expectations, the first and foremost was the family, and when it came to impressing values and providing an example of manhood, the father's influence was paramount.[16] Fathers nurtured, offered moral guidance, and provided solace and companionship for their children. They played many roles within the family: from leading family prayer and setting a moral tone, to instructing children in their lessons and providing examples of many of life's important skills, to teaching them how to play different games and sports.[17] Fatherhood, John Tosh has recently written, blends the requirements of paternal authority with nurture and play.[18]

The basis of this study is the over seventy extant letters Charles Gordon wrote to his son King between 1908 and 1937. These letters were never brief or perfunctory. Even when King was a young boy, the letters were two long pages in length. As King matured and Charles could share more with him, the letters became longer. By the end of the First World War, King was eighteen and Charles's letters were anywhere from a compact four pages, when he was hurried, to twenty-page-long epistles. Although the character of Charles's correspondence to King changed over time, certain features were constant. In all cases they sought to establish contact with King and to renew the ties that were strained with distance.[19] The letters touched on a range of themes, especially personal and family matters and latterly professional activities and current events.

In the early letters, the only references to non-family matters related to Charles's explanation about what he was doing while away so that King could understand the reason for his father's absence. The First World War and King's greater maturity changed the character of the letters. The necessity of maintaining contact with family members and reassuring them of his devotion to them only became more pressing and important for Charles during the extreme uncertainty caused by the war. But Charles also needed to convey some of his thoughts and impressions about the war effort and its consequences. During the last year of the war, when King was eighteen, Charles wrote seven lengthy letters, the most intensive and concentrated of his correspondence, which contained detailed and candid commentary on the current international situation.

A few years after the war, King left the confines of the family home for Oxford University. Charles wrote approximately fifteen letters to King while he was studying in England between 1922 and 1924. While this number of letters strikes one as being limited, other family members kept King abreast of their father's activities in their correspondence. In his sisters' letters, King was informed about Charles's activities and his attempts to discipline their behaviour. Charles was always somehow looming in the background of their correspondence. They told King about how their father struggled with certain aspects of teenage culture, such as dancing, jazz music, and the movies, including those that were based on Connor novels.[20] On one occasion, King's mother wrote expressing her wish that Charles could take a break from his busy schedule and the pressures of completing another novel. But she also admitted that he would have difficulty coping on a holiday at the cottage without King. 'Daddy is very disappointed not to have you home & I do not know how he will manage without you. The lake won't be anything without you.'[21] For King, these letters created a sense of the comings and goings of the family, such that he could still feel he was a part of things. Charles's letters during this period provided King with a detailed picture of postwar Canadian life. They contained lengthy commentaries on labour strife from his vantage point as a member of the Manitoba Council of Industry, which was created in the wake of the Winnipeg General Strike. And from the vantage of the moderator's chair of the Presbyterian Church, Charles provided King with a ringside view of the church-union negotiations taking place with the Methodist and Congregational churches.

When King returned to Canada in 1924, the protracted and sometimes heated and bitter church-union battle was winding down. Charles was on the verge of retirement as the United Church of Canada was finally constituted. After a flurry of letters, in which Charles further outlined the events and personalities surrounding church union, the correspondence slowed considerably. The late 1920s correspondence was limited to a few letters concerning King's struggles as a young minister. More frequent correspondence resumed during the Great Depression of the 1930s. In part, the crisis in King's professional life prompted the more intense and frequent contact. But the events of the economic disaster also prompted Charles to write lengthy and thoughtful letters about labour activism, social welfare, socialist politics, and the worsening international situation. As the gloom of the Depression deepened, Charles's usual optimism dimmed.

This correspondence, therefore, provides a particularly close and intimate glimpse of a father–son relationship. It captures some of the intricacies and emotions of such relationships that cannot be discerned from the ideal construction of fatherhood presented in the prescriptive literature, advice manuals, and other printed sources of the time.[22] Of course, analysing relationships through correspondence alone can only give a partial view. We do not have King's responses to his father's letters. Moreover, the intensity of the relationship is missing. The correspondence does not capture the full range or complexity of their contact or exchanges with each other. For example, the correspondence portrays neither the physical interaction between father and son nor the emotional intensity of particular moments. We do not, for example, get a sense of how anger was expressed or disappointment was communicated. It is difficult to recreate the sense of play and fun that developed between father and son in the correspondence. But to dismiss the letters because of what is missing or not said, to reject them as a literature of silence or omission, would be misleading. The emphasis here is on the experience of fatherhood and the intimate yet sometimes strained nature of father–son relations as seen through Charles Gordon's correspondence.[23]

Questions of power are investigated, especially within the framework of the struggle between a father's desire to have influence and a son's quest for independence. Charles's correspondence to King reflected his ongoing efforts to instil the manly virtues of hard work, discipline, and domestic responsibility, the importance of education, and the necessity of religious conviction. But limits to fatherly advice and influence existed by the twentieth century. Like most fathers, Charles had 'high expectations' of his son, and the reason for these demands rested in his concern with regard to his son's future. Fathers felt responsible for their sons' future welfare. Traditionally, fathers had endowed their sons with land, a business, or even a profession. Boys had been trained or apprenticed under their father's tutelage or a colleague's watchful eye. But in the modern industrial bureaucratic age these patriarchal practices were becoming obsolete. As a result, two realities of modern life confronted fathers: they had little to give their sons except for their wise counsel and their sons' future could not be guaranteed. Fathers had a sense that the world was a demanding, competitive, and sometimes dangerous place. Preparing their sons for the outside world required that they pass on certain qualities of manliness, such as courage, tenacity, resiliency, the work ethic, sound morals, and independence of mind. Attributes such as a good education were crucial.[24] Fathers might steer their sons in a certain direction, as Charles encouraged King to follow him and his father before him into the clergy. But with the declining authority of fathers and greater scope for individual choice in the modern marketplace of occupations, the likelihood of sons complying with fathers was in decline.[25]

Father–son relationships are not static; rather, they change as the father ages and the son grows and matures. Looking at one relationship over a thirty-year period allows us to see how it developed over respective life courses.[26] Transitions in a son's life, such as going away to school, choosing a career path, getting married, and having children focus the father–son relationship in particularly strong ways, and often challenge the relationship and modify its character. Indeed, Charles and King Gordon had a serious difference of opinion over King's career path, specifically as to whether King would remain within the clergy. At no time did the irony of modern fatherhood hit Charles Gordon harder. This dispute, however, did not dissolve the strong and intimate ties of affection and devotion between Charles and King. Similarly, transitions in a father's life from active breadwinner, to retired man, to becoming invalid or dying have a significant impact.

These relationships, although intensely personal and private, were not only matters of the domestic sphere. The questions that caused some difference or dispute between Charles and his son, of the sort Charles had faced with his father, related to their religion. The bewildering religious and cultural upheaval between the mid-Victorian age and the mid-twentieth century meant that there was reaction, rebellion, and ultimately adjustment from one generation to the next. In the sometimes difficult and strained relations between father and son, society's moral, religious, intellectual, and cultural changes were most acutely, and sometimes agonizingly, expressed and realized.

### Charles and His Father

Charles Gordon's 'Ralph Connor' novels offer few clues or insights into his attitudes to or understanding of fatherhood. Fathers are either absent or are shadowy figures in his stories. The exceptions are his

Glengarry books, which were published shortly after King was born. Perhaps the occasion of beginning his own family prompted Charles to reflect on his own childhood and the new phase of life he was embarking upon. In *The Man from Glengarry* (1901) and *Glengarry School Days* (1902) the father-figure appears as a stereotypical Victorian patriarch who is distant, stern, and quick to discipline or admonish family members. In *The Man from Glengarry*, the father-figure was described in terms very similar to Charles's own father, the Reverend Donald Gordon: 'He had coalblack hair and beard, and flashing blue eyes that held people in utter subjection and put the fear of death upon evildoers in the gallery. In every movement, tone, and glance there breathed imperial command' (128). In *Glengarry School Days* a 'stern and stubborn autocrat,' whose demeanour changed only when he led the family prayer, ruled the manse (85). The dominant impression of the fictional Reverend Donald Finch was of a community leader and father who strenuously believed in upholding the patriarchal order. Upon hearing of the mischievous activities of some boys, he 'thought it fit' during his Sunday sermon 'to dwell upon the tendency of the rising generation to revolt against authority in all things, and solemnly laid upon parents the duty and responsibility of seeing to it that they ruled their households well' (116). In these Connor stories the fathers were worthy of respect but not affection or intimacy, as those more tender feelings were reserved for the mothers.[27]

These fictional fathers happen to be ministers, and the depiction of their religious temperament reflects that of Gordon's own father. The Reverend Murray is deeply entrenched in the evangelism of the mid-nineteenth century, as was the Reverend Donald Gordon. His sermons were long and 'passionate denunciations' of immoral conduct, improper thinking, or lax religious devotion. In Connor's account of the Glengarry revival, the preaching of Hughie's father contrasted sharply with that of the visiting professor of theology, whose appeal to the congregation was characterized by 'quiet persistence.' By contrast, the Reverend Murray 'broke forth into a loud cry,' condemning members of the congregation for their inability to control and discipline their children. With ever more intense passion, he cried out: 'Woe unto you! Woe unto you! Your house is left unto you desolate, O lamb of God, have mercy upon us! O Christ with thy pierced hands, save us!' Noticing that his congregation was not moved, the Reverend Murray warned, in starker terms, that they would 'be cursed into everlasting fire' (256–7). Connor fictional fathers were depicted as stern disciplinary figures, and in their role as ministers of the gospel they delivered a message of a harsh, demanding, and judgmental God. In the Connor Glengarry novels, the father – not the mother – created and imposed the rigid atmosphere of religious piety.

The point of this digression into Connor fiction is to suggest that Charles Gordon chose to represent his differences with his father in fiction. We do not know if Charles and his father ever had an open conflict over religious questions. But Charles's formative years were in the late nineteenth century, when a range of social and intellectual challenges were confronting the church and compelling clergy to reconsider their religious beliefs and, more specifically, the nature of their ministry. While Donald Gordon remained rooted in the evangelical certainties of the mid-nineteenth century, Charles preached a social gospel of practical Christianity.[28] Connor novels, which were essentially sermons dressed up in fictional garb, were a modern and entertaining way to reach people with the modern Christian message, shorn of doctrine and emphasizing God's love and forgiveness as opposed to punishment. Despite their differing religious values and temperament, both Charles and his father were both fundamentally preoccupied with preaching the Christian gospel as effectively as possible.

This generational divide between father and son did not result in a breakdown in their relationship. The underlying respect that had developed between them endured. Indeed, Donald Gordon spent the last seven years of his life, while in failing health with bronchial asthma, living with Charles and his family in Winnipeg. During these years Charles recalled the nature of his father's ministry and dogmatic religious faith. One incident, in particular, stuck with him. A leader of the Plymouth Brethren had planned to hold a meeting in Donald Gordon's Glengarry parish. Charles remembered that a large crowd gathered, including his father. At the beginning of the meeting, Brethren tracts were distributed to everyone. After reading it, Donald Gordon tore it up, threw it on the floor, and, according to Charles's recollection, pronounced the tract to be 'not worth saving.' Then he challenged the Brethren leader's authority and ultimately took charge of the meeting by proclaiming its purpose was to worship God. Defying anyone to halt his activities, the Reverend Gordon led the meeting in singing Psalm 100: 'Make a joyful noise to the Lord.' Charles concluded this account on a note of sympathy with his father's position. 'The Brethren gathered up his tracts and left before he began preaching and was heard of no more.'[29] This incident was hardly in concert with Charles's more liberal and tolerant spirit. But it is significant that he chose to recall this incident as an example of what made his father a memorable and admirable figure. Charles's memory of his father remained one of a demanding, stern, judgmental, and even bad-tempered figure. In Charles's mind, he remained a figure of authority and power. Indeed, upon his father's death in 1912, Charles recalled that his father was an old-school minister of the Presbyterian Church. He was a 'fervent and passionate preacher, who expected his word to be law and to rule with an iron rod' with respect to moral questions.[30] In the obituary Charles admiringly concluded that the Reverend Donald Gordon 'in his best days possessed to a remarkable degree the qualities of a great preacher – a passionate enthusiasm, a vivid imagination, and an intense and fervid faith ... He is the last of a band of great preachers.'[31] By 1912 Charles's professional accomplishments in the ministry and the Presbyterian Church had exceeded those of his father, but nevertheless his father still loomed as a powerful and influential presence. Charles still felt that he had to live up to his father's example.[32]

This background on Charles's relationship with his father is significant, for we will see that the tension between the two over religion was repeated in the next generation as Charles also clashed with his son, King, over religion. But a generation later the outcome of the conflict was very different.

### Charles and King Gordon, 1900–1916

Charles Gordon was married in 1899 after a long and difficult courtship with Helen King. Her father, the Reverend John Mark King, had opposed their marriage and did not relent until he was on his deathbed. Children arrived almost immediately after their marriage. We are not privy to any discussions between the newly married couple with respect to family planning, but their haste in having children may have reflected Charles's forty years of age. Financial resources were not a problem. Not only was Charles earning a comfortable salary as minister of the flourishing St Stephen's Presbyterian Church in Winnipeg, but also the royalties from his first two books, *Black Rock* and *The Sky Pilot*, were amounting to thousands of dollars, a sum, in itself, greater than many middle-class incomes of that time. By 1914 Charles and Helen had a large family of six children. Their first-born, King, was their only son, and his birth was followed by those of his sisters Marjorie, Greta, Mary, Ruth, Lois, and Allison.

We first catch a glimpse of Charles Gordon with King through the eyes of journalists who visited the Gordon household/manse in Winnipeg to interview the famous author of the Ralph Connor books. *The Presbyterian* published an account of the interview with the 'father of the Sky Pilot' in its 24 April 1902 issue. Accompanying the article of the Reverend C.W. Gordon was a picture of Gordon holding his infant son on his knee. The photograph leaves the impression of a proud and affectionate father. Another journalist who visited the Gordon home observed, 'Ralph Connor at home playing with his baby boy is altogether normal, natural and lovable.'[33]

Charles was likely more involved or engaged in the domestic sphere and family matters than many men of his generation. His work did not remove him from the home on a daily or regular basis. He was not required to be in the office, factory, or shop following the rigours of the industrial clock. As a professional man, he enjoyed more freedom and mobility. As Margaret Marsh's work has indicated, the masculine culture of domesticity was most developed in the professional and business classes of the modern suburb.[34] For Charles, the manse and family home were at the centre of a great deal of his ministerial activity. He held meetings in his home and frequently worked at his sermons and his novels in his study. During his rounds of pastoral activity, he returned home whenever he could.[35] One of King's fondest memories was riding the sleigh or carriage with his father as he visited members of his congregation. His father's horse was one of the fastest in Winnipeg, King recalled in later life, and therefore these trips, especially on the sleigh in winter underneath mounds of blankets, were real adventures for the young boy.[36]

Charles's professional responsibilities with the Presbyterian Church, which included attending General Assembly meetings and participating on missionary tours throughout the North West, however, took him away from the family home. His numerous public appearances as 'Ralph Connor' to promote his string of best-selling novels also led to frequent departures from the family hearth. Sometimes his absence was extensive. For example, in 1908 he participated in a one-month evangelical crusade with the Chapman-Alexander revival team in Philadelphia, and in 1909 he spent over a month in the coalfields of Alberta and British Columbia attempting to settle a strike that was crippling the coal industry. During the early years of the First World War, he served as chaplain overseas, and toured the United States in 1917 to drum up support for the American entrance into the war.

These absences did not mean that Charles was a distant father removed from the daily life and intimate matters of his family. On the contrary, Charles's letters to King during his prolonged absences were not merely substitutes for his absence from the home, but reminders or continuations of the close relationship that existed at home. The first extant letter from Charles to King was sent in 1908, when King was eight years old. The major theme that dominated Charles's correspondence with his young son was the responsibility that fell to him as the only 'man' in the household during his father's absence. There was no doubt in Charles's mind that males had an important role as the head of the household. The welfare of the family depended not only on the breadwinning skills of the males but also on their willingness to be helpful and loving.

In April 1908, when he was in Philadelphia as part of the Chapman-Alexander evangelical crusade, Charles wrote a letter to King that was full of affection and play and some specific instructions about what King should be doing. To begin with, Charles thanked King for the letter from 'a little boy with blue eyes & short hair.& strong as a little bull,' because it relieved him of his 'terrible loneliness.' Then King was instructed to stop reading the letter and ask his mother to give him 'a hug and a kiss for me.' After that he was supposed to find his sisters and give them a hug and a kiss, and then go and 'kiss the wee sweet tiny baby if she is not asleep' for Daddy. Only after King had extended his father's affections to his sisters could he continue to read the letter, which offered advice about how to live a Christian life. 'Now laddie be a good boy – Care for your mother – Don't think of yourself alone – Jesus thought of other people. Good-bye little man. God bless you and keep you with love.'[37]

As King grew older, Charles's expressions of affection were muted, while mentoring took on a more prominent role. In particular, Charles asked King to report on his schoolwork and encouraged him to do well. Charles continually reminded King that during his absence, King would have to assume the role of the man of the house.[38] He emphasized, 'It will be a little harder for you while I am away. You will have some more responsibility and care for the girls and especially your dear mother. For your mother, I know you will act in my place. Be kind and be thoughtful of her wishes. She has a lot to think of and a lot to worry her.'[39] Writing from New York in 1913, he assured King: 'I know you are trying to do your best to take my place in the family. As you grow up I shall feel … more safe because I know you will grow in your ability to take care of those we both love so much.'[40] Like many other middle-class fathers concerned with respectability, Charles appealed to duty and to religion as a way to establish his paternal authority. In these letters to the youthful King, Charles showed a paternal desire to shape his son's character by inculcating the correct moral and religious values as well as a strong work ethic and a desire for success. In having King attend to his mother and his siblings, Charles was teaching him the virtues of kindness, being affectionate, and putting family first, all necessary qualities in being a man and especially a father.[41] Clearly, Charles was inculcating a strong sense of appropriate gender roles and Christian paternalism in his young son.

King's burden of assuming the role of head of the household and caring for the family became greater when the First World War broke out. Charles volunteered to serve as chaplain to the 79th Cameron Highlanders of Canada, a battalion based largely in Winnipeg. He sailed overseas in May 1915, and the ominous prospect of involvement in the bloody struggle moved Charles to write one of his most senti-mental yet serious letters to King. Of course, Charles never broached the prospect of death, but it seemed to haunt him on his journey. His first wartime letter to King was a retrospective look at their relation-ship and a reiteration of what Charles expected of him. The necessity of assuming the role of the man of the house and being a strong and upright Christian was reinforced throughout the letter.

> You were our first baby dear King and you have your own place in my heart. I want you to know that you have been a great joy to me. You have never caused me a day's anxiety or sorrow. I have always been able to trust you fully and you have never disappointed me. I trust you to do right King boy, according to your conscience. I know you will try your best. You will doubtless make mistakes, but you will be true to your conscience that is God ... keep near in your heart to Jesus. He is closer than I am and he will keep you right. I trust dear mother to you King because I love you. This will mean a lot of self-denial boy – many times you will have to give up your own will & pleasure. Remember mother will need you – your help, your love. Show her your love. Now my boy my dear boy my only son God keep you & make you a good man and great in the service of God. You know I love you but you do not know how much. You will keep this letter always I know. God bless you – Daddy'[42]

In essence this letter passed the torch of familial responsibility to Gordon's son in the event that he did not return from the front. It also made it clear that being willing and able to make sacrifices was at the essence of manhood. Just as Charles and other fighting men were making sacrifices for their country, their sons had to be willing to make sacrifices and step into the breach at home.[43] Charles reminded King that his mother made real sacrifices in bringing him into the world. 'I remember well,' Charles wrote, 'the terrible night and day when she brought you into the world and a young girl she was, but what superb courage, cheer, & patience.'[44] In a later letter, he continued this theme of what dutiful and grateful sons should bestow on their mothers. 'I know children are very apt to forget, apt to be non-understanding. They never can understand the terrible burden and anxiety that mothers (and fathers too for that matter) carry for their children – and it is that burden that clouds the life's sunny sky, and drains the vitality from the heart.'[45]

During this period of heavy family responsibility, King had to consider what university he should attend. On this matter, Charles's advice was detailed and forceful. He wanted King to attend the University of Manitoba because it was small and he thought King would benefit from closer personal touch with professors. He would also be able to foster closer relations with his friends and establish a good foundation for public life in Manitoba, where Charles was hopeful that King would have his future.[46] This letter revealed Charles's apprehension about King's future; but his concern could not be divorced from his worries about his family. His advice about attending the University of Manitoba was designed to keep King close to home, whereby he could continue to look after the family. Charles's desire for his son's success, which meant going his own way in life, had to be balanced with his anxiety about keeping his family together and well cared for. Nevertheless, King's entrance into university marked an important new stage in their maturing relationship. Charles treated King more like a young adult and as someone he could discuss current events with. For example, Charles candidly revealed his underlying fears about the outcome of the war to King, something that he could not do in public because as a public figure he was an integral part of the wartime campaign for recruitment.[47]

After the war the demands on Charles Gordon's time were still significant. He was appointed chair of the Joint Council of Industry, which was created in the aftermath of the Winnipeg General Strike, by the Manitoba government. He was also elected moderator of the Presbyterian Church in Canada, just as the negotiations for church union with the Methodists and Congregationalists were resuming and the bitter controversy over the union within the Presbyterian Church was heating up again. Furthermore, Charles had not abandoned writing novels. In 1915 he had received news from his investment broker that a great deal of his money, proceeds from the best-selling novels, had been lost through the land bust of 1913. His falling fortunes meant that writing became imperative so that he could recuperate his losses. In a few short years, in 1925, he would be sixty-five and required to retire from the ministry. Moreover, his expenses were rising as his older children were entering college. The early 1920s was another period of frenetic activity in Charles's life. One of his colleagues wrote to King and remarked, 'Your father is leading his usual over-strenuous life. He has enjoyed his year as Moderator very much but it has been a very strenuous one and I think he is badly in need of a rest.' This candour about Charles's health suggests that family friends were beginning to look to King to keep an eye out for his father's welfare. Clearly, King was no longer viewed as a boy.

During this period, King went to Oxford University as a Rhodes scholar. Just before he left for England, his father took time away from his busy schedule to accompany King on a seven-day canoe trip on Lake of the Woods. The trip was for rest and recreation, but it also allowed father and son to enjoy some time together while canoeing, an activity they both enjoyed immensely. King's attendance at Oxford marked an important step into independent adult life. Still, Charles made sure that his son was taken care of. He wrote to one of his best friends in England, Sir Ernest Hodder-Williams, the English publisher of Ralph Connor books, introducing King and asking that he make sure his son did not suffer from homesickness. Like any proud father, Charles praised his son's accomplishments and attributes to his old friend. 'He has had rather a brilliant career here in his College and University days; he has taken the top honours in his class, and what I value equally with that, he was elected by his fellow-graduates to the position of Senior Stick.' With respect to King's future, Charles was more cautious and prudent. 'He is a quiet, modest chap, will make no very great splurge but I think he is thoroughly sound and all right.'[48]

Charles continued to offer advice. The pressure of his expectations and his anxieties were constantly below the surface of his letters to King. Like most fathers, Charles realized that it was a fiercely competitive world, and he understood that he had to prepare his son for that cold, stark reality. He tried to keep his letters to King upbeat and positive in tone, but at times they boiled over in outbursts of real concern. On matters of curriculum, he advised King against a traditional 'purely classical course,' as he had taken at University College in the early 1880s, because it would not be 'especially useful for you.' He realized that a modern education in the social sciences would be better preparation for King to compete in the modern world. Charles dispensed more advice about athletics and the necessity of physical exercise. 'Rugger would bring you into competition with men who have specialized all their lives in the game – and besides the need for men in that game is not so great. The boats are very specifically Oxford and would be a great experience. After all what you want is exercise, fun, experience. A star place in athletics would cost more time & energy.'[49] King took up rowing and gleefully reported his times to his father. Charles was thrilled with these results and hoped that King would compete successfully for the Oxford's College 8; but he realized that the competition for that lofty honour was very stiff. Beyond athletics, Charles also approved of King's activities in the Debating Union and the Bach Society. As Charles explained, these activities were particularly valuable because they offered opportunities 'for getting to know men & learning to carry yourself with men.' These intellectual, cultural, and physical activities were character building, in Charles's estimation, and they would prepare King for his purpose in life as much as the classroom. He was most concerned about whether there was any College Christian Organization, where King could carry out some 'definite Christian work.'[50] To be sure that the spirit of God guided King, Charles always asked after his spiritual welfare and attempted to guide him in daily devotions. 'My reading at night,' he closed one letter, 'is still the 121 Psalm. What is yours my boy. Shall I draw up a little schedule so that we can read together?'[51] Charles's selection of 'I lift up mine eyes unto the hills, from whence cometh my help / My help cometh from the LORD,' brought to King's attention, a psalm celebrating God's abiding presence and guidance, was probably not a matter of happenstance. He wanted to be sure that King had remained rooted in the Christian faith.

**The Ministry**

As King's studies at Oxford were nearing their conclusion, Charles discussed matters of his son's future more frankly. The prospect of King following family tradition and becoming a clergyman was at the forefront of Charles's mind. Many of his letters during this period were full of detailed news about church union. But most important, in one letter to his son, Charles explained his approach to the ministry and preaching, and in doing so explained how his career as the fictional writer 'Ralph Connor' related to his ministry. In this letter he was more introspective and explicit than in any other forum in which he was required to comment on his writing. Charles revealed that he often came away with feelings of inadequacy, futility, and defeat in his early years as a preacher. These painful experiences taught him crucial lessons about the ministry, and he thought it was prudent to pass these insights on to King at this moment.

> We are slow to learn that we are dealing mostly with untrained though often acute minds and therefore that we must prepare our stuff accordingly. Our best & most logical line of reasoning is often quite unobserved, passed quite over the heads of our own people, and some little aside, some fool illustration as we imagine sticks, holds and does good. We should prepare as for children – concrete our teaching in illustrations, in story, incident, around personalities. The great preachers – for the most part – ... have this gift. And it can be celebrated & should be. It is humiliating of course, we want to present a line of argument but they want to hear stories. Then again and chiefly our failures teach us the one lesson the preacher will not learn except by a long & painful experience: 'not by might, not by power, but by spirit' we are there to pass on a message we have received that day for that people. That is the essential of great preaching ... And my dear King it is this that gives us the note of authority – and of love. After you have done your best in preparation, facts, organization, and illustration then wait for the life & power that comes from Him whose witness you are ... Try out this on the parables and bring the Parables up to date in 20th century Canadian dross – what I mean – get the pictures vividly true to its own historic setting then make it of today.[52]

Hoping that King would decide to enter the ministry, Charles revealed one of the secrets to understanding not only his literary output but also to understanding his ministry.

In 1925 King began his ministry in the United Church just as Charles was retiring from St Stephen's. He was appointed to supply the church in the Willow River field, a missionary station servicing a backwoods lumbering community, located near Prince George, British Columbia, on the Canadian National Railway line. Immediately, King spearheaded an ambitious campaign to raise the funds for a permanent church building. Recognizing the challenge facing his son, Charles promised King that he would appeal to the people of the Church and Manse Building Fund on his behalf, and he also endeavoured to raise around two or three hundred dollars from friends.[53] In September, when Charles joined his son for the opening ceremonies of the new building, he witnessed the strong bond that had been formed between the young missionary and the community. He was struck by how King's early years in the ministry was startlingly similar to his own. 'It did me a lot of good, I assure you. It revived in my heart some of the tenderest memories that I have. There is no affection like that which is engendered in a common work for our Lord and Master. The missionary gets very little, but in that payment of the heart and spirit he is more than rewarded for the very best and finest service he can render.' The difficulties King faced in this frontier mission field were a haunting reminder to Charles that the problem of securing men and resources for the west was still hindering the work of the church.[54] Charles's trip to King's mission field was a particularly satisfying moment because it seemed that King had absorbed all of his mentoring about Christian values and a suitable career to fulfil a Christian calling.

This period of intense closeness quickly ended when King moved to his next mission station. Between 1926 and 1930, King was stationed at Pine Falls, a company mill town located on the Winnipeg River and adjacent to a Canadian Northern Railway branch line.[55] King struggled with his role as a minister in this company town. He worried about whether he had any positive influence in a community where Abitibi Power and Paper was the dominant force in all aspects of life.[56] Again Charles intervened and provided his struggling son with insights into the difficulties of the ministry. He reminded King that 'uncertainty and dissatisfaction is a natural reaction' during the clergyman's quest to make the 'spiritual and the unseen' real and vital. Charles explained that an effective clergyman would frequently be frustrated. He confessed to King that he often felt 'humiliated and ashamed when thinking of my poverty of spiritual life & power.'[57] In revealing this, Charles was reassuring his inexperienced son that feelings of inadequacy were natural for any clergyman attempting to assert spiritual influence.

Charles's professional mentoring, however, did not alleviate King's doubts. Conflict emerged when King considered leaving Pine Falls and abandoning the ministry. Charles, uncharacteristically, sounded a note of real disappointment. 'The thing that disturbs me most,' he dejectedly wrote, 'is that you seem to doubt whether you are in your

right vocation. How serious that doubt may be I can't judge.' He was
hopeful that King's troubles were a passing phase; and so he tried to
discourage his son from taking any rash action. Charles was torn terribly by King's dilemma. On the one hand, he thought that if King continued in the ministry, then his calling would be reaffirmed. On the
other hand, he recognized that the 'status quo' might become 'impossible.' In a moment when Charles seemed to be losing faith in his son,
he linked abandoning the ministry with cutting ties with both God
and himself.

> Dear boy, your coming into my home taught me more about the heavenly
> Father than all I had known before. That terrible night it was uncertain
> whether you would come to us alive. By my own heart I learned what a
> *Father* meant. And my dear boy our fellowship together has made me
> understand God better. I know a father's desire to help, eagerness to help
> – I know about love. So I am not afraid for you King boy. I would keep
> you with every power I have and so I know the Heavenly Father thinks
> about you. He will show you the way. He will give you the wisdom,
> strength, courage you need to take the way. He knows & he will show
> you. Keep your heart open to Him. He will not fail you.[58]

Like so many devout men of his generation, Charles could not separate the idea of fatherhood from concepts of divine love and caring. He
made a direct link between his relation to King and his understanding
of God. In a sense, during this time of real stress, he seemed to be
reverting to the older patriarchal attitude and style of his father's generation. There was a crucial difference, however. Charles's correlation
of fatherhood with the divine was not defined in the harsh, stern punishing terms of the Victorians. Instead, it was an association of love and
compassion. Still, as Charles sensed King pulling away from his guidance and the Christian ministry, he tried to assert his own will by making reference to divine providence. Differing views about career choice
were igniting a real dispute.

Contrary to his father's expressed wishes, King left the ministry for a
chair in Christian ethics at United Theological College at McGill University in 1931. Charles could not hide his disappointment and warned
King that he had undertaken a particularly challenging task, one much
more difficult than the clergy with its responsibilities of the weekly sermon, worship services, and pastoral work. 'No class of workers,'
Charles informed King, 'gets so much criticism and none so little thanks

and sympathy as the average Professor of Theology. My boy, my boy you will have your share. On the other hand there are rich and great rewards to the real leader of youth in the Church. Looking back over my life's experience my mind rests on very few great leaders in our Colleges.' He could only think of two: Principal Grant of Queen's University and King's grandfather, John Mark King of the University of Manitoba. More significantly, Charles wrote at length about the perils of academic life for true Christian service. In what proved to be a prophetic insight, Charles suggested to King that a chair in a college of the church might be his undoing. A chair could be a 'curse,' he warned in a somewhat humorous fashion, for it was a sedentary job rather than an activist one. 'This is no day for sitters – and at length when he moves the chair sticks to his buttocks. What a sight for the angels – a leader with a chair clinging to him. For God's sake & your work's sake avoid the *Chair*. The academic mind is the disease, which has paralyzed our College men. They so soon get out of touch with life – with men and things – the man who gets out of touch with men gets out of touch with God. For God's dwelling is with men.'[59] King did not completely rebel against his father, for in his mind he had not abandoned a life of Christian service, just the ministry. Clearly he was asserting his own will, establishing an independent identity, and following his own path.

King's new position was soon jeopardized by budgetary problems as the United Theological College and McGill University dealt with the declining revenues brought by the Great Depression. The broad outline of the dismissal of King Gordon from the chair in Christian ethics is well known.[60] Charles's attempt to intervene on King's behalf and his advice regarding the church hierarchy has not been taken into account. When Charles first got the disturbing news that there was 'trouble ahead' for King, he counselled 'equanimity,' especially if the reason for his dismissal was indeed institutional poverty.[61] He advised King to be 'steadfast in your resolve to teach and preach those principles and ethics that you hold to be consistent with the mind of Christ.' According to Charles, King had been thrust into a position of leadership in the battle for 'the right of free speech, the supreme authority of conscience, and the central importance of Christian ethics in all matters affecting the life and work of people.'[62] Charles, however, was frustrated, for he felt that he was left on the sidelines of this great battle. The fact that he had warned his son against taking the chair in Christian ethics was beside the point. The bond of loyalty and deep respect between the two men came to the fore as King was facing this most difficult test of his professional life, and especially his dedication to Christianity. Charles clearly realized that even though he and King had a major disagreement over King's flight from the ministry, they were interested in the same objectives. The difference between father and son was not profound; it was a matter of whether it was necessary to be within the church and ministry to bring about a Christian social order.

King's many friends and those sympathetic to his cause raised sufficient funds to pay his salary, so that he could continue teaching at United Theological College. But the board of governors ultimately decided to terminate the position, essentially firing King. In reflecting on this controversy, some forty years later, King Gordon concluded: 'I doubt if you will be able to get *proof* that the elimination of the chair of Christian Ethics was on account of the political views of its occupant.'[63] At the time, however, Charles was furious and convinced that his son had been fired for his defence of the impoverished, exploited, and powerless in society. For him, the 'true meaning' of the dismissal 'lies deep in the bowels of a treacherous & unscrupulous & disturbed world order represented by a group of worldly minded capitalists.' The whole affair reminded Charles of the battles he had had with the liquor interests in Manitoba some twenty-five years earlier. Despite his anger, Charles realized that it was best for him to work behind the scenes and not to go into print voicing his protest. In private, however he was candid. His son's difficulties began, he insisted, when he championed the cause of the disadvantaged, whether it was the elevator man at McGill who was poorly paid, Montreal's milkmen who worked overly long hours, or the consumers of Montreal who paid too high prices for coal that were set by a local combine of trade. It was not surprising, Charles asserted, that when the United Theological College was ordered to reduce its staff by one that King was selected as the sacrificial lamb. The real cause of King's dismissal, Charles concluded, was his clear articulation of Christian ethics.[64]

Charles, however, did not concede to King on the matter of the church's central role in bringing about a Christian society. The Great Depression had radicalized King and made him an activist in politics. He joined the C.C.F. The more restrained Charles again cautioned King by suggesting that he limit his activism to the League for Social Reconstruction and the Fellowship for a Christian Social Order. 'The political organization that will lead the country on the high road of sound ethical & social thinking may not be the C.C.F. at all,' he warned King. In Charles's estimation it was not a political party that would be the source of social and ethical reconstruction in Canada but the Christian church.[65] On this question of politics, we see that Charles's influence had clearly waned. Charles had implored King not to get directly involved in politics and especially the C.C.F., but in the 1935 federal election, King ran and lost as a C.C.F. candidate in Victoria, BC.[66] As King was becoming more independent and self-confident, despite the setbacks in his career, Charles's role in his life and ability to influence him was in decline and becoming marginal.

### Memory

By the later stages of Charles's life his relationship with King had gone full circle. Instead of Charles dispensing advice and guidance to King, the opposite began to take place. Indeed, the publication of Charles's final book, an autobiography entitled *Postscript to Adventure*, hinged on King's intervention. Charles's health had been failing for two or three years. At Birkencraig, in late August of 1937, just as he had finished the draft of his manuscript, another cold settled in his kidneys, sending him to bed. When he returned to Winnipeg in September he was hospitalized and the doctors decided to operate on his bowel to prevent further congestion of his kidneys. The operation took place on 16 October, just after Charles had sent the completed manuscript of his memoirs to the publisher. While Charles was recuperating after the surgery, King rushed from New York to see him. When King arrived in Toronto en route to Winnipeg, two letters were waiting for him from his father's publishers. King found the time to see John McClelland about the urgent matter of the manuscript, which needed some revision. No one wanted to disturb Charles with the task, for they understood that he was gravely ill. King agreed to read it, and realized 'that a failure to have the book come out now after months of high pressure work would be a great blow to my father besides causing more financial worry which our family has not been free from for a number of years.'[67] As a result, King settled down with the manuscript for the train journey from Toronto around Lake Superior to Winnipeg.

For the most part, King was immensely impressed with the manuscript. It was classic Ralph Connor. As King observed, his father was 'blessed with an extraordinary imagination, or sharpness of observation which leaves tremendously deep and vivid impressions.' While reading the manuscript King was struck by the prevailing characteristics of his father's personality. His irrepressible love of adventure, romantic bent, courage and enthusiasm, and his terrific faith in humanity comes clearly through the many adventures he recounts in the memoir. His father's idealism, King observed while reflecting on the memoirs, 'is rooted in a deeper faith in God – pretty simple and untheological although he knows all that side of it – it has made him attempt the darndest fool things and in a surprising number of cases get away with it. What has kept him young and singularly attractive is a certain gaiety. He will never be remembered as just an 'earnest man,' although never very far away from some 'cause' that is commanding his whole allegiance.'[68] Such keen observations reflect the strong bonds between father and son and the real affection and understanding King had for his father. King turned what in other hands could have been sharp criticism of Charles Gordon's character into charming attributes.

But the memoir also exposed the weakness of the Ralph Connor style. In King's estimation, it was much like the Connor novels, 'like a Breugel landscape, filled with figures and incidents, a discernible pattern, but lacking in the mature depth and perspective which would have been there if the thing had not been written – as all my father's fiction has been written – under extreme pressure.' King's admiration for his father was not above some perceptive criticisms of his writing and ministry. More specifically, King thought that there were two basic things wrong with the manuscript that had to be corrected before it went to press. While acknowledging that he had not realized what an enduring impression the First World War had made upon his father, he thought that the war years received too much attention. Second, and more seriously, too much 'hasty writing' marred the manuscript. 'Sections would have been vastly improved with more time and care. At times the emotional overtones are much too high. Like all highlanders my father's emotional drives are never far beneath the surface.' These first impressions were reinforced on the second day of King's train journey. He concluded that the early sections up to the war were fine, but the later sections needed to be edited and in places rewritten. He hoped his father would rally and be well enough to revise these sections, but he had an ominous 'feeling of a final act.'[69]

Charles rallied briefly but this was short-lived. He died on 31 October 1937. As a result, King had to get the memoirs ready for publication. He worked mostly on those later chapters dealing with post-war world. According to King's rendering, the outstanding aspect of Charles's post-war life was his dedication to the cause of world peace. Three of the final five chapters constituting the final section of *Postscript to Adventure* were about international affairs and the quest for peace. Another chapter concerned Charles's activities with the Council of Industry and his ideas about industrial arbitration. This emphasis on international arbitration and world peace reflected King's growing interest in these matters and, of course, the pressing issues facing everyone as the world was lurching dangerously towards another war. By emphasizing those aspects of Charles's later life that were most important and meaningful to himself, King was, in a sense, bringing his deceased father closer to him. Perhaps King's revision to his father's memoirs was a form of reconciliation – albeit entirely on King's terms. It is significant, however, that King chose not to write extensively on Charles's term as moderator of the Presbyterian Church or his involvement in the church-union controversy that led to the formation of the United Church of Canada. Nevertheless, King had brought the manuscript to fruition so that his father's memory could be preserved.

Of course, a son's determination to shape or protect the memory of his father never ceases. Many years after Charles's death, scholars began to show interest in his life and work. In 1971 Michael Bliss decided to reprint Ralph Connor's *The Foreigner* (1909), a story about immigrant life in North End Winnipeg, in his Social History of Canada series. This series was dedicated to reprinting important texts from Canada's past that had significance for the bourgeoning field of Canadian social history. Ed Rae, of the University of Manitoba, was contracted to write a scholarly introduction. The University of Toronto Press also contacted King Gordon about copyright, and in response King requested 'that in fairness to myself and my sisters, whom I represent as executor for my father's estate, that I should have the opportunity of seeing the introduction in case there are unavoidable inaccuracies of fact and interpretation.'[70] The Press complied with King's request, but when he received Rae's introduction serious difficulties ensued. King found the introduction to be unsatisfactory, for it gave 'a distorted interpretation of [the] book's meaning' and presented an 'untrue picture of [the] social involvement and social philosophy of Gordon.'[71] King's telegram was followed by what amounted to a long sixteen-page long rebuttal or counter-introduction. He asserted that Rae's depiction of Charles W. Gordon as having an 'imperialist, middle class, Anglo-Saxon approach to social problems in the West was ludicrous.' In subsequent, equally detailed correspondence, he outlined his objection to Rae's interpretation that *The Foreigner* was an explication of a 'nativist philosophy rooted in Ontario, Anglo-Saxon, non-conformist ethic, determined to Canadianize the west by pressing the foreigner into its own mold.'[72] On the contrary, King argued, Charles Gordon was a progressive social-gospel minister who championed the interests of the working class and was sensitive to the challenges facing the immigrant people of North End Winnipeg. If anything, King asserted, *The Foreigner* was a celebration of the diversity of cultures that the immigrant brought to Canada.[73] He was also certain that 'Gordon's reputation will certainly withstand Rae's biased attack.'

Things were at an impasse, and King showed little inclination to allow Rae's scholarly introduction to stand uncontested. Despite Michael Bliss's attempts to mediate this dispute by writing a general editor's introduction that outlined the dispute between King and Rae, King was uncompromising in protecting his father's reputation.[74] In the end, *The Foreigner* was not published in the Social History of Canada series. It is clear from this controversy that King was still very much caught up in the idealism of his father's Christian activism. He could not accept the cooler assessment of contemporary scholarship that recognized the limits of Charles Gordon's social-gospel activism or any criticism of his best-selling fiction. What, perhaps, was not known by these adversaries is that *The Foreigner* caused equally intense and irresolvable controversy when it was first published in 1909. While many critics found it to be another typically stirring 'Ralph Connor' story that accurately depicted conditions the West, and especially the challenge of 'Canadianizing' and 'Christianizing' foreign immigrants, others were deeply upset by the book.[75] Charles Gordon received some uncharacteristically bitter criticisms of it. For example, W.H. Riddell, editor of the *Montreal Weekly Star*, was scandalized by the book, charging that it 'shamefully libeled' the Galician people and was 'full of mean and contemptible untruths about' Catholicism.[76] In the pages of the *Winnipeg Free Press* the merits of the novel and particularly its depiction of the Ukrainian community and of the Catholic Church were debated.[77]

## Conclusion

Charles's relationship with both his father, Donald, and his son, King, reflected broader social and intellectual trends. In one family of minis-ters over three generations there existed the struggle between the reli-gious certainty of the mid-Victorian evangelicals and the more liberal understanding of Christianity that characterized the social-gospel generation of the early twentieth century, and finally, a more rebellious desire to pursue Christian goals for society outside the confines of the church during the more secular mid-twentieth century. For Charles Gordon, doctrine was never as important as Christian action or making sure that a liberalized Christian message, shorn of references to sin and a punishing God and the necessity of conversion, was heard throughout society. As a result, Charles was compelled to move outside the pulpit and use the secular media of the novel to make sure his gospel message was received. He remained, however, deeply committed to the church and was a fierce advocate of church union as a means to strengthen the church's presence and apply the teachings of the social gospel effectively. For King, however, remaining within the church was not necessary. He concluded that he could leave the ministry and still carry out Christ's message and mission. Circumstances had changed for King. A range of professional opportunities existed for him that did not exist for his father or grandfather. From one generation to the next, one can detect greater scope for the secular over the religious or sacred.

These tensions among the Gordon men over religious calling or vocation did not fracture the bonds of family. King's rejection of the ministry and defiance of his father's counsel was part of a quest for acceptable boundaries, norms, and options. Unquestionably, King was breaking away from family tradition by insisting that he could serve the Christian gospel outside the ministry and the church. He was asserting his independence and at the same time downplaying his rebelliousness by reasserting links to the family's tradition and religious values. Whether this was a means to assuage his feelings of guilt and remorse or whether he could not resist the powerful family teaching and values cannot be known. What is clear is that family disputes – often between father and son – embodied larger cultural issues. Clearly, the strained relations within families were a fertile ground for the most agonizing expression of moral, cultural, religious, or intellectual change.[78] Often during intense personal conflict between father and son, new values, norms, and roles were worked out. In the case of the Gordon family, and especially in relation to King, we see that the move outside the church was accomplished after much distress and in the most halting and hesitant manner. Still, King's dedication to Christian ideals remained intact. As Stephen Mintz has observed, 'The pattern of family conflict can be viewed as an instrument for maintaining cultural continuity while permitting important modifications and adaptations.'[79] It is through family relations, then, and especially inter-generational conflict, that we can observe how the process of secularization, specifically withdrawing from the church, proceeds – not necessarily in an obvious public way but with a great sense of regret and anguish in the quiet and private confines of family negotiation. Shaking the roots of family tradition, especially religion, and the bonds of family values is exceedingly difficult. Moreover, the story of Charles and King Gordon demonstrates that serious tension over momentous questions and the most treasured family values could not shake the deeper, intimate bonds of affection and the father–son loyalty that tie a family together. For Charles Gordon the bond between father and son was virtually unbreakable. Near the end of his life, while reflecting on the importance of Birkencraig, he wrote, 'No man can keep a boy's heart in him who does not have a boy somewhere in his life. No boy can become the man he wishes to be who does not at critical and desperate moments have a man's hand to clutch and hold to.'[80]

NOTES

1 Library and Archives Canada, MG 30, C241, King Gordon Papers [hereafter KG], vol. 89, file 25, 'Daddy to My Dear Boy,' 11 October 1922.
2 The term 'masculine domesticity' was coined by Margaret Marsh in 'Suburban Men and Masculine Domesticity, 1870–1915,' *American Quarterly* 40, 2 (June 1988), 165–86.
3 These figures are calculated from the numerous royalty reports in University of Manitoba, Archives and Special Collections, MSS 56, Charles W. Gordon Papers [hereafter CWG], boxes 31 and 32.
4 This literature is extensive. See Gail Bederman, *Manliness and Civilization: A Cultural History of Gender and Race in the United States, 1880–1917* (Chicago: University of Chicago Press, 1995); J.A. Mangan and James Walvin, eds, *Manliness and Morality: Middle Class Masculinity in Britain and America, 1800–1940* (New York: St Martin's Press, 1987); Michael Roper and John Tosh, eds, *Manful Assertions: Masculinities in Britain since 1800* (London: Routledge, 1991); and Clifford Putney, *Muscular Christianity: Manhood and Sports in Protestant America, 1880–1920* (Cambridge, MA: Harvard University Press, 2001). For Canada, see Michael Moss, *Manliness and Militarism: Educating Young Boys in Ontario for War* (Toronto: Oxford University Press, 2001).
5 Mark Kimmel, *Manhood in America: A Cultural History* (New York: Free Press, 1995). Fuller discussion of this aspect of Roosevelt's cultural significance are

in Bederman, *Manliness and Civilization*, 170–215 and Sarah Watts, *Rough Rider in the White House: Theodore Roosevelt and the Politics of Desire* (Chicago: University of Chicago Press, 2003).

6  CWG, box 3, fd. 4, Theodore Roosevelt to Gordon, 21 June 1906, regarding *The Prospector*, and box 5, fd. 7, Theodore Roosevelt to Gordon, 4 January 1915, regarding *The Patrol of the Sun Dance Trail*.

7  Daniel Coleman, *White Civility: The Literary Project of English Canada* (Toronto: University of Toronto Press, 2006); Clarence Karr, *Authors and Audiences: Popular Canadian Fiction in the Early Twentieth Century* (Montreal, Kingston: McGill-Queen's University Press, 2000); Keith Walden, *Visions of Order: The Canadian Mountie in Symbol and Myth* (Toronto: Butterworths, 1982); and Moss, *Manliness and Militarism*, 82–3.

8  On the relationship between the social gospel and the cult of masculinity, see Susan Curtis, 'The Son of Man and God the Father: The Social Gospel and Victorian Masculinity,' in Mark Carnes and Clyde Griffen, eds, *Meanings for Manhood: Construction of Masculinity in Victorian America* (Chicago: University of Chicago Press, 1990), 67–78.

9  'The flight from domesticity,' a late-nineteenth-century rebellion against the confines of the home and family, has been most cogently argued by John Tosh in *A Man's Place: Masculinity and the Middle Class in Victorian England* (New Haven, London: Yale University Press, 1999), 170–94.

10  Similar arguments are implied in two recent studies of fatherhood in post-1945 Canada. See Robert Rutherdale, 'Fatherhood and Masculine Domesticity during the Baby Boom,' in Lori Chambers and E. Montigny, eds, *Family Matters: Papers in Post-Confederation Family History* (Toronto: Scholar's Press, 1998), 309–33 and 'Fatherhood, Masculinity, and the Good Life during Canada's Baby Boom, 1945–1965,' *Journal of Family History* 24, 3 (July 1999): 351–73. Chris Dummit, 'Finding a Place for Father: Selling the Barbecue in Postwar Canada,' *Journal of the Canadian Historical Association*, new ser., 9 (1998): 209–23.

11  This image is employed by John R. Gillis in the opening sentence of his discussion on fatherhood. 'Fathers occupy a very modest place in our symbolic universe – always at the threshold of family life, never at its center.' See Gillis, *A World of Their Own Making: Myth, Ritual and the Quest for Family Values* (New York: HarperCollins, 1996), 179.

12  This irony is also pointed out in Anthony Rotundo, *American Manhood: Transformations in Masculinity from the Revolution to the Modern Era* (New York: HarperCollins, 1993), 281–3.

13  Gillis, *A World of Their Own Making*, 179, 194.

14  CWG, box 30, fd. 1, 'The Crooked Tree,' long version, no date.

15  See Robert MacDonald, *Sons of Empire: The Frontier and the Boy Scout Movement, 1890–1918* (Toronto: University of Toronto Press, 1993).

16  Anthony Rotundo, 'Learning about Manhood: Gender Ideals and the Middle Class Family in Nineteenth Century America', in Mangan and Walvin, *Manliness and Morality*, 43.

17  The literature on fatherhood includes Stephen Frank, *Life with Father: Parenthood and Masculinity in the Nineteenth Century American North* (Baltimore, London: Johns Hopkins University Press, 1998); Shawn Johansen, *Family Men: Middle-Class Fatherhood in Early Industrializing America* (New York, London: Routledge, 2001); and Robert Griswold, *Fatherhood in America: A History* (New York: Basic Books, 1993). The historiography of fatherhood in Canada is still scanty. See note 10 above and Cynthia Comacchio, *The Infinite Bonds of Family: Domesticity in Canada, 1850–1940* (Toronto: University of Toronto Press, 1999).

18  John Tosh, *Manliness and Masculinities in Nineteenth Century Britain: Essays on Gender, Family, and Empire* (London: Pearson Longman, 2005), 5; Neil Sutherland, *Growing Up: Childhood in English Canada from the Great War to the Age of Television* (Toronto: University of Toronto Press, 1997), 53–9.

19  For a cogent discussion of the value of correspondence in understanding the dynamics of family history, see Françoise Noel, *Family Life and Sociability in Upper and Lower Canada, 1780–1870* (Montreal, Kingston: McGill-Queen's University Press, 2003), 7–11, 173–87.

20  This broader family correspondence in the King Gordon Papers is extensive, and the number of letters reaches in excess of a couple of hundred. Unlike the correspondence from Charles, that from his sisters and his mother does not begin until he leaves home in 1922. On adolescence, see Cynthis Comacchio, *The Dominion of Youth: Adolescence and the Making of Modern Canada, 1920 to 1950* (Waterloo: Wilfrid Laurier University Press, 2006).

21  KG, box 89, file 3, Helen Gordon to King, 1 July 1923.

22  Cynthia Comacchio, 'A Postscript for Father: Defining a New Fatherhood in Interwar Canada,' *Canadian Historical Review* 78, 3 (September 1997).

23  On the importance of a historical understanding of men's relationships and the experience of manhood, see Karen Harvey and Alexander Shepard, 'What Have Historians Done with Masculinity? Reflections on Five Centuries of British History,' *Journal of British Studies* 44, 2 (April 2005) and John Tosh, 'Masculinities in an Industrializing Society, Britain 1800–1914,' *Journal of British Studies* 44, 2 (April 2005). See also Frank, *Life with Father*, 6.

24  See Stephen Mintz, *Prison of Expectations: The Family in Victorian Culture* (New York: New York University Press, 1983) and John Tosh, 'Authority

and Nurture in Fatherhood: The Case of Early and Mid-Victorian England,' *Gender & History* 8 (1996): 48–64.

25 John Tosh, 'The Old Adam and the New Man: Emerging Themes in the History of English Masculinities, 1750–1850,' repr. in Tosh, *Manliness and Masculinities*, 61–82.

26 On the value of the life-course approach to understanding gender, see Veronica Strong-Boag, *A New Day Recalled: Lives of Girls and Women in English Canada, 1919–1939* (Toronto: Copp-Clark, 1988). Shawn Johansen adopts the same life-course approach, in *Family Men*. The pioneering theoretical article on the life-course or life-cycle approach to history is Tamera Hareven, 'Cycles, Courses, and Cohorts: Reflections on the Theoretical and Methodological Approaches to the Historical Study of Family Development,' *Journal of Social History* 12 (1978): 97–109.

27 One can capture a glimpse of the Rev. Donald Gordon's ministry session records. See Presbyterian Church Archives (Toronto), Accession 1993-4023, Session Records of the United Congregations of Indian Lands, Kenyon and Roxboro, 1853–71.

28 See Brian Fraser, *The Social Uplifters: Presbyterian Progressives and the Social Gospel in Canada, 1875–1915* (Waterloo: Wilfrid Laurier University Press, 1988) for an assessment of Gordon and his Presbyterian contemporaries and their commitment to the social gospel.

29 CWG, box 1, file 3, Sketch no. 3.

30 *Winnipeg Free Press*, 12 February 1912.

31 CWG, box 1, file 2, no title, n.d.

32 Such veneration of mid-Victorian fathers by their sons was a commonplace sentiment among many famous writers; see Lee Kremis, 'Authority and Rebellion in Victorian Autobiography,' *Journal of British Studies* 18 (1978): 107–30.

33 Both these articles are found in CWG, box 53, fd. 1, Scrapbook, 1898–1905.

34 Margaret Marsh, 'Suburban Men and Masculine Domesticity, 1870–1915,' in Carnes and Griffen, *Meanings for Manhood*, 111–27.

35 On the domestic orientation of the clergy, see John Tosh, 'Domesticity and Manliness in the Victorian Middle-Class: The Family of Edward White Benson,' in Roper and Tosh, *Manful Assertions*, 44–73; and John Tosh, 'Methodist Domesticity and Middle Class Masculinity in Nineteenth Century England,' in R.N. Swanson, ed., *Studies in Church History* 34 (1998).

36 See King's memories of domestic life with his father in the CBC interviews of the 1960s, KG, vol. 92, file 'Ralph Connor CBC Sunday,' 155–6, 208, 221.

37 The early correspondence between Charles and King is in KG, box 89, file 18.

38  KG, file 18, 'Daddy to My Dear Boy,' 5 June 1909; file 19, 'Your Daddy to My Dear Boy,' 27 June 1911.

39  KG, file 20, 'Your Daddy to My Dear Boy,' 21 February 1912.

40  KG, file 20, 'Your Daddy to My Dear Boy,' 5 February 1913.

41  Johansen, *Family Men*, 87–108.

42  KG, file 20, 'Daddy to My Dear King,' 31 May 1915.

43  KG, file 21, 'Your Daddy to My Dear King,' 7 July 1917.

44  KG, file 22, 'Your Father to My Dear Boy,' 4 December 1918.

45  KG, file 21, 'Your Daddy to my Dear Boy,' 4 January 1919.

46  KG, file 21, 'Your Daddy to My Dear Boy', 16 October 1916.

47  Ibid.

48  CWG, box 23, folder 9, 'Charles W. Gordon to Hodder-Williams,' 4 July 1921.

49  CWG, vol. 89, file 24, 'Your Daddy to My Dear Boy,' 4 November 1921.

50  KG, file 23, 'Your Daddy to My Dear King,' 12 December 1921.

51  KG, file 23, 'God keep you, Daddy to Dear Old Boy,' 11 October 1920.

52  KG, file 27, 'Your Daddy to My Dear Old Boy,' 15 December 1924.

53  CWG, vol. 89, file 28 'Your Daddy to My Dear King,' 29 May, 14 July 1925.

54  CWG, box 5, fd. 6, C.W. Gordon to Dr Edmison, 21 September 1925.

55  This description is based on J. King Gordon, A Discussion of the Industrial and Social Conditions of Pine Falls, 'A Company Town Owned and Operated by the Manitoba Paper Company'; KG, vol. 6, file 1.

56  Ibid.

57  KG, box 89, file 29, 'God Bless You Daddy to My Dear King,' 18 May 1926.

58  KG, file 30, 'Your Father to My Dear Boy,' 4 January 1929.

59  KG, file 31, 'Yr Daddy to My Dear King,' 4 April 1931.

60  See Michiel Horn, *Academic Freedom in Canada: A History* (Toronto: University of Toronto Press, 1999), 114–17.

61  KG, vol. 90, file 1, 'Your Daddy CWG to My Dear King,' 20 March 1934.

62  Ibid., 'Daddy to My Dear King,' 11 May 1934.

63  In assessing this controversy Michiel Horn has suggested that 'there is no hard evidence that Gordon was let go for his opinions or activities and there is a good deal of evidence that the college deficit provided the grounds for the abolition of the chair.' Horn, *Academic Freedom in Canada*, 116. King's observation was included in a letter to Michiel Horn, 377n110.

64  CWG, box 1, fd. 10, C.W. Gordon to Charles Clayton Morrison (editor, *The Christian Century*), 8 November 1934.

65  For Charles's letters on the necessity of reform see KG, file 31, 17 December 1931; 27 December 1931; file 33, n.d. [c. 1932–3?].

66  For King's involvement in the L.S.R. and his political activities, see Michiel Horn, *The League for Social Reconstruction: Intellectual Origins of*

*the Democratic Left in Canada, 1930–1942* (Toronto: University of Toronto Press, 1980), passim.

67 KG, vol. 92, file 5, King Gordon, 'En Route Winnipeg,' All Hallowes Eve, 1937.

68 Ibid.

69 Ibid.

70 KG, vol. 92, file 17, King Gordon to R.I.K. Davidson, 15 October 1971.

71 KG, vol. 92, file 19, King Gordon telegram to Jean Wilson, 25 November 1972.

72 KG, vol. 92, file 17, King Gordon to R.I.K. Davidson, 3 April 1973.

73 KG, vol. 92, file 19, King Gordon to Jean Wilson, 1 December 1972.

74 KG, vol. 92, file 17, Michael Bliss to King Gordon, 3 July 1973.

75 One of many positive reviews appeared in *The Presbyterian Witness*, 27 November 1909. See also *The Globe*, 20 November 1909.

76 CWG, box 4, file 3, W.H. Riddell to C.W. Gordon, 10 March 1910.

77 See *Winnipeg Free Press*, 6–28 January 1910.

78 This applies to another famous Canadian clerical family. See K.W. McNaught, *A Prophet in Politics: A Biography of J.S. Woodsworth* (Toronto: University of Toronto Press, 1959), and Mark Johnson, 'The Crisis of Faith and Social Christianity: The Ethical Pilgrimage of James Shaver Woodsworth,' in R.J. Helmstadter and Bernard Lightman, eds, *Victorian Crisis in Faith: Essays on Continuity and Change in Nineteenth Century Religious Belief* (Stanford: Stanford University Press, 1990), for J.S. Woodsworth's discussion of theology and Methodist piety with his family, including his clergyman father, while he slowly gravitated away from the moorings of the church. A similar observation has been made by Susan Curtis in 'The Son of Man and God the Father: The Social Gospel and Victorian Masculinity,' in Carnes and Griffen, *Meanings for Manhood*, 78.

79 Mintz, *Prison of Expectations*, 88.

80 CWG, box 30, fd. 1, 'The Crooked Tree,' short version.

# 8 Casual Fornicators, Delinquent Dads, Young Lovers, and Family Champions: Men in Canadian Adoption Circles

VERONICA STRONG-BOAG

Fathers of every sort, in contrast to birth and adoptive mothers, are often shadowy figures in accounts of adoption. While women's role as parents has been regularly taken for granted as an important measure of their capacity as adults and citizens, men too have been judged by their contribution to the welfare of daughters and sons. Canadian scholars such as Cynthia Comacchio and Robert Rutherdale are now charting the critical outlines of the history of fathers, which, as with so much else, is marked by the frequent fault lines of difference.[1] Evidence surviving in popular, child-welfare, and legal records, although limited, also permits us to consider the various fathers in the adoption circle. On the one hand, many representations have been essentially negative, stressing the failure to accommodate to normative ideals of respectability and discipline.[2] On the other, there are recurring, if less frequent, images of responsible paternity, of men who include parenting among the duties they are prepared to shoulder. Like male residents in Ontario's Victoria Industrial School for Boys or British Columbia's post–Second World War communities,[3] fathers in adoption circles were ultimately measured by their capacity for breadwinning: this was the leitmotif of hegemonic masculinity in Canada from at least Confederation on. While emotional and other contributions to children's well-being might be cited, material support was the first requirement if men were to gain approval. For all intermittent references to other ties between dads and offspring, 'the reality was that fatherhood came to be associated almost exclusively with its material aspects.'[4]

Drawing on my larger study of the evolution of adoption in English Canada in the nineteenth and twentieth centuries,[5] this chapter examines four recurring images of Canadian birth and adoptive fathers.

These I have characterized respectively as 'casual fornicators,' 'delinquent dads,' 'young lovers,' and 'family champions.' These tidy phrases cannot of course sum up the totality of any type of paternal experience. Time, geography, and specific communities produced many types of actual fathers, who might well over a lifetime demonstrate any or all aspects of these ideal types. These terms do, however, convey the range of ways that birth and adoptive fathers emerge in public discussions in Canada in the nineteenth and twentieth centuries. The first highlights the common theme of sexual licence; the second conjures up breadwinning failures and sometimes far worse; the third points to young fathers believed to be caught up in a moment of inexperience, even of romance; and the fourth aims to capture the observations of responsible fatherhood that surface in accounts of both birth and adoptive dads. Only the last version received full social approval. The first three expressions of masculinity might be termed non-hegemonic (or, in common parlance, unrespectable and even abnormal). 'Casual fornicators,' 'delinquent dads,' and even 'young lovers' were marked by the deficiency of their family relations, and sometimes much more. Perceived domestic failure helped define individuals, as Nancy Christie has so effectively argued, as marginal and deviant within the community at large.[6]

In discussions of adoption, all four images are particularly closely associated with biological paternity. Although they rarely drew the same attention as birth mothers, birth fathers always attracted some interest, since male failure, whatever its cause, was presumed to lie close to the heart of the child-raising crisis that necessitated the resort to adoption. Until the end of the twentieth century, adoptive fathers in contrast emerged far less commonly in public records. As members of heterosexual couples acquiring new progeny, men have been largely taken for granted. Nevertheless, even before the appearance of gay dads in the 1990s and beyond attracted unprecedented attention, some adoptive fathers have always been visible, predominately as domestic champions, but occasionally too as delinquents in the hard work of raising children. This chapter considers first the commonplace core criteria for responsible modern Canadian manhood and then the representation of donor (biological) and beneficiary (adoptive) fathers in the late nineteenth and twentieth centuries.

## Standards for Canadian Manhood

Paternal shortcomings and merits of every kind have been closely connected with fears about sustaining individual and national productivity, vitality, and discipline. It is far from surprising that Michael Bliss, who went on to become one of Canada's most influential historians of men in business, medicine, and politics, pioneered in drawing attention to commonplace anxieties surrounding the outcome of male sexuality. His 1970 essay 'Pure Books on Avoided Subjects: Pre-Freudian Sexual Ideas in Canada'[7] introduced the twin themes of control and licence, respectability and the fall from grace, that have subsequently preoccupied Canadian scholars of masculinity.[8] Ironically enough, although national leaders such as Joseph Flavelle, William Osler, and Canadian prime ministers appear to owe at least some part of their success to their ability to sublimate physical desires,[9] Michael Bliss's early sex educators largely appeared as spoil sports and martinets. In an expansive spirit reminiscent of much of the 1960s, 'Pure Books' ultimately seemed more sympathetic to a politics that equated sexuality with pleasure and society with repression. Since that early study, which might well have portended a different career trajectory for its author, who was instead encouraged to continue his doctoral work on Canadian businessmen,[10] feminist perspectives have considerably complicated the portrait of Canadian masculinity. Scholars like Karen Dubinsky, Joan Sangster, and Steven Maynard have reminded us that women and men regularly court somewhat different outcomes in their encounter with sexuality.[11] Michael Bliss's 1970 recognition that respectability has been highly dependent for men, as for women, on expressions of sexuality deemed appropriate by the authorities of their time, not to mention by subsequent historians, remains nevertheless a benchmark exploration in the Canadian history of gender.

Coverage of fathers in Canadian adoption circles has reflected dominant assumptions about preferable, often assumed to be normal, conduct for male adults. Like the boys subjected to lectures from pioneer sex educators, good men were expected to govern themselves carefully. Weak men and weak fathers succumbed to physical desires with little thought of consequences; the strong did not. For many social critics, restraint in sexual matters was tied to discipline in life generally. More particularly, it was believed to underpin material, not to mention moral, accomplishment. Thus it followed that responsible men fathered no more children than they could hope to raise comfortably. Measured by the standard of economic support, most biological parents in the adoption circle have been deemed sexually irresponsible and thus slackers in some of life's hardest work.

While middle-class experts of every sort have been most visible in linking respectability to material well-being, they were not alone. By the closing years of the nineteenth century, as Cynthia Comacchio has observed, 'the male-breadwinner ideal was becoming integral to working-class notions of respectability.'[12] Both native and foreign born Canadians experienced the imperatives of this moral vision. 'Canadianization' as it developed after Confederation demanded so-called normal families in which men laboured hard outside homes and women preferably within, with parenting duties frequently divided along gender lines. Racialized men, notably those with Aboriginal, African, and Asian ancestry, encountered a particularly harsh spotlight.[13]

When biological fathers failed the breadwinning test of worthy masculinity, whether intentionally or accidentally, they might well precipitate children and their mothers into the hard hands of private and public authorities. If sexual intercourse and reproduction were followed by apparent financial delinquency, these men were vulnerable to assessment as impulsive, intemperate, and idle, qualities that recalled male Canadians evaluated in the context of encounters with the criminal justice system. Such judgments were especially likely to be made of fathers from the working-class and racialized minorities, just those folks who also more commonly faced Canadian judges. The particular structural circumstances that made it more difficult for poorer Canadians everywhere and in every decade to meet the standards of middle-class experts were routinely ignored.

Beneficiary fathers have in contrast frequently possessed class and racial advantages that set them apart from male donors. To be in a position to make additions to households immediately signalled the passage of one crucial test of responsible manhood. The economic means to assume duties considered properly those of birth fathers or those that would otherwise fall to child-welfare authorities or private charity distinguished adopters right from the beginning. Such Canadians might not be fertile, but they possessed other highly valued qualities associated with hegemonic masculinity. The centrality of male breadwinning was repeatedly underscored by the continuing preference, often requirement, of adoption agencies until the last years of the twentieth century that prospective adoptive mothers not work outside the home. Women's ability to dedicate themselves to domesticity confirmed that their husbands were good providers, heads of their households, and would-be responsible parents.[14] In some ways, the choice to adopt, especially when it was publicly acknowledged, as it was increasingly after the Second World War, elevated such men to the high status of 'communal fathers,' those whom Robert Rutherdale has

importantly depicted in another context as contributing 'useful familial influences to the whole community.'[15] These citizens claimed
important public space, roles, and authority as 'family men' that bach-
elors and the childless in general would have had much more difficulty in asserting. Whatever the disturbing or distressing questions it
raised about fertility, adoption's affirmation of the acceptance of adult
responsibilities offered important sources of prestige. Real men were
not distinguished by sperm count.

Records describing birth and adoptive fathers introduced Canadians
who were identified as having stumbled or succeeded at one of the critical tests of manhood. Those who were considered little more than a
source of DNA faced censure. Those who lived up to the code of responsible breadwinning, even when they could not biologically reproduce,
emerged as the clear champions in the masculinity department.

**Representations of Birth Fathers**

Birth fathers have had a variety of relationships to birth mothers. Some
have been only brief encounters, sometimes violent and unmarked by
commitment or affection. Some were relatively permanent, a result of
courtship, common-law unions, and legal marriage, and sometimes
marked by love and respect. Until the late twentieth century, unwed
parenthood placed men in a unique legal position regarding offspring.
Whatever the reason for not marrying their sexual partners, they had
only one legal connection to their offspring, the obligation of financial
support, and only then if paternity was acknowledged or could be
proven. The mother alone was the legal guardian. Only her consent
was necessary for the surrender of youngsters. In most instances,
mothers and children could inherit from one another but fathers had
no equivalent relationship.[16] One scholar has succinctly summed up
the common relationship: '"You have no rights, only obligations."'[17]

Canada's most extensive study of adoption, Paul Sachdev's *Unlocking the Adoption Files*, placed such birth fathers firmly on the margins of
the adoption story. While acknowledging the father as a 'principal protagonist' at the beginning of the path to adoption, Sachdev and his
assistants largely shared informants' assessment of him as a 'phantom
figure.' One birth mother summed up the commonplace indictment:
'Birth father is not a person in my estimation.' In general, adopters,
adoptees, and birth mothers 'were either opposed or ambivalent'
about releasing information about adoptees to biological fathers.[18] The

responses of Sachdev's Newfoundland sample reflected widespread assumptions about male disinterest and irresponsibility. As one authority has further noted, Canadians have generally been convinced both that it was 'unnatural' for any woman to wish to surrender a child and that it was equally peculiar for unwed dads to want to parent.[19]

Observers of birth fathers have been regularly prone to single them out as uncaring and delinquent, sometimes less negatively as young lovers, and much less frequently as domestic champions. Among the most abhorred has been the rapist. In the early 1990s one Ontario case set forth the extent to which such malefactors strayed from masculine ideals. The equality demands of the *Charter of Rights and Freedoms* had raised the general question of whether the consent of all natural fathers, like that of birth mothers, was needed for adoption. Not surprisingly, among those women to resist such claims was one rape survivor who vehemently rejected any presumption of equality. She had not consented to intercourse and the perpetrator ought to have no rights of consent over the resulting infant. After some deliberation, the courts concluded that paternal agreement to the transfer of guardianship and custody should be dispensed with in such cases, since 'the remote chance that a rapist might wish to acknowledge and assume responsibility for the child he fathered, bears no realistic proportion to the government objective of providing an expeditious and final adoption.'[20] While violence against women might be sufficient in some quarters to deny perpetrators the title of 'real men,' the measure of entitlement here was the unlikelihood of rapists' willingness to provide materially and otherwise for the results of their sexual actions.

Men who paid no heed to the consequences of their actions were damned as casual fornicators who brought their entire sex into disrepute. Like many of those described by Karen Dubinsky, such fathers might not be formally identified for public disgrace, or held legally accountable, but they were not readily ranked among the respectable even when they were supposedly 'seduced' by those they made pregnant.[21] The fact that many fathers, as with those served with paternity suits in Ontario over the course of the twentieth century, either fled provincial jurisdiction or insisted upon adoption further confirmed their general unworthiness.[22]

Men's determination to escape familial obligations could be especially visible when it came to the military. Canadian and American bases in Newfoundland during and after the Second World War, like those elsewhere across the nation and around the world, presented a special challenge to local women involved in sexual relationships and a context provocative of adoption.[23] As the film *Seven Brides for Uncle Sam* (NFB, 1997) movingly conveyed, Americans at Fort Pepperrell became experts at loving and leaving. Newfoundland authorities quickly came to reckon the costs in unwed pregnancies. As they learned, 'putative fathers are largely Servicemen, and herein lies the greatest problem, because nearly all of them have departed and have been discharged,' leaving behind mothers and children to 'become public charges.'[24] Like their civilian counterparts in Hamilton from 1859 to 1922, many such mid-twentieth-century men viewed the off-spring of encounters they frequently held as casual as little more than potentially expensive encumbrances. For such reluctant progenitors, adoption provided just one more way of sidestepping responsibility for conception.[25] Shored up by its association with a pre-eminently male institution, the masculinity of servicemen appeared in no need of affirmation by the performance of responsible paternity. Indeed, 'zip-less' sexual adventures promised an alternative to respectable hege-monic masculinity with its investment in breadwinning and its burdens. As sociologist R.W. Connell has outlined so convincingly, men are imbedded in situations that offer a variety of masculine codes, and sexual irresponsibility is one option.[26]

By the later decades of the twentieth century, men who offered sperm for artificial insemination could be said to have rather inadvertently joined the unprepossessing company of casual fornicators whose names have frequently been lost to progeny. However essential their contribu-tion to the creation of families, they have commonly been regarded as no more than a necessary evil that recipients best hid from posterity. Observers might associate these birth fathers with crass money-making, as well as perhaps with altruism, but the searchers who emerged in the 1990s also clearly hoped for reputable antecedents. Optimism fuelled recurring stories of medical interns, lawyers, and even Nobel Laureates. Such invisible patriarchs might have been relatively unthinking, even mercenary, in dispensing the stuff of offspring, but they had potential qualities that might well be treasured later.[27]

Known dads who refused to pay the piper for their pleasure fostered fewer romantic fantasies. Their malfeasance was often associated with the direct mistreatment of wives. Such was true of one Ukrainian farmer after the First World War who, upon the death of his over-worked wife in childbirth, was portrayed by an Anglo-Celtic critic as brutal in his immediate search for a young replacement whom he would, presumably, similarly abuse. When no one proved foolish enough to become his bride, seven sons and daughters were summarily dispatched to an institution, where two soon died. The fate of the rest was unspecified, but readers were left to hope they might be properly Canadianized at the hands of more responsible fathers.[28] Drinking, drugs, unemployment, promiscuity, and violence were all commonly credited with the failure of such 'worthless men' to support progeny and mothers.[29]

Court decisions often voiced the recurring condemnation. In 1913 the Manitoba judiciary considered the case of a man who had filed a writ of habeas corpus for a daughter placed by his deserted wife in the home of a 'well-to-do-farmer.' She paid her child's room and board from her wages as a domestic in a boarding house. Obvious industry and self-sacrifice clearly stood her in good stead when she claimed cruelty and lack of support in opposing the claim of her spouse. The birth father himself lacked permanent housing in Canada and planned to remove his daughter to his own parental home in Wales, but provided no evidence of the feasibility of this proposal. Despite the presumption of paternal entitlement, the judges decided that the child should remain with her foster family. The birth parents were given restricted access but no control or custody.[30] Other problematic dads, such as journalist Victor Malarek's wife-beater father in post–Second World War Montreal, were graded similarly low by child welfare authorities. Assault and dependence on a waitress wife for subsistence confirmed the senior Malarek's overall inadequacy. His sons paid the penalty when they were apprehended by child welfare and brutally fostered in other families and institutions.[31]

Claims of rehabilitation, as with one BC recovering drug addict, who had largely ignored his seven-year-old daughter since her birth and then attempted in the 1980s to recover her custody from her aunt and uncle, did not necessarily compensate for a damning record of neglect.[32] At much the same time, Newfoundland courts similarly dispensed with the requirement for consent of another delinquent dad who had hardly looked back when he abandoned his eighteen-month-old offspring. Her happiness and good adjustment with her stepfather were believed jeopardized by the claimant, whatever the latter's promises to the contrary.[33] In the 1990s the suit of another Newfoundland birth father who had ignored his former wife's efforts to help him foster ties with their child and never paid support, 'although he clearly had the means to do so,' similarly failed. Judges again interpreted his petition as a threat to his daughter's 'stability and emotional security.'[34] The material and other care of a stepfather promised much better. Biology once more proved no guarantee of good conduct.

Yet for all the grand host of outwardly wayward Canadians whose shortcomings were regularly assessed as directing girls and boys to other homes, some birth fathers in the adoption circle have always been recognized as endeavouring to assume the proper duties of worthy men. Some sympathy for young lovers whom misunderstandings and aggrieved parents might have separated, at least for a time, or for whom financial obligations proved overwhelming, supplied a recurring theme in many commentaries. Although Barbara Melosh, a leading American scholar of adoption, claimed in 2002 that 'to date, not a single birth father has published a full-length memoir, and few men claim the name "birth father" publicly,'[35] Canada nonetheless supplies examples of such confessions by former young lovers who might escape some of the opprobrium usually applied to delinquent dads. In 1989 the former Rentalsman for the province of British Columbia published *My Search for Catherine Anne: One Man's Story of an Adoption Reunion*. Many years after his life as an undergraduate at the University of Toronto, he discovered to his dismay that he had fathered a child who had been surrendered for adoption.[36] A somewhat different story, but filled with similar regrets, was filed by the deputy chief news editor of the *Vancouver Sun*. He had been one of two star-crossed teens, pregnant at sixteen and seventeen, who chose a 'perfect home' for their newborn. Twenty-three years later, in 2003, he sought his daughter out in the belated hope 'of making things right.'[37]

Growing public openness about such previously private matters signified a critical shift in the response to unwed dads in the last decades of the twentieth century. Although one legal scholar concluded in 1986 that 'the road to unwed fatherhood is all but impassable,'[38] Canadians increasingly contested that fate. Challenges to tradition and law, which had long acted to curb paternal feelings and rights, increased dramatically after the 1960s and 1970s. Even as they focused increasingly on the plight of teen mums in these years, child-welfare authorities moved beyond their familiar interest in financial support to grow more concerned about the fortunes of young dads. As Manitoban social workers observed in 1960, unmarried fathers were now 'generally assumed' to have many of the 'same emotional problems' as their partners.[39] When psychological explanations for the fall from sexual grace became increasingly popular, young parents of both sexes emerged as ripe for rehabilitation. As Simma Holt, a BC journalist and later Liberal MP, argued: 'To the boy, this experience is one of ego identity; the child is part of himself. Despite the difference in the nature of their possessiveness towards this child, the strong natural bond of flesh and blood is with the boy as much as with the girl. But there are no social workers, counselors, nurses, or doctors to help him.'[40] The dereliction from adult duties, such as three-fifths of Toronto birth fathers cited in one study, who failed to spend any time at all over four weeks with teen mums, was increasingly credited to psychological maladjustment and less to moral failure. The result for offspring might of course be much the same.[41]

After the Second World War, court decisions showed growing sympathy for young lovers caught up in events beyond their control. In 1950s Ontario, young Dutch immigrants struggling to make the transition to maturity found themselves the parents of twins and handed them over at birth to their family doctor to place with a well-to-do couple. Almost immediately, pressed hard by their families, they reconsidered the surrender. Eventually the provincial Court of Appeal ordered the return of their offspring. The economic prospects of the repentant birth father had clearly improved; the young truck driver had moved his family from a trailer to a 'modest apartment' and he could now be reckoned as a possible candidate for worthy fatherhood.[42] In the mid-1980s a teen emigrant from Vietnam found herself pregnant in Alberta, but shame kept her apart from her Canadian-born boyfriend. She fled to a home for unwed mothers and surrendered her baby. The young father, however, was not prepared to acquiesce. Aided by his 'strong and supportive family,' he won her back, got married, and together they successfully initiated a legal challenge to the loss of their infant to adopters.[43] In 1993 *Chatelaine* featured the story of the struggle of an unwed student to oppose the adoption of his son. While initially uninterested in fathering, he too succumbed to his family's conviction that blood kin should raise children. The result forced the birth mother to rescind the open adoption and introduced continuing conflict over custody, access, and support. Whatever the inspiration for his intervention or the damage, the young man demonstrated, at least belatedly, some willingness to meet the standards of hegemonic adult masculinity.[44]

In the face of especially hard times, sometimes precipitated by widowing, divorce, or unemployment, Canadian fathers, like those elsewhere, have had a long history of passing youngsters around the extended family, to friends, and to institutions for shorter and longer periods of respite.

This general tendency, which I have elsewhere termed 'interrupted relations,' has also been observed by Bettina Bradbury and Diane Purvey in
their studies of Canadian orphanages.[45] Such acts were not necessarily
those of parental slackers. When better times or older youngsters promised help, responsible fathers might well attempt to retrieve progeny.
This was not always easy. Orphanages sometimes farmed boys and girls
out to other families variously desirous of youngsters and suspected the
motives of blood relatives. Recipients might be reluctant to give up additions to their households. Many legal cases testified to recurring paternal
efforts to reconnect with offspring. In 1906, for example, a recent widower gave his newborn to neighbours, who later argued that the transfer
was intended to be permanent. He rejected this interpretation, telling
pre–First World War courts that he had told the foster parents that they
could only have the child until she '"could run with his other children."'
Successful retrieval was made immeasurably easier by the fact that not
only had his daughter regularly visited her blood siblings but that her
birth father now possessed a housekeeper and a twenty-three-year-old
niece as well as older sons and daughters for assistance. At least as
importantly, he, like the foster family, was also reckoned 'well-to-do and
may even be called wealthy.' Despite the fact that his neighbours had
cared for her without reimbursement for seven years, the father was
acquitted of abandonment and regained his daughter.[46]

The shifting climate of opinion in the late twentieth century was
especially supportive of paternal efforts to resist any relegation to the
sidelines. In 1972 the nation's leading mass-circulation magazine, the
Star Weekly, heralded the tone with its article 'Father Knows Best,'
which celebrated divorced dads living together with their four kids,
aided by a housekeeper. There was no hint of a sexual relationship and
their celebrated cooperation was credited, ironically enough, to the fact
that their ex-wives were good friends.[47] In the same decade, in an initiative that would become almost common place, a 'putative father'
tried to force the Toronto Children's Aid Society to recognize his right
to 'notice of wardship proceedings with respect to his illegitimate
child.' In a token of changed sentiments, a lower court supported his
claim, although the Supreme Court of Canada eventually reversed that
decision in 1973: ultimately he was not deemed a parent under the
law.[48] While that negative conclusion was confirmed by others elsewhere, [49] the times were nevertheless on his side.

By 1975 BC's Royal Commission on Children and Family Law
acknowledged unmarried fathers' efforts 'to have a voice in planning for

their children' and indicated that some at least were 'also willing, and able, to raise their children as single parents.'[50] 'Nineteen years later, the province's panel to review adoption legislation agreed that birth fathers deserved legal recognition.[51] Like those in Australia, where the 1980s saw something of a rush of applications for custody of offspring by both Aboriginal and newcomer birth fathers,[52] Canadian courts slowly and uncertainly extended paternal rights. In 1986, in the case of 'O'Driscoll v. McLeod,' the BC Supreme Court concluded that 'a natural father and his child born in and out of wedlock shared a legal relationship from which legally enforceable rights and obligations flowed.' A year later, the same province produced the ruling that legislation's failure to require paternal consent to adoption contravened the Charter of Rights and Freedoms.[53] In 1988, however, the Ontario Divisional Court debated and then rejected claims by a biological father that the Charter guaranteed him equality in custody.[54] Other decisions in the 1990s were more favourable, as when the BC Supreme Court allowed an unwed father the right to 'apply for custody, guardianship or access in spite of the mother's refusal to allow him to acknowledge paternity,' and another court in Newfoundland permitted a petitioner to shift his parenting responsibilities to his sister and brother-in-law, a request that was clearly viewed as a responsible solution.[55]

Opposition to proposed stepfather adoptions also provided opportunities to assert responsible paternity. In one case, typical except for its particularly happy ending, a birth father opposed adoption by the mother's new husband, fearing that 'the order would abrogate his access rights given under an earlier Court order.' The Alberta judge encouraged resort to a family counsellor, who won agreement to continued access after adoption of the seven-year-old boy by his mother's new partner. The result appeared to please everyone, although the mother and her husband confessed that the proposal 'first came as a shock to them.' It was more than that, since, as the judge acknowledged at length, continuing access breached a fundamental presumption that adoption severed all such ties. This break from much practice was easier because the birth father possessed 'some measure of economic success in his life and has indicated his desire of providing for and assisting Ronald, as his only child, during his lifetime and through his estate.'[56] Occasional legal cases where birth fathers applied with new wives to adopt the offspring of previous unions could also present men as champions of domestic responsibility. Courts listened to fathers characterize themselves, sometimes successfully, as the chief caretaker, sometimes in the face of birth mothers who could be dismissed as 'harmful and disturbing to the children.'[57]

Of course, not all applicants were successful in their appeals. Racialized identities sometimes appeared to weaken claims to the worthiness of hegemonic masculinity. In the 1990s an unmarried birth father of Jamaican origin sought custody against the wishes of the White mother who had given the child up for adoption. His acknowledged 'fitness' for responsible parenting, even when combined with 'racial and cultural reasons' which meant that the daughter would 'be more readily accepted and integrated into the milieu provided by her father' failed, however, to translate into full authority. The judgment, in recognition too of increased support for shared parenting of various sorts, awarded the father custody, but he had to share guardianship with the adoptive parents and the birth mother.[58] Significantly less fortunate was a Black father from Mississippi who unsuccessfully petitioned an Alberta court to retrieve his child, surrendered to Canadian adopters by its mother. The additional complication of borders added to racial disadvantage in undermining his case for responsible parenthood.[59] The 'best interests of the child' doctrine regularly favoured adopters already in place, all the more so when birth mothers did not join forces with paternal claimants.

Such varied decisions in the last decades of the twentieth century clearly evoked the complicated and contentious nature of individual cases before Canadian courts. They also revealed unprecedented consideration for the rights of unwed birth fathers and some recognition that 'lack of access could have devastating emotional consequences for fathers.'[60] Not surprisingly, Newfoundland in 1999, like other jurisdictions in the same decade, first made legislative reference to 'birth fathers.' No longer were they an invisible presence in adoption law.[61] More than ever they were credited with possible claims to respectable masculinity.

**Representations of Adoptive Fathers**

Until very recently, particular invisibility has cloaked the vast majority of male adopters. Most public records have been almost silent about their contribution. Their female partners have always been viewed as the key players in initiating and sustaining parental relations. Whereas adoptive mums have had to pass muster in the eyes of adoption authorities, their legal heterosexual partners have faced far less scrutiny. Good would-be fathers largely sufficed if they supplied the critical material foundation for expanded households. Once they had, as became increasingly necessary in the last decades of the twentieth century, submitted their economic credentials to professional study of the home, they thereafter for the most part stepped to the sidelines in the larger public drama. Safely on the margins, they did not have to endure reminders about possible infertility nor in fact be asked to take on the same day-to-day responsibilities of care that were largely assumed to be proper for women.

Pre-eminent designation as breadwinners did not necessarily imply emotional detachment.[62] Material success could involve heartfelt embrace of parental duties. As Cynthia Comacchio has rightly observed, however, the commitment to breadwinning required most fathers to be 'absent from the home for the better part of their children's waking hours' and thus supplied a major 'paradox of modern fatherhood.' This was the 'inherent tension between the worldly success essential to being a good father, and the good father's essential domestic involvement.'[63] Adopters, like other fathers, had to find some way of accommodating income earning with the twentieth century's growing enthusiasm for male emotional and physical engagement in child-raising. They did, however, begin with something of an advantage with regard to public opinion. Merely by agreeing to add strangers to their households, they already scored high marks in a financial-worthiness test that other men had presumably failed.

The significance of their contribution was confirmed by the fact that men have regularly been judged more reluctant to welcome new offspring. Would-be mothers have always been reckoned the chief champions and beneficiaries of adoption. Men were commonly judged less dependent on offspring for self-realization. Some degree of special paternal reticence was also presumed to originate with shame over supposed infertility. As one adopter explained to his adult daughter, '"No man likes to think that he's infertile. It makes him less masculine. It's nice to know you can procreate."'[64] Some clinical assessments have further concluded that male adopters have also felt less close to and successful with youngsters in general and needed more assistance in parenting than their biological counterparts.[65]

A 1961 study of twenty-seven new fathers 'ranging in background from bus driver to university professor' typically identified wives as both inspiration and driving force in adoption. One man stated quite bluntly: '"Most adoptable children are illegitimate and the idea of nurturing someone's else's mistake repelled me."' Agencies everywhere repeated stories of husbands who insisted on harder-to-get girls lest the family name be tarnished by an 'outsider.' The study's author tried to reassure his audience, insisting that 'agencies had no perfect babies so they don't expect to find perfect fathers.'[66] Whatever the encouragement, however, some men's reservations lingered: Canada's dads have routinely been evaluated as having fewer of their needs, as opposed to those of their female partners, met by adoption. Thus, merely by acquiescing, if no more enthusiastically than that, men in fact demonstrated a certain meritorious self-sacrifice. In effect, by prioritizing the claims of would-be mothers and fatherless youngsters, they almost automatically qualified as good men.

Whether moved by their wives' desires or their own, many Canadian men have, however, ultimately proved willing, even determined, to parent youngsters born to others. As Canadian historians such as Cynthia Fish, Jack Little, and Robert Rutherdale have demonstrated, fathers have frequently invested strong emotions in paternal roles.[67] Many male adopters desperately wished for the opportunities and status that paternity promised. Sometimes acts of adoption could be intensely practical. The Second World War brought forward a host of servicemen who endeavoured to complete adoptions so that military allowances would help support youngsters.[68] Material benefits springing from legal recognition were not the only attraction. Like the fictional well-to-do bachelor lawyer who was portrayed rescuing a Canadian niece before the First Great War, adopters might well feel that youngsters in their homes heralded 'light and joy and laughter.'[69] One male adopter addressing Canadians in 1930 spoke of personal shortcomings and tragedy but also of transcendence:

I have experienced a good many troubles, and yet I have been very happy. There are six children in my family, although the eldest ones would be offended if I called them children now. They are not really all mine. I acquired one or two of them under various circumstances during my journeyings. The eldest is a young man of twenty-six. The baby is a little chap of four. Neither of these two came to my wife or myself by natural means. In between these two are four others, two girls and two boys, and they all run in together and form the happiest family I ever saw. When I go to my work every morning I have the right feeling in my heart.[70]

Five years later a rather less emotional confession came from the adoptive father of a toddler. While his series describing the 'experiment' of procuring a brother for his biological daughter, 'Diana,' for the mass circulation women's magazine *Chatelaine* sometimes seemed disconcertingly clinical, the author concluded ultimately that 'John is very much part of ourselves' and 'we love John. That is not our achievement. It is his.'[71] Decades later a successful grocer and adoptive parent of two boys and a girl in post–Second World War Prince George, British Columbia, testified to the commitment that could be ignited in the course of getting to know youngsters. While he had been active in local affairs, which Robert Rutherdale has interpreted as community fathering, and an excellent provider, he still claimed as his '"single biggest regret"' the failure to be still more involved in the lives of his sons and daughter.[72] His relations with them supplied a critical measure by which to judge his life as a whole.

For all their fears of inadequacy, some adopting dads, like the fictional Matthew Cuthbert, the foster parent of Anne of Green Gables, clearly flourished in their interaction with youngsters. Some stepfather claimants before the courts supplied further evidence of the importance that could be attached to such ties. While their desires could not always be readily distinguishable from those of biological mothers who normally initiated adoption proceedings, three would-be fathers found themselves in circumstances that allowed them to demonstrate their own commitment. In the 1960s and 1970s one BC step-parent fought to continue involvement in the life of a child whom his wife brought into and out of her marriage with him. He insisted on continuing relations with his informally adopted son.[73] In another instance, this time from the Maritimes, the birth mother divorced her first husband in 1976, obtaining custody and support for her son. In April 1977 she remarried and financial assistance ceased. Soon after, she began adoption proceedings with her new partner. In December 1977 she suddenly died. The widower nevertheless chose to continue the legal action and attempted, as authorized by the decision of a lower court, to proceed without the consent of the birth father. The latter appealed. The Supreme Court of Nova Scotia concluded, in a majority decision, with one dissenter, that the death of the 'natural parent, who would have normally protected the child from future uncertainties,' combined with the claimant's occupation as a salesman which frequently kept him on the road had to be set against his 'sincere love' for the child. The birth father's appeal won the day: it was deemed in the best interests of the son to have 'a father on reserve' should the stepfather 'die or change.'[74]

Another case in Ontario in 1990 similarly suggested a depth of feelings on the part of a would-be adopter. Here a stepfather whose relationship with the birth mother had broken down in the course of adoption again wished to continue the acquisition of parental rights. Since his circumstances were rather different, his request met a happier fate than that of his counterpart in the Maritimes. The presiding judge concluded that 'the step-father was the only father the child had ever known and fulfilled the role of father in every way except for the biological aspect of it.' In particular, he cited 'the step-father's interest in the child's life' and the fact that the boy did not know he was not the biological offspring. The child's 'best interests' were, he concluded, best served by recognizing effective paternity.[75]

Growing acceptance of transracial parenting in the last decades of the twentieth century provided further opportunities for adopters to demonstrate paternal commitment. White fathers of minority children, whether Aboriginal, otherwise native-born, or international, clearly violated long-standing preferences for matching, which among other outcomes might help camouflage infertility. By deliberately flouting commonplace assumptions of normalcy, which were often infused with racism, a few more progressive Canadians publicly professed different standards. Like David Kirk, the influential Canadian scholar of adoption and adoptive father of youngsters of African heritage, and others who surfaced in the popular press,[76] such iconoclasts often appeared to embrace a more inclusive national politics. When leading public figures like journalist Pierre Berton and politician Jean Chrétien also added an African-Canadian daughter and a Native son respectively to their households in the 1960s, some part of the Canadian mainstream had clearly embraced adoptive fatherhood as a badge of honour.[77] Such trans-racial adoptions offered the potential for extending community fathering into the national realm of multiculturalism.

By the 1990s the surge in support for fathering cautiously extended to include legal recognition of gay dads. While it has always been relatively easy to find female adopters, such as novelist Mazo de la Roche and her cousin Caroline Clement,[78] it has been harder to discover male couples of any kind raising children with official approval. While cases of male adopters without female partners sometimes surface in early records, as with two First World War farming brothers from Ontario who rescued a brother and a sister, they were highly unusual.[79] For the most part, opportunities awaited the emergence of a late-twentieth-century gay and lesbian rights movement that was prepared to add parenting to the political and personal agenda. Lesbians led the way, but would-be fathers also emerged to wage their own campaigns for recognition as worthy custodians of youngsters.[80]

In 1996 the province of British Columbia became the first jurisdiction in the world to pass legislation allowing same-sex spouses to adopt as couples. By 2003 the Toronto Children's Aid was reported as placing twelves youngsters with gay parents. As one admiring observer commented, 'The wave of gay men wanting to become parents is the ultimate expression of being out of the closet.' She singled out the example of a thirty-three-year-old new dad who had broken up with a partner over his desire to parent and then proceeded to make arrangements with a surrogate mother in London, Ontario. He would have been applauded by Toronto counterparts flocking to a course called 'Daddies and Papas 2 B' at much the same time.[81] When the *Georgia Straight*, a generally progressive Vancouver weekly, embraced the boldness of a Lower Mainland gay couple in adopting an African-American son from Chicago in 2004, fatherhood had clearly come a long way.[82] The obvious material comfort of these BC suburbanites also reminded everyone that successful breadwinning stood would-be fathers in good stead. Ultimately, sexual orientation appeared somewhat less important than financial capacity. In any case, queer dads, like lesbian mums, increasingly demanded a broader definition of good parenting. The households they championed stood in the forefront of the radical future of the family foretold by some contemporary advocates of adoption.[83]

Although adoptive dads, including gays, overwhelming emerge as family champions in public accounts, especially in the later decades of the twentieth century, they too have produced failure and tragedy. Some surrogate fathers of young 'home children,' the offspring of British poverty who migrated to the dominion from the mid-nineteenth century until after the Second World War, emerged as brutal.[84] Even blood ties and religious faith did not guarantee safety, as with the nieces beaten and starved by their clergyman uncle, who was also their foster father, in Ontario in 1898.[85] Nor did adoptive children escape the sexual abuse that was so regular a part of some natural families. One adoptive father who confessed to sexually assaulting his charge for a decade evoked a dreadfully familiar pattern. His victim, however, seized an option unavailable to birth daughters. In 1994 she convinced the BC Supreme Court to overturn the 1980 transaction that created kinship with her abuser.[86] First Nation adoptees, who appeared in significant numbers in Canada in the 1960s and 1970s, may have been especially likely to attract predators such as a Kansas cross-border adopter who sexually molested Manitoba-born Cameron Kerley.[87] Ultimately, such abusers might pass the breadwinning test but they betrayed hegemonic ideals of fatherhood that also investigated heavily in care and protection.

In the last decades of the twentieth century, a fathers' movement emerged to campaign for extended paternal rights.[88] As Canadian legal scholar Susan B. Boyd has carefully noted, this movement has sometimes been deeply misogynist. Too frequently its demands have appeared more intended to assail feminists and women in general and reassert male power than to address injustice and take day-to-day responsibility for children's overall well-being.[89] Yet, for all such reactionary tendencies, many men, today as in the past, have invested heavily in meaningful roles in parenting. A legion of good fathers have assumed that caring for daughters and sons by birth and by adoption is a critical part of responsible adulthood.

In the process of becoming fathers, Canadian men have demonstrated many versions of masculinity over the decades. Some were clearly dangerous to youngsters. Casual fornicators and dead-beat and delinquent dads compromised many futures, as did sometimes young lovers and even supposed family champions. Many men, however, struggled hard to become supportive and loving parents to a variety of offspring. By the end of the twentieth century, many signs confirmed the unprecedented popularity of adoptive fatherhood as one version of successful masculinity. One Vancouverite celebrated his new status by inaugurating a set of stories celebrating the daring of Chinese girls like his daughters. In the process, he demonstrated how fiction and fact might combine to challenge biology as destiny.[90] Such men emerged as proud representatives of the community fathers whose contributions have generally bettered both private and public life. Such adopters were fully paid-up members of a fraternity in Canada as elsewhere that took parenthood very seriously as one of the most rewarding ways of being human.

NOTES

My thanks to Angus McLaren, Robert Rutherdale, and Chris Shelley for comments on an earlier version of this chapter. I also very much appreciate the research support of Nicholas Clarke, Stephanie Higginson, Heather Latimer, Lorie MacIntosh, Amy Salmon, Melanie Scheuer, Anna Treadwell, Susy Webb, and Almas Zakiuddin in the course of my study of adoption in Canada. I also owe much to the financial encouragement provided by UBC's Hampton Fund, the SSHRCC, and the Killam Program of the Canada Council. Finally, I would like to thank my doctoral supervisor, Michael Bliss, whose prose style became an abiding inspiration after we first met in his third-year Canadian history class at the University of Toronto in 1968.

1 See, for example, Cynthia Comacchio, 'Bringing Up Father: Defining a Modern Canadian Fatherhood, 1900–1940,' in Lori Chambers and Edgar-Andre Montigny, eds, *Family Matters: Papers in Post-Confederation Canadian Family History* (Toronto: Canadian Scholars' Press, 1998), 289–308 and Robert Rutherdale, 'Fatherhood and the Social Construction of Memory: Breadwinning and Male Parenting on a Job Frontier, 1945–1966,' in Joy Parr and Mark Rosenfeld, eds, *Gender and History in Canada* (Toronto: Copp Clark Ltd, 1996), 357–75. The best overall treatment of debates among Canadian historians and others about the shifting and diverse nature of family roles, including that of fathers, is supplied by Nancy Christie and Michael Gauvreau, eds, *Mapping the Margins: The Family and Social Discipline in Canada, 1700–1975* (Montreal and Kingston: McGill-Queen's University Press, 2004); see esp. the 'Introduction' by Nancy Christie, 3–24. See also the early and influential discussion of the 'missing man' by John Demos in 'The Changing Faces of Fatherhood,' in *Past, Present, and Personal: The Family and the Life Course in American History* (New York: Oxford University Press, 1986), 41–67.
2 See Demos, 'Changing Faces of Fatherhood,' whose phrase 'father as abdicator' (63) very much captures the negative images considered here.
3 See Bryan Hogeveen, 'You will hardly believe I turned out so well': Parole, Surveillance, Masculinity, and the Victoria Industrial School, 1896–1935,' *Histoire sociale / Social History* 37, 74 (November 2004): 20–7 and Robert Rutherdale, 'Fatherhood and the Social Construction of Memory.'
4 Cynthia Comacchio, 'Bringing Up Father,' 304. See also Laura Johnson and Rona Abramovitch, *'Between Jobs': Paternal Unemployment and Family Life* (Toronto: Social Planning Council of Metropolitan Toronto, 1986).
5 See my *Finding Families, Finding Ourselves: English Canada Confronts Adoption from the 19th Century to the 1990s* (Toronto: Oxford University Press, 2006).
6 Christie, 'Introduction,' 15.
7 Canadian Historical Association, *Report*, 1970, 89–108. Child-advice books of every sort have been chock full of recommendations for self-discipline. See also the influential volumes by Canadian authors William E. Blatz and Helen M. Bott, *Parents and the Pre-school Child* (New York: W. Morrow and Co., 1929) and their *The Management of Young Children* (New York: W. Morrow and Co., 1930).

8  See, *inter alia*, Sandy Ramos, '"A Most Detestable Crime": Gender Identities and Sexual Violence in the District of Montreal, 1803–1843,' *Journal of the CHA*, n.s., 12 (2001): 27–48, 39–40; Steven Maynard, 'Rough Work and Rugged Men: The Social Construction of Masculinity in Working-Class History,' *Labour / Le Travail* 23 (Spring 1989): 159–69; and Joy Parr, 'Gender History and Historical Practice,' *Canadian Historical Review* 76, 3 (September 1995). See also Mark Moss, *Manliness and Militarism: Educating Young Boys in Ontario for War* (Toronto: Oxford University Press, 2001) and Angus McLaren, *The Trials of Masculinity: Policing Sexual Boundaries 1870–1930* (Chicago: University of Chicago Press, 1997).

9  See, *inter alia*, Michael Bliss, *A Canadian Millionaire: The Life and Business Times of Sir Joseph Flavelle, Bart., 1858–1939* (Toronto: Macmillan, 1978); *William Osler: A Life in Medicine* (Toronto: University of Toronto Press, 1999); *Right Honourable Men: The Descent of Canadian Politics from Macdonald to Mulroney* (Toronto: HarperCollins, 1994); and *Northern Enterprise: Five Centuries of Canadian Business* (Toronto: McClelland and Stewart, 1987).

10  This was later published as *A Living Profit: Studies in the Social History of Canadian Business, 1883–1911* (Toronto: McClelland and Stewart, 1974).

11  See Karen Dubinsky, *Improper Advances: Rape and Heterosexual Conflict in Ontario, 1880–1929* (Chicago: University of Chicago Press, 1993); Joan Sangster, *Regulating Girls and Women: Sexuality, Family and the Law in Ontario, 1920–1960* (Don Mills: Oxford University Press, 2001); and Steven Maynard, 'The Maple Leaf (Gardens) Forever: Sex, Canadian Historians and National History,' *Journal of Canadian Studies* 32, 2 (Summer 2001): 70–105.

12  Comacchio, 'Bringing Up Father,' 293. On the 'growing hegemony of the bourgeois family pattern among Canadian working classes,' see also Dorothy E. Chunn, 'Boys Will Be Men, Girls Will Be Mothers: The Legal Regulation of Childhood in Toronto and Vancouver,' in Nancy Janovicek and Joy Parr, eds, *Histories of Canadian Children and Youth* (Toronto: Oxford University Press, 2003), 188–206. See also Colin Howell's argument that 'the language of masculinity often transcended class divisions' in 'A Manly Sport: Baseball and the Social Construction of Masculinity,' in Parr and Rosenfled, *Gender and History in Canada*, 200.

13  See, *inter alia*, Franca Iacovetta, 'Making "New Canadians": Social Workers, Women and the Reshaping of Immigrant Families,' in Franca Iacovetta and Mariana Valverde, eds, *Gender Conflicts: New Essays in Women's History* (Toronto: University of Toronto Press, 1992), 261–303, and Iacovetta, *Such Hardworking People: Italian Immigrants in Postwar Toronto* (Montreal and Kingston: McGill-Queen's University Press, 1992). See also Adele Perry, *On the Edge of Empire: Gender, Race, and the Making of British Columbia, 1849–1871*

(Toronto: University of Toronto Press, 2001) for its important discussion of how race, notably 'whiteness' and 'aboriginality,' informed all discussions of gender competencies.

14 See Rutherdale, 'Fatherhood and the Social Construction of Memory,' 362–3. See also Veronica Strong-Boag, 'Canada's Wage-Earning Wives and the Construction of the Middle Class, 1945–60,' *Journal of Canadian Studies* 29 (1994): 5–25 for its discussion of the debates about 'working wives.'

15 Rutherdale, 'Fatherhood and the Social Construction of Memory,' 367. He has adapted this term from E. Anthony Rotundo's discussion of 'communal manhood' in *American Manhood: Transformations in Masculinity from the Revolution to the Modern Era* (New York: Basic Books, 1993), 365.

16 On the legal situation before the abolition of distinctions between the children of married and unmarried relationships see A.L. Foote, 'Family Organization and the Illegitimate Child,' in D. Mendes Da Costa, ed., *Studies in Canadian Family Law*, vol. 1 (Toronto: Butterworths, 1972), 45–66.

17 See Lori Chambers, '"You Have No Rights, Only Obligations": Putative Fathers and the Children of Unmarried Parents Act,' in Chambers and Montigny, *Family Matters*, 115–33.

18 Paul Sachdev, *Unlocking the Adoption Files* (Lexington, MA: Lexington Books, 1989), 147, 159.

19 Elizabeth S. Cole, 'Societal Influences on Adoption Practice,' in P. Sachdev, ed., *Adoption: Current Issues and Practices* (Toronto: Butterworths, 1983), 18–19.

20 'Re Lorena Jacqueline K. (No. 2) Feb. 19, 1992 (Ontario Provincial Court),' in Douglas W. Phillips, Ruth J. Raphael, Douglas J. Manning, and Julia A. Turnbull, *Adoption Law in Canada: Practice and Procedure* (Toronto: Carswell, 1995), 6–43. On the role of the Charter in family law see Susan Boyd, 'The Impact of The Charter of Rights and Freedoms on Canadian Family Law,' *Canadian Journal of Family Law* 17, 2 (2000):, 293–332.

21 On the complications and the misunderstandings of sexual relations in which women as well as men have exerted power see Karen Dubinsky, '"Maidenly Girls" or "Designing Women"? The Crime of Seduction in Turn-of-the-Century Ontario,' in Iacovetta and Valverde, *Gender Conflicts*, 27–66 and Dubinsky and A. Givertz, '"It was only a matter of passion": Masculinity and Sexual Danger,' in Kathryn McPherson, Cecilia Morgan and Nancy Forestell, eds, *Gendered Pasts: Historical Essays in Femininity and Masculinity in Canada* (Toronto: Oxford University Press, 1999).

22 Chambers, '"You Have No Rights, Only Obligations,"' 18.

23 On some of the implications of military bases see Saundra P. Sturdevant and Brenda Stoltzfus, *Let the Good Times Roll: Prostitution and the U.S. Military in Asia* (New York: New Press, 1992).

24 Newfoundland Provincial Archives, Files of Secretary of the Commission of Government, GN38, S6-1-7, folder 10, 'Child Welfare Act 1944,' Copies of Reports of Division of Child Welfare [typescript copies], Report of period January 1st to March 31st inclusive, no. 1 – 1946, 4.

25 Lori Chambers and John Weaver, '"The Story of Her Wrongs": Abuse and Desertion in Hamilton, 1859–1922,' *Ontario History* 92, 2 (Autumn 2001): 107–26. On the failure of many fathers to pay maintenance orders, see Andy Wachtel and Brian E. Burtch, *Excuses: An Analysis of Court Interactions to Show Cause Enforcement of Maintenance Orders* (Vancouver: Social Planning and Research, United Way of the Lower Mainland, 1981).

26 See R.W. Connell, *Masculinities: Knowledge, Power and Social Change* (Berkeley: University of California Press, 1995) and *Gender* (Cambridge, UK: Polity; Malden, MA: Blackwell Publishers, 2002).

27 On possible dangers for offspring, see Canada, Royal Commission on New Reproductive Technologies, *Final Report*, vol. 1, especially p. 42 with its reference to 'genealogical bewilderment.' On searchers see Susan McClelland, 'Who's My Birth Father,' *Maclean's*, 20 May 2002, 20–5, with its UBC student in search of her genetic father, a medical intern, and the award-winning Canadian documentary 'Offspring,' which featured the search of its director, Torontonian Barry Stevens, for his genetic father, in this case a lawyer. See also the story of Nobel laureate sperm in David Plotz, *The Genius Factory: Unraveling the Mystery of the Nobel Prize Sperm Bank* (New York: Random House, 2005).

28 Rose A. Hambly, 'A New Work of Mercy,' *Maclean's*, 15 March 1921, 64.

29 L.E. Lowman, 'Mail-Order Babies,' *Chatelaine*, April 1932, 26.

30 'Re Evans,' *Dominion Law Reports* (henceforth *DLR*), (1914), 218–23.

31 See Victor Malarek, *Hey Malarek!* (Toronto: MacMillan, 1984).

32 See 'Decotiis v. Lundquist [1986] W.D.F.L. 1681 (B.C.S.C.),' in Phillips, Raphael, Manning, and Turnbull, *Adoption Law in Canada*, 4–95.

33 'B. (C.) v. B. (R.) (1991), 91 Nfld & P.E.I.R. 271, 286 A.P.R. 271 (Nfld. Prov. Ct.),' in Phillips, Raphael, Manning, and Turnbull, *Adoption Law in Canada*, 4–113.

34 'G. (S.) v. G. (A.) (1991), 113 N.B.R. (2d) 158, 285 A.P.R. 158 (Q.B.),' in Phillips, Raphael, Manning, and Turnbull, *Adoption Law in Canada*, 4–111.

35 Barbara Melosh, *Strangers and Kin: The American Way of Adoption* (Cambridge, MA: Harvard University Press, 2002), 245.

36 Barrie Clark, *My Search for Catherine Anne: One Man's Story of an Adoption Reunion* (Toronto: James Lorimer, 1989).

37 Randy Shore, 'The First Supper,' *Vancouver Sun*, 27 October 2003, C1.

38 Lynn Kettler Penrod, 'Adoption in Canada,' Master of Laws thesis, University of Alberta, 1986, 258.

39 Welfare Council of Greater Winnipeg, 'Study of Services to Unmarried Parents in Manitoba,' 1 September 1960, 8. See also the indication that fathers were a recent concern in Alberta: *In the Matter of the Child Welfare Act, 1965*. Hearings held before His Honour Judge H.S. Patterson, Chairman Frank J. Fleming, Esq., and Mrs. W.F Bowke, vol. 3, at the Court House, Calgary, on 9 and 10 March 1965, 590.

40 Simma Holt, *Sex and the Teen-age Revolution* (Toronto: McClelland and Stewart, 1967), 93.

41 Harry MacKay and Catherine Austin, *Single Adolescent Mothers in Ontario: A Report of 87 Single Adolescent Mothers' Experiences, Their Situation, Needs, and Use of Community Services* (Ottawa: Canadian Council for Social Development, 1983), ix.

42 'Re Maat and Maat, Maat' and 'Maat v. Hepton and Hepton,' *DLR* 7 (1957), 488–502.

43 See 'P. (L.) v. H. (D.J.) (1986), 69 A.R. 327 (Q.B.), (reversed in part 1987), 10 R.F.L. (3d) 418, 55 Alta. L.R. (2d) 227, 81 A.R. 276 (C.A.),' in Phillips, Raphael, Manning, and Turnbull, *Adoption Law in Canada*, 4–50 and 5–51.

44 Anonymous, 'Whose Baby Is It, Anyway? Whose Rights Should Prevail, Mom's, Dad's, or the Adoptive Parents'?' *Chatelaine*, February 1993, 41–3.

45 'Interrupted Relations: The Adoption of Children in Twentieth-Century British Columbia,' *BC Studies* 144 (Winter 2004): 3–28; B. Bradbury, *Working Families: Age, Gender and Daily Survival in Industrializing Montreal* (Toronto: McClelland and Stewart, 1993); and D. Purvey, 'Alexandra Orphanage and Families in Crisis in Vancouver, 1892–1938,' in R. Smendych, G. Dodds, and A. Esau, eds, *Dimensions of Childhood: Essays on the History of Children and Youth in Canada* (Winnipeg: University of Manitoba Legal Research Institute, 1990).

46 'Smith v. Reed,' *DLR* 17 (1914), 59–63.

47 Tom Alderman, 'Fathers Know Best,' *Star Weekly*, 11 March 1972, 7–9.

48 'Children's Aid Society of Metropolitan Toronto v. Lyttle,' *DLR* 34 (1973), 127

49 'Re D.F.T. et al. and Attorney-General of Nova Scotia,' *DLR* 94 (1979), 680–6.

50 BC Royal Commission on Family and Children's Law, *Fifth Report* (March 1975), 90 and 6.

51 Margaret Lord, *Final Report to the Minister of Social Services of the Panel to Review Adoption Legislation* (July 1994), 57–8.

52 Audrey Marshall and Margaret McDonald, *Many Sided Triangle: Adoption in Australia* (Carlton South, Vict.: Melbourne University Press, 2001), 87.

53 'O'Driscoll v. McLeod (1986), 10 B.C.L.R. (2d) 108 (S.C.),' in Phillips, Raphael, Manning, Turnbull, *Adoption Law in Canada*, 4–9.

54  Kerry J. Daly and Michael P. Sobol, *Adoption in Canada* (Guelph: University of Guelph, May 1993), 81–2. For another negative decision see the case of 'Hobbs (Buck) v. Coradazzo (1984), 40 R.F.L. (2nd) 113, 54 B.C.L.R. 303 (B.C.C.A),' in Phillips, Raphael, Manning, and Turnbull, *Adoption Law in Canada*, 4–8.

55  'H.(R.) v. B.T. (1991) 36 R.FL. (3d) 208, 84 *D.L.R.* (4th) 24 (Ont. Prov. Div),' in Phillips, Raphael, Manning, and Turnbull, *Adoption Law in Canada*, 6–44.

56  'Re Smith and Koch,' *DLR* 67 (1976), 315.

57  'Re Sharp (1962), 40 W.W.R. 521, 36 D.L.R. (2d) 328 (B.C.C.A.), affirming (1962), 38 W.W.R. 257 (B.C.S.C.),' in Phillips, Raphael, Manning, and Turnbull, *Adoption Law in Canada*, 4–88.

58  'M. (C.) v. H. (H.), [1990] W.D.F.L. 1141 (Alta. Q. B.),' in Phillips, Raphael, Manning, and Turnbull, *Adoption Law in Canada*, 6–59.

59  See 'Waddell v. Hunter (1993) 48 R.F.L. (3d) 203, 84 B.C.L.R. (2d) 104 (S.C.)' and 'S. (J.W.) v. M. (N.C.) (1993), 10 Alta. L.R. (3d) 395 (Q.B.), affirmed (1993), 50 R.F.L. (3d) 59, 12 Alta. L.R. (3d) 379, 145 A.R. 200 (sub nom. D. (H.A.) v. M. (N.C.)), 55 W.A.C. 200 (C.A.), leave to appeal to S.C.C. refused (1994), 1 R.F.L. (4th) 60 (note), 15 Alta. L.R. (3d) lii (note) S.C.C.),' in Phillips, Raphael, Manning, and Turnbull, *Adoption Law in Canada*, 4–10 and 4–85.

60  Chambers, '"You Have No Rights, Only Obligations,"' 116.

61  Newfoundland Statutes, 1999, chap. A-2.1, An Act Respecting Adoptions, p. 215.

62  See John Demos's early reminder in 'The Changing Faces of Fatherhood' (46) that duty need not exclude affection.

63  Cynthia Comacchio, '"Postscript for Father": Defining a New Fatherhood in Interwar Canada,' *Canadian Historical Review* 78, 3 (September 1997): 395.

64  Michelle McColm, *Adoption Reunions: A Book for Adoptees, Birth Parents and Adoptive Families* (Toronto: Second Story Press, 1993), 60.

65  See Nancy J. Cohen, James Duvall, and James C. Coyne, 'Characteristics of Post-Adoptive Families Presenting for Mental Health Service,' in *Final Report* (Newmarket, ON: Children's Aid of York Region, January 1994), iv.

66  Nathan Dreskin, 'Why Fathers Are the Hardest to Adopt,' *Star Weekly*, 11 February 1961, 3.

67  See Cynthia S. Fish, 'Images and Reality of Fatherhood: A Case Study of Montreal's Protestant Middle Class, 1870–1914,' PhD thesis, McGill University, 1991; J.I. Little, 'Introduction' to *Love Strong as Death. Lucy Peel's Canadian Journal, 1833–1836* (Waterloo: Wilfrid Laurier University Press, 2001); and Robert Rutherdale, 'Fatherhood and Masculine Domesticity during the Baby Boom: Consumption and Leisure in Advertising and Life Stories,' in Chambers and Montigny, *Family Matters*, 309–33.

68  See BC, Superintendent of Neglected Children, *Annual Report for the Year Ending 31 March 1940*, 2.

69  Nora Tynan, 'The Christmas Baby,' *The Canadian Magazine*, 1907–8, 168. For a similar fictional portrayal see Lilian Leveridge, 'The Bachelor and the Baby,' ibid., November 1909–April 1910, 347–52.

70  A Social Service Worker, 'The Stupid Side of Social Service,' *Chatelaine*, August 1931, 6. See also Godfrey and Martha Bilton and the orphan Andy in Beryl Gray's short story 'The Stowaway,' *Chatelaine*, March 1932, 19, 51–3, in which a responsible father helps his wife overcome the loss of three children to illness by bringing home Andy, whom she nurses through scarlet fever. See also, for a similar general division of responsibilities along expressive-instrumental lines, but a divide that men are prepared to challenge in times of need, Jessie May Burt, 'Adopted,' *Chatelaine* April 1933, 14–15, 36–8.

71  James Wedgwood Drawbell, 'Experiment in Adoption,' *Chatelaine*, May 1935, 94 and 'Experiment in Adoption,' ibid, January 1935, 6–7, 35; February 1935, 18–19, 30, 46, 53; March 1935, 20, 32, 42, 44–5; April 1935, 26, 51–2, 65.

72  Rutherdale, 'Fatherhood and the Social Construction of Memory,' 356.

73  'Re McWhannel et al and Kerr,' *DLR* (3d) 46 (1974), 625–9.

74  'Re Wolfe and Cherrett,' *DLR* 89 (1979), 673.

75  Re F. (J.R.) (October 25, 1990), Dec. No. A32/89 (Ont. Prov. Ct),' in Phillips, Raphael, Manning, and Turnbull, *Adoption Law in Canada*, 6–44.

76  See esp. H. David Kirk, *Shared Fate: A Theory and a Method of Adoptive Relationships* (Port Angeles, WA, and Brentwood Bay, BC: Ben-Simon, 1984). On Kirk himself see Strong-Boag, *Making Families, Making Selves*, passim. For other examples see also Paul Grescoe, '"A Daughter – Or a Symbol?"' *Star Weekly*, 10 May 1969, 2–3, 4, 6; and P.A. Nowlan, 'Big, Happy and Varied: One Sackville Family's Story,' ibid., 10 March 1973, 6.

77  See Pierre Berton, *My Times: Living with History, 1947–1994* (Toronto: Doubleday, 1995) and Lawrence Martin, *Chrétien* (Toronto: Lester Publishing, 1995).

78  See Joan Givener, *Mazo De La Roche, The Hidden Life* (Toronto: Oxford University Press, 1989).

79  See Ethel M. Chapman, 'Could You Adopt a Baby?' *Maclean's*, December 1919, 116.

80  See Tom Warner, *Never Going Back: A History of Queer Activism in Canada* (Toronto: University of Toronto Press, 2002), esp. chap. 10, 'Legal Recognition of Same-Sex Relationships'; and David Rayside, 'The Fight for Relationship Recognition in Ontario,' in his *On the Fringe: Gays and Lesbians in Politics* (New York: Cornell University Press, 1998), 141–78. See also Suzanne M. Johnson,

*The Gay Baby Boom: The Psychology of Gay Parenthood* (New York: New York University Press, 2002).

81 Margaret Philip, 'Gaybaby Boom,' *Globe and Mail*, 3 May 2003, F4–5.

82 Colin Thomas, 'Babies without Borders,' *Georgia Straight*, 22–9 January 2004, 17–18, 22.

83 For discussion of adoption's radical potential see Judith S. Modell, *Kinship with Strangers: Adoption and Interpretations of Kinship in American Culture* (Berkeley: University of California Press, 1994), 237–8.

84 See, *inter alia*, Joy Parr, *Labouring Children: British Emigrant Apprentices to Canada, 1869–1924* (Toronto: University of Toronto Press, 1994).

85 'A Vicar Goes to Prison,' *Toronto Star*, 22 October 1898.

86 'Re Ontario Birth Registration No. 66-05-035455 (June 21, 1993), Doc. No. A930432 (B.C.S.C.), summarized at [1993] B.C. W.L.D. 1868 (B.C.S.C.),' 6-7 and 'Re Ontario Birth Registration No. 66-05-035455, RE (January 26, 1994), Doc. No. AD40033 (B.C. S.C.),' in Phillips, Raphael, Manning, and Turnbull, *Adoption Law in Canada*, 6-7-8.

87 Ray Aboud, 'A Death in Kansas,' *Saturday Night*, April 1986, 28–39.

88 See Barbara Hobson, *Making Men into Fathers: Men, Masculinities and the Social Politics of Fatherhood* (London, New York: Cambridge University Press, 2002).

89 See Susan B. Boyd, *Child Custody, Law, and Women's Work* (Toronto: Oxford University Press, 2003), esp. chap. 6.

90 Steve Whan, 'The Story behind the Stories,' *Rice Paper* 8, 4 (Fall 2003): 36–7.

# 9 Writing Religion: Some Influences on Twentieth-Century Developments in Canadian Religious History

BRIAN F. HOGAN

During the twentieth century Canadian religious history slipped its apologetic and hagiographic moorings to sail into the challenging seas of modern scholarly inquiry and critical discourse. This essay reviews some of the influences that stimulated a more research-oriented approach to such writing.[1] It is based on extended exposure to the field over the last forty years.[2] And it is inspired by developments in the cultural history of reading and writing, as epitomized in the *History of the Book in Canada* project.[3] At century's end the public, formal role of organized religion was less prominent than at the beginning. Still, religious activity, structures, and thought remained more than marginal to the life of citizen and country. For most, religion retained its enduring allure. For them it provides the normative narrative for engaging and negotiating life's passages. For many, particularly among the ranks of 'new' Canadians, religion provides the crucial context for encountering and interpreting cultural experience and expression. It accomplishes these tasks while continuing its traditional role of moderating gaps between persons, family, ethnic group, and larger society.[4]

The introductory section argues for the significance of the new, critical religious history within the Christian tradition. This form of research and writing, as opposed to the reductionist efforts too regularly trumpeted in dogmatic, enthusiastic, or ideological representation, is the essential handmaiden of memory. The opposite of accurate reconstructions, of course, are distorted representations, with their vitiating repercussions for all religious truth claims. In both the short and long term, such disproportionate, even deceptive, misrepresentations culminate in the loss of integrity and credibility. The following section, reflects on the enduring tension between faith and reason, and on factors that have skewed the relationship in the recent period. Consequently, I consider first the causes and then the central themes of the new critical history, including an accelerating concern for anthropology within religion with its attention to context. This points, finally, to the essay's conclusion concerning a right reading of religion. The article focuses on the Christian experience while acknowledging the significance of other faith traditions.

The central argument of this essay, the significance of accurate representation, flows from developments within Christian theological anthropology over the last two centuries. Theological investigation has increasingly tilted in the direction of exploring, at ever more refined levels, the complex of issues attending the human person as knowing, believing, relating, and, simply, being. Within the larger ambit of Christian theology, the focus on issues of anthropology expresses a monumental shift in emphasis. The change represents a turn away from religion understood almost exclusively as concerned with the transcendent – the sacred and divine seen as mystical and mysterious, perceived only as through a glass darkly – to religion understood as essentially and immediately concerned with the immanent implications of what it means to be a believing person, culture, and society.

The role that anthropology has recently played in modulating Christianity is strikingly reminiscent of that played by the social gospel a century ago, itself stimulated by the initial stirrings of the turn towards the created order in biblical and theological scholarship. Taken with Roman Catholic social teaching, the practices and discourses of the social gospel were likewise aimed at a renewed understanding and commitment to the service of the human person, within the full context of culture, place, and period. Practically, these concerns have propelled religious questions and inquiry into every corner of contemporary social, political, and economic activity and debate. This tendency runs counter to the secularist assumptions that emerged with the Enlightenment tradition. According to this tradition religion, within a modern society, is properly a private matter, rather marginal to the main activities of life and society, and should remain so. To the contrary, religious groups increasingly wrestle with the implications of faith beliefs for every area of human endeavour, including the social, the political, and the economic.

There exists, thus, a natural connection between the subject of this essay and the early work of Michael Bliss. His essay on the response of the Methodist Church to the First World War provides a striking example of just how quickly the religious imperative, in the face of momentous events, can be swayed, even sacrificed, on the altar of expediency. But above all, his extended service as the initiating editor of the University of Toronto Press's Social History of Canada series drew attention to many texts that exemplified a maturing encounter with exactly the kinds of issues referred to above. Moreover, the concerns addressed in these texts have fuelled a large part of Canadian social debate, and legislative activity, across the century with respect to such issues as health care, poverty, social welfare, education, and gender inclusiveness. The successful effort to recapture these texts, several decades later, provided fresh impetus and insight for contemporary investigations in Canadian social history.

The social-gospel texts insist on the essentially social nature of religious belief. Their inclusion in the social-history series underlines the fact. Their authors tried to be more or less objective, rather than descending to the hyperbole and propaganda that has characterized too much religious discourse. They did not, of course, eliminate exaggeration and distortion, but they did temper public debate by heightening expectations of civility and focusing on significant questions of immediate social consequence. Common social concerns threading through these texts helped to bridge sectarian divides and laid the foundation for a more tolerant society. In turn, this society has exhibited a welcoming attitude towards the increasingly heterogeneous mix of cultures and faiths that now defines its complexion.

An important dimension of nurturing this complex commonweal is the ability to chronicle its complexity in accurate and measured manner. Faithful representations of religious purposes, accomplishments, and failures as evidenced in the social-gospel experience and in continuing Canadian social-justice initiatives are a crucial component in the necessary, if seemingly Sisyphean, effort to craft such narratives. Where religion can draw on its root reserve as an essentially regulating enterprise, in the sense of providing communication and connection, it can serve itself and the broader commonweal. Calling on its own best tradition, the dedication to truth, it has the capacity to contribute significantly to the construction of larger narratives that, while more unifying than fragmenting, will hardly be uniform.

In short, the development of critical, research-based religious history is of crucial importance both for religious groups themselves and for society as a whole. At their worst, religious groups confronted with real or perceived attacks by the 'other' have exhibited an appalling and destructive penchant for dogmatic, literalist, and fundamentalist approaches to human and social problems, and they have betrayed their first principles. What results is the loss of integrity and credibility. At its best, religion witnesses to the human desire and capacity for connectivity, cohesion, and continuity, at personal and communal levels. Here, religious principles regularly recall individuals and groups to new levels of critical self-regard and re-direction. Reflection on the importance of first principles, such as the dignity of the person, serves as a powerful corrective to the ingrained human tendency towards self-interest, greed, domination, and exploitation.

To sum up this introductory section, it can be said that good, solid, historical writing deliberately eschews literalism, dogmatism, and the many distortions characterizing ideological rhetoric and advocacy. While all historians are tasked with the responsibility of accurately remembering, recreating, and representing the past, religious historians can arguably be held to an even higher bar of expectation with respect to accuracy of fact and balance of interpretation. The intent of this essay is to trace the evolution of higher standards and expectations, and to account for their implementation among religious historians, over the course of the century.

## Context – Religion's Transitions

In 1900 religion was Canada's central social reality. The Sabbath ruled: labour, leisure, and commercial pursuits paid obeisance to the dictates of a calendar moulded on the liturgical year.[5] Sunday was kept sacred for rest and worship. It was so recognized and protected in the law of the land, which foreclosed, in most instances, such leisure pursuits as sports activities, the cinema, and the theatre. Most major holidays were based on religious feasts or 'holy days.' Some measure of religious ritual was present as an integral part of most public events. Religious architecture dominated the cultivated landscape of both rural and urban Canada. In some areas, such as Quebec, health care, educational activity, and social services were almost totally subject to religious bodies. In almost all areas they were strongly influenced in origin and form by customs and codes derived from the Judaeo-Christian tradition. That tradition strongly informed the legal structures of the country, and also provided the primary content and direction for manners and morals.

In 1900 much religious writing took the form of apologetics. A defensive character derived from the potent mix of a triple endowment: first, the Reformation with its heritage of theological and social separations and conflict within Western Christianity; second, the Enlightenment with its insistence that rationality was the dominant, really domineering, aspect of human anthropology, with a derivative neglect of the affective, spiritual, and physical dimensions; and third, the apotheosis of expressive nationalism and capitalism with attending, and aggressive, linguistic, ethnic, racial, and tribal features. Too frequently across the century these aligned with a variety of reactive and bellicose ideological systems with a fateful affinity for militarism.

The strength of these three influences changed over the century. The multiplication of ecumenical and inter-faith initiatives assisted a gradual transition away from the aggressive apologetics and assertive missiologies characterizing the early period. This trend also helped to temper the third influence – tribal, racial, ethnic, and linguistic quarrels – which were themselves on the wane after 1970, notwithstanding their fresh resurgence in a variety of post-modern moments. As for the second influence, the relationship between faith and reason has been a constant, frequently difficult, attendant of the Christian religious tradition. But whereas in 1900 faith was ascendant, by 2000 its public place had diminished considerably. While the number of citizens who did not claim religious ties tripled between 1961 and 1991, Canadians remained wedded to the idea, at least, of religion. Some 88 per cent of respondents in the century's concluding census continued to claim such affiliation. Yet numbers alone are hardly the whole story. A generation's downward trend in regular communal observance suggests that religious ritual was honoured as much, or more, in the breach as in the observance at century's end. Still, the statistics denote a stubborn national insistence on at least a notional adherence, which is strongest in the Atlantic area of the country. It diminishes towards the West, to the point of lowest affiliation on the Pacific coast.

There can be no doubt that religion slipped from serving as the primary cultural phenomenon for many, even most, established ethnic groups. Still, it maintains a significant place, especially in marking such key transitional points as birth, marriage, and death. Illustrating the perception of the diminished role of religion is the example of the monumental *Canada Year Book, 1994,* which celebrated the seventy-fifth anniversary of the establishment of Statistics Canada. The seven-hundred-page, double-columned, oversized text refers to religion in only two places, devoting a total of twenty-seven lines to some brief, if informative, generalizations on an activity that continues to demonstrate a commanding institutional and associational presence.[6] This negligible coverage suggests significant cultural cleavage. It is impossible to imagine either government or the people tolerating such tokenism a century earlier.

Most Canadians, then as now, place themselves within the Judaeo-Christian tradition.[7] The primary cultural tension was between Protestants, viewed as central to the national narrative, and Catholics, viewed as less so. Limning this primary tension, exacerbated by the country's dominant linguistic cleavage, was the gradually increasing presence and significance of a broad variety of other religious groups. For its part, Canada's Jewish population was small in size, and mostly restricted to a few large urban areas, but it was also well established and represented institutionally and culturally.[8] There was far less organizational coherence or cultural expression among representatives of other world religions. But the seeds were already sown. Several such traditions had an established presence by the third quarter of the century and were of escalating significance in the final. Catholics also increased numerically. Among the curious discontinuities of the century is the fact that while religious enthusiasm and practice has declined within much of the 'established' culture, many more recent arrivals have shown an amazing affinity for the spiritual. Many of the newcomers, whose numbers increased with the end of the Second World War, and grew exponentially with adjustments in Canada's immigration laws in the late 1960s, came with intact experience and expectations of religion as an integral part of personal and social contexts. For many of these peoples, including Portuguese, Italians, Poles, Eastern Europeans, Central and South Americans, Filipinos, Indians, Goans, Vietnamese, Koreans, and Middle Easterners, religion plays a similar role for the bonding of people, culture, and community as it had earlier for French and British arrivals. For large numbers of these so-called 'new' Canadians, places of worship retain pride of place as vibrant spiritual, educational, and social centres.

It is within this context – decreasing religiosity and increasing diversity of religion – that we can best understand and interpret the change in attitude that occurred within the academy. At the outset, scholars seemed to be accelerating their distance from religion, though religion did retain a ceremonial role. By mid-century the distancing had evolved to an outright hostility in many parts of the Western world, especially in Communist countries. Simultaneously, religion disappeared from the educational curricula, a transition accomplished by the late 1960s. Complaints soon emerged that students were no longer capable of accessing their cultural tradition. There was a growing ignorance of fundamental scriptural texts and stories. Literary, historical, philosophical, and political texts replete with the characters, conflicts, values, and tensions established in the Hebrew and Christian scriptures were now experienced as 'awesome' in the worst possible sense.[9]

During the third quarter of the century, however, a counter-reaction began, characterized by a decreasing antipathy to religion within the academy. It gradually evolved to a general curiosity about religion as a phenomenon worthy of academic investigation. This transition spurred, and was in turn encouraged by, the establishment of departments of religion in many Canadian universities beginning in the 1960s.[10] Within a generation almost all major Canadian universities supported such activity. These departments exhibited a particular interest in world religions other than the Christian. In rather short order a basic attitude of hostility to religion evolved to one of probing inquiry. In the final quarter of the century this development kept pace with a gradual growth in religious observance generally. This embrace of religion as a legitimate area of inquiry nevertheless retained a prickly edge. On the one hand, religion was now resurrected, newly baptized, as an area worthy of academic inquiry. On the other, much of academia maintained its aversion to the methods, tasks, and terminology of theology, the traditional intellectual activity of 'doing religion' within the Western context. Ironically, such activity had been the very cradle of academia. The tension continues to distinguish university life.[11]

A final remark in this regard. Much of the notable progress that has distinguished twentieth-century religious historical writing must be attributed to the influence of the academy. It is true that the writings of Stephen Jay Gould, among others, have clearly illustrated science's propensity for the blindly dogmatic.[12] But it is also true that science has evolved a quiver of self-corrective procedures to tame and contain such tendency. History as an exercise in apologetics, ideology, jingoism, and propaganda still exists, of course. The difference is that the criteria for distinguishing and constraining such distortion are now clearly established wherever academic freedom obtains. The concern here is to chart and credit the higher standards of historical writing that have evolved and generally prevail. By mid-century, most religious historians were developing their formative skills within university rather than seminary environments. Their work quickly came to reflect the increasingly rigorous standards of the academy. As the century progressed, these persons and standards progressively permeated even church-affiliated institutions as normative. This was a positive development.

It is sufficient here to conclude that slippage in formal observance has been accompanied by more analytical self-examination. Such slippage, and the thinning of financial resources, quickened the desire to identify causes. These concerns provided powerful motivation for more discerning explorations of relationships between life within and without the sanctuary. It is especially noteworthy that such investigators are no longer restricted to the ranks of designated clerical hierarchies, but extend to many lay observers. In fact, by century's end, the vast majority of such researchers and writers were from the ranks of the laity, a complete turnaround within the century. This is a distinctly notable departure within the tradition, of elemental, though unexamined, consequence.[13] Here there is a compelling conundrum. The public role of religion has increasingly diminished since the 1960s, and formal observance has declined. Simultaneously, there has been a quickening level and sophistication of critical interest in the historical, social, and cultural role of religion.

## Factors Influencing the Growth of More-Critical Religious Writing

There were many routes to a more-critical religious writing. Taking a very broad perspective, the Renaissance and scientific revolution raised standards of evidence and logical argumentation. What emerged was an objective style of discourse, distinguished more by logical analysis than rhetorical device. Such discourse stimulated the establishment of standards by which investigators could measure the value and veracity of investigative techniques, methodologies, and conclusions. In turn, such standards and practices assisted in identifying and separating out truth claims based in fact and reality from those located in realms of fantasy, folklore, ideology, legend, superstition, and the outright fictive.

Much of this activity took place in voluntary societies dedicated to the investigation and advancement of specific areas of knowledge. Such societies, epitomizing modernity, have contributed greatly to advances in the hard sciences. They played a similar role in virtually every area of human knowledge. These self-regulating groups promoted research, critiqued methods, tested hypotheses, and compared results. They provided venues that favoured the exchange of ideas in the context of vigorous debate. As with meetings, so with publications: articles, reports, reviews, bulletins, and journals all embraced progressively rigorous editorial procedures.

The empirical method has produced astounding results for human progress and longevity, but it has also had the effect of exaggerating the rational faculty. Culturally, this tendency contributed to a serious diminishment of the value and place of other dimensions of human being and knowing, including the intuitive, mythical, and religious. What resulted was a seriously truncated anthropology. In turn, the diminished sense of person foreclosed a holistic epistemology. To some degree, rationalism's hostility for religious thought constituted a reaction to the profound sectarian passions that characterized much religious thought throughout modernity, from the wars of religion through to the lesser fires surrounding the Guibord Affair or the *Jesuit Estates Act* in late-nineteenth-century Quebec. The great scandals, the splits and separations within Christianity, were accompanied by a steady stream of vituperative exchanges between ecclesial entities. A repetitive diet of most un-Christian behaviours contributed to alienate many people from Christianity within the culture. One of the primary places of fracture was the academy. The previous, medieval period experienced a clear collaboration between altar and academy, tested frequently but abiding through time. The established tension between faith and reason was now weakened under the double assault of defensive, apologetic, religious literalism and aggressive, dogmatic, scientific rationalism. As the twentieth century dawned, the split between religion and science, and the scientific method, was an established phenomenon in the West.[14]

The social gospel saw the beginnings of something more fruitful. A broad recognition of the daunting tasks confronting a credible representation of religious belief was well established early in the century. Novel methodologies and departures in biblical and theological studies accompanied, and precipitated, these inquiries. This was, essentially, a historical accomplishment, recapturing elements of the deepest tradition of Christianity as against more recent assaults and accretions. It encouraged a desire for closer rapport and collaborative effort. What emerged was a deliberate desire to be less apologetic and aggressive, less defensive and hostile, and more tolerant. These shifts in fundamental attitudes stimulated and supported a novel theological departure, ecumenism, and, later, inter-faith dialogues. The result was a vast extension of areas for cooperative undertakings in the economic, political, and social spheres. Increasingly, Christians, and other religious groups, perceived that there were far fewer divisive issues than recent historical experience suggested.

The Catholic Church participated in this movement at the turn of the century, but broadly speaking, for Catholics it required the work of many decades to shuck off the cast of defensive separation that had progressively encapsulated the church after the sixteenth century. The Second Ecumenical Council of the Vatican, 1961–5, the first full council of that church since the sixteenth-century Council of Trent, provided the moment of emergence from the church's chrysalis stasis. This monumental sea change for Catholicism was firmly grounded on the rock of modern historical investigations.

The Vatican Council was but one moment in the continuing struggle to bridge the gap between faith and reason that proved to be a key challenge for all churches. The bridging was accomplished, in great part, through the introduction of a series of structural innovations, three of which I will consider here: the development of modern archives and of archivists trained in the proper care and maintenance of religious records; the preparation of teachers and preachers in the renewed categories of biblical, historical, ethical, and pastoral studies, equipped with the new historiographical methodologies; and the emergence of professional historical societies.

The teachers, preachers, and scholars imbued with the new critical spirit both fuelled and drew fuel from the proliferation of archives and professional historical societies. An interesting example of the elemental relationship that exists among archivists and historians is provided by the Canadian Baptist Archives, located at McMaster Divinity College in Hamilton. The Baptists of Ontario and Quebec established the Canadian Baptist Historical Society in 1865. That society founded the Canadian Baptist Archives, active for five years and aggressively soliciting manuscripts and memoirs before fading from view. Four decades later, in 1912, a reconstituted historical committee was again at work. Archival and historical endeavours achieved a new level of professional organization and institutionalized security as established by the historical committee after the Second World War. The appellation chosen in 1961 was the Canadian Baptist Historical Collections, adjusted a decade later to the Canadian Baptist Archives. Supervision was entrusted to an employee of the McMaster Divinity College.[15]

The historical societies, as the primary vehicles for scholarly discourse, provide the best perspective from which to view the emergence of the new critical religious history. Throughout the century, many societies devoted to the field were founded and flourished. Such societies offered a meeting place for professionals and amateurs to exchange ideas, papers, and research interests. They provided entry to the discipline for graduate students to test nascent oral and writing skills, along with an introduction to established members, research projects, and contacts for future research and employment. They supported the development of bulletins, journals, reviews, and, latterly, websites, to facilitate communication. Most important, they promoted the establishment of more rigorous academic and editorial standards for research and writing. Along the way, they offered academic prizes and scholarships, and honoured historical accomplishment, as a means of encouraging work in the discipline. They served to bridge specialized fields within the societies and between individuals in cognate professional areas. Finally, they were connecting points for like societies in other countries, nurturing the web of critical exchange that characterized the century. The societies modified the adversarial character of appropriate advocacy while honing skills to a finer edge. While so doing, they managed, mostly, to mollify internal anxieties concerning the abandonment, or diminishment, of vital dimensions of ecclesial traditions. The cumulative effect has been to lessen, greatly, the distance between religious and academic worlds.

Among such organizations, the Canadian Society of Biblical Studies (CSBS) is significant for several reasons. The Hebrew and Christian scriptures constitute the seminal texts for religious experience, expression, and reflection within all Jewish and Christian communities. Arguably, they are the most thoroughly studied texts in human history. The CSBS describes itself as 'the oldest humanities academic society in Canada. The Society provides a meeting place for those interested in all aspects of the academic study of the Bible – Hebrew Bible, Septuagint, New Testament – in its literary and historical context.'[16] The CSBS, like many of the societies mentioned here, holds its annual meetings in conjunction with other academic disciplines in the Congress of Canadian Learned Societies sponsored by the Canadian Federation for the Humanities and Social Sciences (CFHSS). This creative mix generates cross-fertilization among fields of learning. While the CSBS does not sponsor a specific journal, its membership supports access to other professional societies and their journals.

The Canadian Catholic Historical Association and La société Canadienne d'histoire de l'Église catholique (CCHA/SCHÉC) are two distinct entities, with separate executives, under a common umbrella organization, Historia Ecclesiae Catholicae Canadensis (HECC). They were created within the first year of its establishment. The presidency of this organization rotates between the two societies. The HECC also oversees the publication of articles accepted by each society in an annual journal, edited separately for each association. The immediate stimulus for the founding of the society was provided by the annual meetings of the American Historical Association (AHA) and the American Catholic Historical Association (ACHA), which chose Toronto as the venue for the celebration of their golden jubilee gatherings in 1932. The CCHA, formally founded in June 1933, has retained its incorporated name, though the title of its publication has changed over the years. Initially named *Report/Mémoires/Rapport* (1933–65), in 1966 the annual was re named *Study Sessions / Sessions d'étude*. The English section retained that appellation until 1984, when it became *Historical Studies*. For the 1990 volume SCHÉC changed its title to *Études d'histoire religieuse*.

From the initial 1933–4 publication the journal was professionally prepared and printed in typeset, bound format. It was primarily concerned with the publication of papers delivered at the annual meeting and treating of some dimension of Catholic history. During the final quarter of the century the publication policy shifted to focus exclusively on Canadian subjects. Further to enhance critical objectivity *Historical Studies* adopted a peer-review policy in 1988 and showed increased interest in welcoming papers other than those delivered at the annual meeting. In 2005 the editors adopted the 'double-blind' format common to academic publications as a means of advancing this objective. A second publication, the CCHA *Bulletin*, was introduced in the late 1980s, appearing in Spring and Fall editions that run between ten and twenty pages. It contains short articles, extensive book reviews, information about the society and the activities of its members, and news of other conferences, research projects, and the activities of cognate societies at home and abroad.

The 1964 volume of *Study Sessions / Sessions d'étude* included a new feature introduced by Michael M. Sheehan, 'A Current Bibliography of Canadian Church History.' The bibliography provided ease of access to the expanding literature in the field. Further, it served to track emerging sub-fields and specialties. The title was later adapted to 'Canadian Religious History,' thus reflecting the long-standing inclusive nature of the bibliography. The bibliography averages some thirty pages per year arranged within some nineteen categories. Its methodology, and the distribution of tasks to cover distinct geographical and thematic areas, is detailed in 'A Manual for Canadian

Religious Bibliography Collaborators.'[17] The silver anniversary of the founding of the societies occasioned the compilation of an integrated index to the contents of the first twenty-five volumes. This accomplishment was repeated to mark the golden anniversary, with the provision of indexes for each article in each language.[18] In 2004 Richard LeBrun completed the preparation of all English-language texts since 1933 for electronic access on the CCHA website, making the society one of the most 'wired' in Canada.

Initially, the CCHA and SCHÉC combined annual meetings in one location. Later the CCHA chose to hold its annual assembly with the gathering of the Congress of Learned Societies, while the French side remained with a stand-alone format. This choice enabled meetings of the SCHÉC to circulate among both smaller and larger Quebec centres, and thus to explore and encourage regional and local expressions of their subjects of study. Executive members meet once or twice a year to attend to HECC affairs. The societies held joint sessions on two occasions, in 1966 and in 1983, at St Paul University in Ottawa, to celebrate the silver and golden anniversaries of their founding. The later assembly led to the publication of a double volume of articles.

One of the great strengths of professional societies is their practice of periodically evaluating undertakings, matching intentions against accomplishments, noting strengths, weaknesses, new developments, and desirable directions. Michael Sheehan's presentation at the golden jubilee celebration of the two societies exemplifies this dimension of societal strength. He returned to the original intent of the societies, noting that 'the encouragement of research, the preservation of significant survivals from the past and the work of publication find equivalent statement in the French and the English versions.'[19] He traced the work of the societies, comparing CCHA choices and emphases with those of the older American Catholic Historical Association. In so doing he referred to self-critical assessments as a regular feature of the societies' work.[20]

In many ways the 1983 gathering, and the publication of the double volume, marked both the coming of age of Catholic history and a take-off point for such writing as a mature scholarly discipline. The quality of research and writing reflected in the articles profiles the advanced state of the discipline. Early sections dealing with the history of the societies, and reflecting on sources and historiography, epitomize a level of scholarly discourse impossible to imagine five decades earlier. A certain synergy had been attained, precipitated in great part by persons professionally prepared and established according to the highest contemporary standards. These now found a novel level of critical interest and reception within cognate disciplines across the academy. In the 1970s the CCHA's meetings began to include a joint session with members of the Canadian Society of Church History. This departure accompanied and supported the writing of religious history beyond narrowly sectarian lines, to include broader perspectives and considerations. Modelling this type of inclusive review, and without the rancorous edge formerly characterizing such writing, was the century's single effort to trace the whole history of Canadian Christianity. The Ryerson Press three-volume *History of the Christian Church in Canada (1966–1972)* reflected the novel character of writing in the field at the level of a major monograph.

There exist a rather large number of such sectarian societies at national and regional levels. Some have achieved a significant level of historical scholarship with the support of interested professionals. Among others, an inclusive list would include associations concerned with the Anglican, Lutheran, Mennonite,[21] Methodist, and Presbyterian traditions.

A fourth association of established prominence, with a mandate beyond the sectarian, is the Canadian Society of Church History (CSCH), founded in 1960. This is 'a non-denominational association dedicated to promoting and encouraging research in the history of Christianity, particularly the history of Christianity in Canada.'[22] The society, which meets annually with the Congress of the Humanities and Social Sciences, provides the central academic venue for religious historians to develop contacts and to exchange information on new and on-going areas of historical research. Commencing in 1967, papers presented at the conference, and submitted for distribution, were circulated to members in typescript format, stapled and taped, under the title of CSCH *Papers*. In 1991 the society adapted the title to read CSCH *Historical Papers*. By then the annual was presented in a regular-sized, bound journal format, providing for much easier cataloguing and retrieval. As with form, so with substance: the quality, breadth, and depth of materials have improved with the years, guided by ever more exacting editorial attention.

And, as with the CCHA, so with the CSCH. Members have welcomed the discipline of critical self-reflection and evaluation as a means of assessing and stimulating work in the field. In volume 10 (1979), John Moir reviewed 'The Canadian Society of Church History – A Twenty Year Retrospect,' while in the next annual three of the field's senior practitioners reflected on future challenges and opportunities.[23] The 1985 *Papers* carried two articles, by Thomas McIntire and Paul Dekar, echoing this thematic that emerged from a special forum dedicated to 'The Teaching of Religious History: Methods and Problems.'[24] That issue, marking the silver anniversary of the society, also carried a cumulative index of the published papers, prepared by John Moir and Paul Laverdure. In its first twenty-five years the society had published fifteen volumes of papers, totalling some seventy-two articles.[25] The four articles gathered from the 'Symposium on Objectivity and Commitment in Scholarship,' and published in the 1988 volume, indicate the continuing commitment to methodological and historiographical issues. Similarly, they exhibit a strong commitment to established criteria for measuring judicious scholarship while attending to appropriate dimensions of advocacy.

Beyond the Christian tradition, there is the Association for Canadian Jewish Studies (ACJS) / Association d'études juives canadiennes. This organization was established in 1976 as the Canadian Jewish Historical Society / Société d'histoire juive canadienne. 'Its goals are to encourage scholarly research in Canadian Jewish history, life and culture through academic disciplines. It is a national Association with an established headquarters in Montreal.' The ACJS is affiliated with historical organizations and institutions functioning at local and regional levels. A robust example of such regional organization is the Jewish Historical Society of Western Canada, founded in 1968, which has actively solicited materials relating to the settlement and expression of Jewish life. In 1999 the society was amalgamated with a museum and a Holocaust education centre to form the Jewish Heritage Centre of Western Canada. The association is a constituent organization of the Canadian Jewish Congress, and holds its annual meeting and conference in conjunction with the Congress of the Humanities and Social Sciences. The national publication representing these interests was the *Canadian Jewish Historical Society Journal*, vols. 1–10 (1977–88). In 1993 it was superseded by *Canadian Jewish Studies / Études juives canadiennes (CJS/ÉJC)*, the organ of the Association for Canadian Jewish Studies.[26]

A sixth organization, of dominant accomplishment and weight in the field, is the the Canadian Society for the Study of Religion / Société Canadienne pour l'étude de la Religion (CSSR / SCÉR), founded as a companion society to three existing associations: the older Canadian Society of Biblical Studies, the more recent Canadian Society of Church History, and the Canadian Theological Society. In 1971 these four bodies founded the Corporation for Studies in Religion / Corporation cana-dienne des sciences religieuses and initiated *SR: Studies in Religion / Sci-ences religieuses*, mandated to publish articles in the areas referred to above. *SR* is published seasonally. The corporation also publishes sev-eral series of books corresponding to certain sub-specialties. The society follows established standards for scholarly publishing in its academic work. An agreement between La Société Québécoise pour l'étude de la Religion (SQÉR) and the Canadian Society for the Study of Religion / Société Canadienne pour l'étude de la Religion (CSSR/SCÉR) was reached in 1991 in which the two organizations established a set of pro-tocols detailing their future relationship. In 2007 the CSSR/SCÉR serves as an umbrella organization for seven societies dealing with aspects of religious studies in Canada. Among its stronger points is its charter com-mitment to the whole field of religious research and reflection, thereby serving as a welcoming venue for writers across all faith traditions. A second telling feature is the reflective attention the society has paid to the evolution of Canadian religious studies. Publications in this area pro-vide a valuable historical record.[27]

The lead editorial in the first number of *SR* explained that the journal was intended to replace the *Canadian Journal of Theology*. It described the crucial distinction between theological and religious studies. At this time, the editorial explained, religious studies departments were now success-fully established within Canadian academia. The new organ was intended to reflect the broader concerns that these departments embod-ied, inclusive of, but not restricted to, the concerns of established organi-zations representative of Judaeo-Christian traditions. Within the Christian tradition 'first order theology' has been understood to be the actual practice and experience of the faith tradition. 'Second order theol-ogy' consisted of critical reflection on this experience. This distinction assists in illuminating the governing tension that now obtains in relations between altar and academy. The 'altar' fears that academic reflection on religion might be reduced to second-order theology. In other words, religious-studies activity could become, or rather, inherently is, an exer-cise of a strictly rational dimension. In the Christian tradition such activ-ity is considered to be authentic and integral only when connected to the life-blood of praxis, the heart of the matter. Severed from the sensible and expressive, it follows that such inquiry must, at base, repeat the funda-mental modern error of reducing the human to the rational.

For its part, the academy remains wary of first-order praxis as intrinsically uncertain and resistant to logical examination. At any moment religion can – in fact, by its very definition naturally must – encourage and exhibit behaviours beyond the strictly rational. Quite apart from anxieties induced by the exertions of enthusiasts, fundamentalists, and literalists, religion, from this viewpoint, is perceived to be a congenitally volatile mix, a very movable feast indeed. How then successfully to examine, comment on, and critique the phenomenon in a manner respectful of the standards of the academy? It is all too aware of the excesses and destructive expressions of religious movements and persons over the centuries, not to mention the last decades. In response, the academy exhibits a clear desire to shy away from any activity that might be perceived as supportive of anything less than clear, logical, defensible, in short, sensible activity. Still, rather to the surprise of many secular scholars, and confounding their prediction that religious studies would soon be confined to the terminal labours of pathology, religion resumed vigorous vitality towards the new millennium, particularly within North America.

The experience of religious studies departments over a generation exposed the essentially tautologous nature of the tension. An increasing recognition of the inherent values represented by each has given birth to a growing mutual, if wary, respect. As a result, over these decades a slow dance has evolved between elements of altar and academy in search of a more inclusive resolution. The budding relationship reflects a wary circling towards cautious embrace. It is like that of the proverbial porcupines, amorous of intent but mindful of past, prickly encounters. Over these decades, too, a double development has further shifted the grounds for the relationship. For their part, seminaries and theological schools, generally, have adopted exacting levels of scholarship, and far more transparent standards and practices.[28] On its side, the academy has been influenced by movements within culture and by the heightened awareness of the limits of the rational that have accompanied post-modernity. The combined effect is the promise of more reasonable exchanges into the future. This important achievement has been fostered in no small part at the cross-over points and labours of societies and of journals such as *SR*.

The extent and impact of these new, fruitful relationships have been further fuelled by other kinds of interactions: the local and the interdisciplinary. Beyond history, critical reflection requires exploration of developments in such disciplines as anthropology, ethnography, psychology, and sociology. These, and others, now have sub-disciplines concerned with the investigation of religious activity and influence at one or more levels. Their professional societies, journals, and other publication activities mirror that interest. Moreover, these professional interactions have been institutionalized at local levels across the country, in varying degrees. These expressions have led to the development of formal relations among university communities and contiguous seminaries and theological schools, particularly at the level of graduate research–based programs. In Vancouver, Toronto, Halifax, and many places in between, such relations have now been functioning for several decades.[29] All told, there has been enormous expansion of reasonable, critical discourse at myriad levels, a development that bodes well in the increasingly eclectic and globalized Canadian landscape.

## Seven Thematic Influences on Religious Historical Writing

This section considers seven central (but hardly exhaustive) movements and moments expediting twentieth-century religious writing: feminism, social theology, ecumenism, the Second Ecumenical Council of the Vatican, globalization, the march of 'isms,' and the shift to the subject.

First and perhaps foremost is the novel regard directed towards women, a regard both internal and external to women. While it is by no means only positive, it is overwhelmingly so. It is multi-faceted and irreversible and only just beginning. Many Christians perceive it as reflecting the engaging, empowering, and counter-cultural gaze of Jesus Christ, as related in scriptural accounts, and as almost immediately attenuated and alienated through successive cultural accretions and myopic structural expressions. In the first half of the century, women were enfranchised and recognized as full persons before the law. In the middle decades, spurred by war, they entered the public sphere and professions in increasing numbers. Along the way they came to enjoy a fuller voice, place, and connection within most religious groups, some of whom welcomed them to the ministries of service, celebration, and administration at every rank. Many Christian and Jewish groups were pioneers in perceiving, receiving, and expressing the implications of this regard. Others still struggle with a progressively improbable posture and dynamic. On the one hand, they profess the equality of every human person; on the other, they shore up structures of exclusion precluding the possibility of such recognition by entrenched denials of voice and role. The explicit anachronism constitutes a level of cognitive dissonance that is increasingly puzzling and invincibly alienating.

With the emergence of feminist and women's studies, research and writing around this theme was of primary significance in the twentieth century. Religious recognition and incorporation of this theme, or resistance to it, has been a defining trope of the time. The increased presence of women in the academy has been matched within the ranks of religious historians, archivists, and librarians. Women have encouraged new questions, perspectives, and research interests. Among academics who claim religion as their primary area of research and writing, Phyllis Airhart, Brigitte Caulier, Nancy Christie, Alison Prentice, Elizabeth Rapley, Elizabeth Smyth, and Marguerite Van Die are of established notice.

A second central thematic is the development of social theology and social ethics. This began with the social gospel, being characterized by cross-fertilization between the ivory tower and the practical order. This innovation found a progressively prominent place within Christianity and it quickened the transition from abstract, propositional theology to theological inquiry based on pastoral experience and perception, privileging praxis over theory. The movement welcomed the insights, methodologies, and critiques that the social sciences brought to religious inquiry and social commentary. These new tools provided a novel set of optics for both internal and external regard and evaluation.

Over the course of the century, the churches, albeit often with great reluctance, incorporated new forms and levels of self-reflection and critique. They often discovered internal contradictions that were deeply entrenched within administrative, theological, and operative levels of ecclesial life. Examined within a Gospel context and tradition, the subordinated role of women in church and society was one of the major areas illuminated as intolerable. But there were many others. Foremost were burning issues of militarism, racism, and genocide; religious, ethnic, and linguistic conflict; political and economic exploitation and injustice; and, generally, social and human development, including a host of medical, relational, and reproductive issues. All of these provided grist for mills that most found too slow in the grinding to satisfy the thirst for equitable social lives and structures, in short, lives rooted in justice initiatives.

The increasingly fruitful interactions between church, academy, and society are well illustrated by the work of Michael Bliss. On the one hand, he studied the social gospel himself in his earliest writing, itself some of the earliest academic scholarship on the topic. On the other hand, he founded and edited the University of Toronto Press's Social

History of Canada series between 1971 and 1977, when twenty-nine (of fifty-five total) titles were published. Perhaps the defining feature of the series was its recovery of the most generative texts of the social-gospel movement, texts that fundamentally shaped the country's social consciousness. Moreover, they framed the field for issues and platforms across the centre-left field of Canadian economic and political life well into the final quarter of the century, and their republication knitted together the century's two movements towards sociological thinking. The fifth title in the series was Nellie McClung's *In Times Like These*, written in 1915, a call for women's rights. In several other of her sixteen books the progenitor of Canadian feminism employed a common vehicle of the social-gospel movement, the novel, to explore a wide variety of social issues in compelling format. The succeeding title in the series, Herbert Brown Ames's *The City Below the Hill* (1896), utilized rudimentary sociology to provide a damning indictment of the conditions of poverty in one of Montreal's most blighted industrial districts. Bliss's monograph *Plague* later revisited the area, and many of the same issues, in his examination of the 1885 smallpox epidemic.[30] Works such as *The Wretched of Canada: Letters to R.B. Bennett, 1930–1935*, the first of the series and introduced by the Bliss himself, J.S. Woodsworth's *Strangers within Our Gates* (1909), Salem Bland's *The New Christianity* (1920), and F.R. Scott's *The League for Social Reconstruction: Social Planning for Canada* (1935) reflect the range of concerns, and the lasting imprint, that the movement made on church and society. Social theology continued to bear fruit late into the twentieth century, including the liberation theology of the mid-1970s, and it finds more recent expression in such internationalist movements as Christian Peacemakers.

A third generative movement was ecumenism, the desire for reunion of the Christian churches. The century's single most significant religious event, the 1925 creation of the United Church of Canada from the union of Congregational, Methodist, and Presbyterian churches, resulted from the marriage of ecumenism and the social gospel. Ecumenism cut off at the root layers of suspicion and hostility. Confronted by modernity, the churches' basic intent was to regroup in support of the primary mission of Christianity, the promotion of the Gospel. At bottom, the movement was driven not by complaisant attitudes of accommodation, nor by reaction against galloping secularist assumptions. The stimulus was much more elemental, a mission response based on vivid theological perception of fundamental Christian principles. This understanding stimulated religious organization and expression in support of human communities that would be fundamentally civil, equitable, and just across their social and economic structures. The process of coming to this understanding, and of then proceeding through the stages of responding to the tasks that lay beyond the realization, was enormously complex. At every turn, critical historical inquiry and reflection served to shepherd and support the endeavour. Full union did not prevail, but ecumenism dissolved generations of distrust and detritus. During the last decades of the century the lessons of ecumenical exchange among Christian churches began to be applied to a maturing range of interfaith dialogues.

The fourth theme worthy of mention here is the Second Ecumenical Council of the Vatican, convened in Rome for four sessions, from 1962 to 1965, after some five years of massive preparation. It represented an unprecedented scale of global participation, self-evaluation, critique, and renewal. Further, it signalled a coming to terms with modernity, with an attendant rethinking and re-phrasing of religious thought and expression, from liturgics and catechetics to biblical and theological inquiry. For Catholics the event marked a definitive turn from theology as primarily a deductive exercise to a more engaging, inductive, and empirical task, responsive to context and privileging praxis.

Protestant and Catholic social theology paralleled and informed one another through the century. The roots of the Vatican II experience lay in a variety of structures and activities loosely termed 'social Catholicism,' beginning with the late-nineteenth-century pastoral developed by Pope Leo XIII. The departure point was his revival of the Thomistic tradition within Catholicism. Catholic scholars renounced the static memorization of propositional texts, which had increasingly characterized, and traumatized, the tradition over the last centuries, and instead embraced theological methodologies reflecting the dynamic Thomistic methodology of critical, inclusive, theological inquiry, responsive to time and place. The broad historical labours associated with this effort gave birth to renewed confidence, a confidence that enabled the church to proceed beyond its reflexive hostility to new approaches and methodologies within biblical and theological studies.[31] What resulted were much more vibrant pastoral practices. The Council precipitated Canada's premiere theological event of the century, the Canadian Centennial Theological Conference, which convened at the University of Toronto in August of 1967. It was organized and hosted, on behalf of the Catholic episcopacy, by the Pontifical Institute of Medieval Studies (PIMS), located at the University of Toronto. Some of the greatest luminaries of contemporary Christian and Jewish scholarship were present.

Articles by Canadian scholars such as Fernand Dumont, Eugene Fairweather, Arthur Gibson, Bernard Lonergan, Roderick MacKenzie, Anton Pegis, and J.M.R. Tillard reflect the primary premise of the two volumes that resulted from the congress, that is, that contemporary theology had completed its long march from a deductive to an empirical science, the primary focus of modern scholarship. Throughout, the content and foci of the volumes represent the influence and impact of historical scholarship across the several disciplines constituting modern theological inquiry.[32] It was no accident that the Institute of Mediaeval Studies served as host. For more than a generation it had given vibrant example of meticulous attention to the canons of contemporary scholarship in its treatment of texts and contexts. The example was of immense significance for advancing historical and theological sciences within Catholic, and other, institutions. And the influence stretched well beyond the boundaries of North America. PIMS provided one of the most critical testimonies of Catholicism's capacity to recover its tradition of commitment to exacting scholarship.

The Council was, immediately, the work of the Roman Catholic Church. Its reflections, however, reverberated throughout the world. In large part it represented catch-up, and in many ways it was prophetic. In virtually all ways it was recognized as propaedeutic for the complex of pastoral tasks associated with 'going out to the whole world,' not in some aggrandizing imperialistic manner, as of yore, but fired with an inclusive and complete anthropology, respectful of the cultures and faiths of other peoples. Finally, it embraced a broad pastoral committed to the construction of peaceful human communities based on principles of justice and service. It was followed by a generation of papal and ecclesial statements addressing every conceivable political, economic, and justice issue in the modern world. Of immediate interest to this essay, there is universal agreement that the Council's accomplishments would not have been possible without the historical research and recovery of the previous century across virtually every area of the Christian tradition. Such scholarship was, not infrequently, interdisciplinary and ecumenical, as in the case of contemporary biblical tools and translations.

The intellectual awakening that culminated in Vatican II was married to a dynamic praxis. Such praxis was responsive to the predicaments and concerns of the century. And it was expressive of categories proposed by such philosophical movements as the existentialist, personalist, and phenomenological. From these predicaments and movements the scholarly effort received continual challenges and stimuli stemming from wars, ideologies, mushrooming demographics, and a confounding amalgam of aesthetic, medical, economic, and social irruptions. To them it contributed strategic scriptural and doctrinal data for critiquing and confirming such activities as appropriately integral to the tradition, or not.

The combined concerns of social theology and ecumenics, and the maturation of theological consciousness represented by Vatican II, contributed to a novel awareness of, and sympathy for, issues within the global arena. Globalization was a belated but nonetheless fundamental facet of twentieth-century religious thought and experience. Briefly, this included an attempt to escape from the strictures and structures of an essentially Mediterranean Christianity and an overly Eurocentric mindset, and to attempt to be more inclusive of the perceptions, experiences, and cultural constructs of other peoples. The theological expression of globalization consciously eschewed aggrandizement and encouraged alternative and novel attempts to think about religion and to organize structures and expression. It deliberately favoured the marginal and disenfranchised as central to the religious enterprise. All of this assisted the growth and development of interfaith dialogue and the very early stages for conscious reflection on the implications of living in one world with many faiths. Such dialogue and experience is not nearly as advanced as the ecumenical. But this area of writing reflects considerable development from the interpretive framing of such works as Charles Gordon's *The Foreigner* (1909) and J.S. Woodsworth's *The Strangers within Our Gates* (1908), on the cusp of the period, sympathetic though their intent.

Much of the comment, concern, vitality, destruction, and print of the twentieth century flowed from and focused on the amalgam of 'isms' that constitute a sixth thematic. These expressions appear to be legion. They have exhibited a repetitive pattern of excess and destruction. Singly, and in combination, these movements constituted an enervating wave of assaults on the fundamental integrity of the Western humanistic tradition. Frequently, they presented alternative world views in which religion and the mytho-poetic had diminished, if any, place. They have engendered continuous review and response in religious writing. The death throes of imperialism and colonialism through the first quarter of the century generated world war, inaugurating a century of militarism and massive violence. The inexactness, inadequacies, and exploitative greed of capitalism continued through the century. However, it exhibited far more resilience and capacity for self-correction and creative contribution than anticipated, particularly where corralled within the critical matrix of democratic regulation and legal market-place. Communism, fascism, Nazism, even consumerism, engendered religious crusade, and consumed oceans of ink. As with nationalism earlier, Marxism itself, and myriad expressions of socialism, were embraced as essential handmaidens to the religious imperative of build-ing a better world, reflective of the inaugurated kingdom. At the oppo-site extreme, they were vilified as seeds of the demonic, typifying the long legacy of invidious catalysts successively scarring the human land-scape. The march of the 'isms' generated a series of theological reflec-tions and pastoral responses, beginning with those of the social gospel.

Finally, the twentieth century exhibited a 'shift to the subject,' a tec-tonic trend of inclusive and incalculable consequence. The shift contin-ued a movement begun with the long-drawn-out demise of feudalism as an ordering of society distinctly hierarchical and patriarchal, and as highly reductive of person, at the levels of both rights and responsibili-ties. It was greatly encouraged by the Reformation and strongly influ-enced by multiple legacies of the Enlightenment. It has found expression in a broad range of political, legal, personal, and social enti-tlements enshrining 'rights' of every kind. Lastly, it has accelerated with the categories of post-modernity. Here there is novel regard for the particular, a sceptical eye for the meta-narrative as purblind, and a focused favouring of the marginal. The trend pushed the boundaries of the personal, as over against the social, towards some ultimate point, where the communal centre might well dissolve. Within the Judaeo-Christian tradition these influences combined to foster recovery of a fuller anthropology recognizing and claiming the biblical testimony of the human as 'made in God's image and likeness.' Recovery of the full implications of this revelation, particularly the focus on individual freedoms, has led to a renewed emphasis on the primacy and dignity of person. Overall, this trend has been highly touted by both church and culture. Conversely, dimensions of the post-modern moment, par-ticularly, have engendered strikingly negative reactions by some Chris-tian and other groups, placing many of the achievements of the above thematics in problematic, even parlous, circumstance. Balanced histor-ical scholarship will continue to be crucial in the long-term response to comprehending, interpreting, and catechizing the complex of issues attending this defining movement of the shift to the subject.

In the philosophical and theological fields, the shift was exhibited in a series of changed foci. These ranged from the transcendent to the immanent, the deductive to the empirical, and from community as all to person as primary. And they have probably engendered as much reactive prose as supportive. Attempts to explore and to order these new perceptions were rooted at basic levels of inquiry within such fields as anthropology, epistemology, and ontology. The 1970s witnessed a recombination of many of the formative concerns explored in the philosophical schools of the century, particularly existentialism, personalism, and phenomenology, with the categories of social theology. These were poised for the new departures expressed in political, liberation, feminist, and ecological theologies.

At almost every stage, the explosion of information and human knowledge outstrips efforts to organize and order critical reflection at the level of fine-tuning required by the rationalist categorizations of modernity. Increasingly, therefore, religious reflection is required to return to the grounded reality provided by some few fine principles within the tradition and then to test these at new levels of perception as providing an interpretive framework sufficiently fluid for engaging the challenges of the time within the ambit of fundamental – though not fundamentalist – religious teaching. Failing this formative task, the religious impulse successively falls prey to the seductive conclusion that error has no rights. In turn, this view degenerates to the converse, perverse, reading that right has no error. At this remove the heretic, or the other, is seen as always and only wrong. Of course, any action directed against such a person, up to and including demonization and termination, is religiously reconciled. Over against such posture of terminal righteousness, too common to the century, are examples of a countervailing presence represented by such leaders as Mahatma Gandhi, the Dalai Lama, Martin Luther King, Desmond Tutu, and Pope John XXIII. For the latter, the lens of a life lived against the blind violence of the first half of the century encouraged a significant departure from the time-honoured practice of righteous condemnation. He saw this as basically antithetical to the fundamental catechesis counselled by Christian teaching – lives of service, characterized by charitable activities and justice initiatives by way of reconciliation. His refusal to employ the vehicle of *anathema* at the Second Ecumenical Council of the Vatican was respected, though not without testing, by his successor and the Council itself. This recovery of the implications of an aphorism of Augustine, 'better a mind believing than a body bending', repudiates religion as refuge for crusade, ideology, triumphalism, and dominance; in fact, for any status other than celebration and service.

The thematic of the human person, his/her needs and rights, privileges, and responsibilities, authenticity and integrity, and the tension between selfless service and self-fulfilment has fuelled much of the century's reflection. It promises to remain the focus into the future, expressive of the enduring pull of person as primary within the necessary nexus of community. The tension mirrors the fundamental torque of Christianity. That is, the proclamation of a Messiah simultaneously human and divine, existing within a Trinitarian community of three persons, one God. The shift to the subject is the central insight of the century, doing much to explicate the other key thematics explored here, such as the novel perception, place, and self-regard of woman.

## Conclusion

For both person and community the discipline of critical self-reflection has featured prominently among the constants of Christianity. It has been expressed in myriad ways, including the formal Sacrament of Reconciliation (Penance) and mandated forms of spiritual counselling and direction. A wide varieties of liturgical, contemplative, meditative, retreat, and journalizing practices are prefaced by a moment of consciousness-examen for clarification intended to generate internal movements of contrition, conversion, and commitment to amendment. The moment is considered essential for the integrity of whatever acts of adoration, thanksgiving, supplication, or worship might follow. In short, self-knowledge as a healthy prelude to purgation and procedure on some more unitive way, within and without, has been an expected and highly respected part of the tradition. In fact, in most religious traditions self-knowledge is regarded as the basic departure point for authentic religious experience and credible expression. The point, of course, is not to diminish person or group. It is to build on the rock of certain self-knowledge rather than the swamp of illusion or self-delusion, occurrences too common to human affairs.

Bliss's review of the Methodist Church in the First World War provides striking illustration of just how wildly suggestible, and changeable, human beings and groups can be, even the best of them. Further, it reveals just how potent the religious impulse can be when married to emotive cause as crusade. The 1914 flip from pacifist proclivity to enthusiastic militarism occurred at warp speed. And this among the most rational, logical, and intelligent of citizens. And hardly just Methodists. Events of the century suggest that the example is all too typical behaviour. Within two decades many of Germany's leading theologians, the dominant schoolmasters of Christianity, would embrace the very worst features of National Socialism with startling vengeance. Correspondingly, religious leaders across the world adapted to the anti-Nazi crusade in almost seamless manner. And the Red Scare after that, when *kill a commie for Christ* expressed a credible response for followers of the Prince of Peace, righteousness eviscerating any sense of irony. Similar studies could range through the ranks of Catholics, Sikhs, Hindus, Jews, Muslims, and other faith groups, and find like response. In the face of threat and conflict, principle, perspective, and proportion seem regularly to fail. The limbic mind ascending, fear transcends and hormones trump belief with invincible facility. Currently, the incredibly popular *Left Behind* series effectively utilizes the most compelling of literary devices to convey a theological pastoral expressive of the most sensational dimensions of the apocalyptic motif. The series exploits violent conflict and focuses on destructive retribution to project a cosmology of ultimate despair, for all but a favoured fractional remnant. In many ways, the depiction is but a variant of repackaged nineteenth-century Social Darwinism manifesting the most pathological face of muscular Christianity. It is, and deliberately so, the antithesis of the social-gospel tradition, particularly as represented in literary form, and as concerned with personal salvation in the context of social amelioration. The series shocks. And it provides striking illustration of the need for solid and engaging historical scholarship across the landscapes of literary, scriptural, theological, and, most important, pastoral studies. The series might well be dismissed as a passing phenomenon of minor moment – except, of course, for the reality of the fresh-scrubbed face of dispensational premillennialism, the present pivotal point for much of American culture, politics, and diplomacy. It is a particularly potent brew. Solid history is hardly the total antidote. It does, however, provide firm grounding, established example, and certain criteria for testing the attractions, enthusiasms, and trials of the moment against the well-trod trails, and betrayals, of the tradition.

In the course of the century the writing of religious history has evolved from a level of pious advocacy, too easily exploited in moments of exceptional stress, to that of scholarly discipline. The evolution has occurred as the result of events and prods both internal and external to the churches. Where advanced, critical historical inquiry is seen to fuel refined, reflective correction for a right reading of religious passages. Where stymied, religion regularly exhibits a tendency to slip into stasis moments of locked rooms and hearts prefacing lockstep. The argument here is that such inquiry is vital to assist individuals and communities to transcend defensiveness, denial, and fear. And to establish clarity and conversion for engaging the many levels of reconciliation required by both personal and political passage through time. Michael Bliss's work on religion, and more generally his lifelong dedication to both rigorous academic scholarship and to writing books and newspaper articles for the widest possible public, exemplifies the contribution that such reflection can make to taming and containing an ingrained penchant for disproportionate representation and response.

In many ways the ministry of memory represented by historical labours exemplifies the corrective discipline of self-reflection. In so doing it provides a bulwark against hubris and tendentious disposition. If the labour seems Sisyphean, it is so in the ritualistic sense characterizing most teaching and preaching. Accurate, critical, and creative reconstruction and representation are constitutive of the establishment of engaging, enduring, and vital havens for humanity. Such representation is necessary to develop the discerning habit of perceiving the possible and necessary through the emotive fog of the moment. In the course of a century historians have ground the lens ever finer. The result is a more translucent optic for communities and culture to perceive that 'beauty, ever ancient, ever new.'

## NOTES

1 Unless modified, references are to twentieth-century Canadian religious historical issues and events. Similarly, 'Catholic' identifies the Roman Catholic Church or its members.

2 In 1963 Michael M. Sheehan initiated the annual *A Current Bibliography of Canadian Church History* project. It is published in *Historical Studies / Études d'histoire religieuse*, the journal of the Canadian Catholic Historical Association and La société canadienne d'histoire de l'Église catholique. This writer was responsible for its compilation from 1975 to 1992. In 2006 he completed the first edition of a cumulative database of some 20,000 items identified in the annuals: *A Bibliography of Canadian Religious History / Une bibliographie d'histoire religieuse du Canada, 1964–2005, BiCRH/BiHRC: 1* is available in three interactive formats: WordPerfect, Word, and PDF, either on CD or online at the website for the CCHA. A review of the field is found in Brian Hogan, 'Religious Bibliography in Canada, 1962–1992,' in *Third National*

*Conference on the State of Canadian Bibliography,* Charlottetown, PEI, 1992
(Toronto: Bibliographical Society of Canada and the Association of Canadian Studies, 1994), 393–414.

3 To prepare a summary review of twentieth-century religious publishing,
'Print and Organized Religion in Canada,' for the third volume, published
2007 (Toronto: University of Toronto Press), required reflection on religious
writing as a whole. What resulted was a series of templates intended to provide an initial organizational structure for all such writing.

4 An engaging exploration of the secular vs sacred debate can be found in
Stuart MacDonald, 'A Review of Dr. Reginald Bibby's Book: *Restless Gods:
The Renaissance of Religion in Canada,*' 2003. See website of the Presbyterian
Church in Canada (PCC), 'Current Realities,' Autumn 2005, http://www
.presbyterian.ca.

5 A recent examination of the Sabbatarian movement is Paul Laverdure, *Sunday in Canada: The Rise and Fall of the Lord's Day* (Yorkton, SK: Gravelbooks,
2004), xiii, 253.

6 *Canada Year Book, 1994* (Ottawa: Minister of Industry, Science and Technology, 1994), 82, 102. Statistics show an astounding 9.4% drop in religion as
occupational employment between 1989 and 1991 (211).

7 Ibid., 108.

8 The Jewish population, at 17,000 in 1901, had increased to 156,000 by 1931.
A strongly literate culture, Judaism has historically been committed to
intellectual pursuits. A reflection of this, including Canada's role in the
expression and recovery of Yiddish as a living language, is found in Adam
G. Fuerstenberg, 'Jewish Writing,' *The Canadian Encyclopedia* (1988), 2: 1109.

9 An established similar complaint dealt with diminished familiarity with the
classical Greek and Roman heritage.

10 An outline of this development is provided in Harold Coward and Roland
Chagnon, 'Religious Studies,' *The Canadian Encyclopedia* (1988), 3: 1850–1.
Reflecting interest in scriptural questions, as well as the heritage of Empire,
departments of Near Eastern Studies, or their equivalent, had existed for
some time. The 1951 creation of the Institute of Islamic Studies at McGill
University, however, represented a new departure.

11 See, for example, W.F. May, 'Why Theology and Religious Studies Need
Each Other,' *Journal of the American Academy of Religion* 52 (1984): 748–57.

12 Stephen Jay Gould, in *The Mismeasure of Man* (New York: W.W. Norton,
1981), provides graphic illustration of the limits, or abuse, of rational discourse. His historical review of the misuse of science to undergird the ideology of racist theories highlights one dimension of culture's capacity for
fixation on the fictive. The conclusion of the volume, however, illustrates

the enduring strength of the scientific method's capacity for self-critique, when the determination is present, or develops over time, to identify and debunk skewed views engendered by velleity and sustained by either ideology or outright villainy.

13  This change is dramatically evident among Catholic academics. In the early 1960s the Catholic Theological Society of America accepted only clerics as members. A generation later the vast majority of its members were from the ranks of the laity. A large portion of these were women. In the Western world in the last half-century, the preponderance of theological expertise passed from the minds of clerics to those of the laity.

14  A fine overview of this topic can be found in Gary B. Ferngren, ed., *Science and Religion: A Historical Introduction* (Baltimore: Johns Hopkins University Press, 2002), 401.

15  See website for the Canadian Baptist Archives: http://www.macdiv.ca/ students.baptist archives.php (Autumn 2005). Telephone conversation, Dr Gordon Heath, archivist and historian, McMaster Divinity School, 19 December 2005.

16  See website of the Canadian Society of Biblical Studies, http://www.ccsr .ca/csbs (Autumn 2005).

17  Brian F. Hogan, 'A Manual for Canadian Religious Bibliography Collaborators' (1993), 25.

18  Lucien Brault, comp., *Index to the Transactions of the Canadian Catholic Historical Association* (Hull, QC: Leclerc Printers, 1960), 248. Canadian Catholic Historical Association, *Index to the volumes of 'Report' (1959–1965), and 'Study Sessions' (1966–1983) of the Canadian Catholic Historical Association* (n.d.), 81, 91.

19  Michael M. Sheehan, C.S.B., 'Study Sessions of the Second Fifty Years,' CCHA *Study Sessions* 50 (1983): 59–71.

20  Sheehan identified these instances of this type of text: Arthur Maheux, 'Où en sommes-nous en fait d'histoire de l'Église canadienne?' *Rapport* 26 (1959): 13–18; Michael Sheehan, 'Considerations on the Ends of the Canadian Catholic Historical Association,' *Report* 30 (1963): 23–31; 'Table ronde' ('une discussion autour des objectifs poursuivis et à poursuivre par notre Société'), *Sessions d'étude* 38 (1971): 85–98; John K.A. O'Farrell, 'The Canadian Catholic Historical Association's Fortieth Anniversary: A Retrospective View,' *Study Sessions* 40 (1973): 61–8; Gaston Carrière, 'Les quarante ans de la Société Canadienne d'Histoire de l'Église Catholique,' *Sessions d'étude* 40 (1973): 25–32. Later instances of this type of review are Mark McGowan, 'Life outside the Cloister: Some Reflections on the Writing of the History of the Catholic Church in English Canada, 1983–1996,' CCHA *Historical Studies* 63 (1997): 123–33; and Brian Clarke, 'Writing the History of Canadian

Christianity: A Retrospect and Prospect of the Anglophone Scene,' CCHA *Historical Studies* 63 (1997): 115–22.

21  A reflection of activity within one denomination is found in Lawrence Klipenstein, 'Canadian Mennonite Writings: A Survey of Selected Publications, 1980–1995,' in *German-Canadian Yearbook*, vol. 14, ed. Hartmut Foeschle (Toronto: Historical Society of Mecklenburg, Upper Canada, 1995); Harry Loewen, 'Mennonite Literature in Canadian and American Mennonite Historiography: An Introduction,' *Mennonite Quarterly Review* 73, 3 (July 1999): 557–70; and Ted D. Regehr, 'Historians and the Mennonite Experience,' ibid., 443–69.

22  See website of the Canadian Society of Church History: http://www.Augustana.ca (Autumn 2005).

23  John Moir, 'The Canadian Society of Church History – A Twenty Year Retrospect,' CSCH *Papers* 10 (1979): 76–98; N. Keith Clifford, Paul Dekar, and John Webster Grant, 'Church History of Canada, Where from Here?' CSCH *Papers* 11 (1980): 1–10, 11–20, 21–5.

24  Thomas McIntire, 'Teaching Religious History in Three Academic Settings: Complexes of Correlations' and Paul Dekar, 'The Teaching of Religious History: Methods and Problems,' CSHC *Papers* 16 (1985): 79–87; 88–93.

25  Paul Laverdure, 'Preface, *Cumulative Index of* the CSCH, *Papers*, 1960–1984,' in CSCH, *Papers* (1985), 2.

26  See website of the Association for Canadian Jewish Studies: http://fcis.oise.utoronto.ca/~acjs (November 2005). *CJS/ÉJC* 1–11 (1993–2003).

27  Even apart from major monographs focusing on this work by region see, for example, Paul W.R. Bowlby, *Religious Studies in Atlantic Canada: A-State-of-the-Art Review*, The Study of Religion in Canada, vol. 6 (Waterloo, ON: Wilfrid Laurier University Press, 2001); William Closson James, 'Religion-and-Literature Studies in Canada: Then and Now,' *Studies in Religion / Sciences Religieuses* 30, 2 (2001): 193–205; Harold Remus, 'Religious Studies in Ontario, 1992 to 1999: State-of-the-Art Update,' *Studies in Religion / Sciences religieuses* 28, 2 (1999): 197–208. In Quebec a like attention is exhibited in Jean-Marc Larouche and Guy Ménard, eds, *L'étude de la religion au Québec: Bilan et prospective* (Sainte-Foy, QC: Presses de l'Université Laval, 2001).

28  In North America the Association of Theological Schools (ATS) has played a historically unprecedented role in this process.

29  Among these institutions, the Toronto School of Theology stands out as being of significant consequence well beyond Canada's borders. The complex level of interaction and integration with the University of Toronto that this body, and its constitutive parts, represents, is unique.

30 Michael Bliss, *Plague: A Story of Smallpox in Montreal* (Toronto: HarperCollins, 1991). The book regularly treats of the role of religious beliefs and leaders while exploring the negative consequences for the city attending linguistic and religious cleavages.

31 The 'simple' peasant pope, John XXIII, provided one of the most dramatic expressions of this sense of confidence in a moment of exceptional public candour. His opening speech at Vatican II was directed immediately to the 2200 cardinals and bishops gathered in St Peter's Basilica. In it he clearly chastised his primary counsellors as pursuing their administrative functions in too timorous a manner: 'In these modern times they can see nothing but prevarication and ruin. They say that our era, in comparison with past eras, is getting worse, and they behave as though they had learned nothing from history, which is, nonetheless, the teacher of life.' In two brief paragraphs Pope John effectively encapsulated the philosophical and theological accomplishment of the preceding century. He then laid down the primary principle for proceeding through the enormous complex of issues and tasks ahead. Not without tensions, it was that sense of confidence in grace as operative in this time and place, as through history, that provided the essential dynamism which characterized the Council. 'Pope John's Opening Speech to the Council, 11 October 1962,' in *The Documents of Vatican II*, ed. Walter M. Abbott (New York: Guild Press, 1966), 710–11.

32 Lawrence K. Shook, ed., *Theology of Renewal*, vol. 1, *Renewal of Religious Thought*; vol. 2, *Renewal of Religious Structures* (Montreal: Palm Publishers, 1968), 380, 480.

# Health and Public Policy

# 10 Personality, Politics, and Canadian Public Health: The Origins of Connaught Medical Research Laboratories, University of Toronto, 1888–1917

CHRISTOPHER J. RUTTY

On the eve of the official opening of the Connaught Antitoxin Laboratories and University Farm, some twelve miles north of the University of Toronto campus, the October 1917 issue of the *Canadian Journal of Medicine and Surgery* began a news item as follows:

> Down in an obscure corner of the basement of the Medical Building of Toronto University a great and important public work is carried on. It is great because there is no limit to its expansion. It is important because it is the most outstanding effort of Government organization on this continent to stop, with a scientific barrier, the encroachments of disease that claim a high mortality. And it is unique because its service is free as air and entirely untrammeled with red tape.[1]

From its humble origins in a backyard laboratory and stable in downtown Toronto in 1913, Connaught Antitoxin Laboratories soon evolved into the cornerstone of Canada's public-health infrastructure and a key player in the national and global control of many infectious and other diseases. Connaught is best known for its major contributions to the research, development, and large-scale production of an unusual range of biological products, including diphtheria toxoid, insulin, pertussis vaccine, heparin, penicillin, a variety of combined vaccines, and the Salk and Sabin polio vaccines, as well as its major contributions to the global eradication of smallpox.[2]

Connaught's central role in the insulin story is described in Michael Bliss's *The Discovery of Insulin*, albeit at the time he researched that seminal work, Connaught's archives had not yet been collected and catalogued. Bliss could thus only discuss Connaught's contributions in

limited detail, and hint at the major part the Labs would play in the
subsequent developments in insulin research, production, and distribution in Canada and globally. Little had been published on the history of Connaught Laboratories in 1982 when *The Discovery of Insulin*
appeared beyond a few short articles and a 1968 book by Connaught's
second director, Robert D. Defries, *The First Forty Years, 1914–1955:
Connaught Medical Research Laboratories, University of Toronto*.[3] However, in 1991–2, by the time I began to research my PhD thesis on the
Canadian polio story, under Michael Bliss's supervision, Connaught's
archives had been organized to a significant degree and I was able to
immerse myself in them to document Connaught's key role in the
polio vaccine story.[4] In the process, I discovered the broader and
largely untold history of the Labs and its significance to the evolution
of Canada's public health system. A postdoctoral fellowship that
focused on the history of Connaught, coupled with almost ten years of
providing historical research and creative and consulting services for
Connaught itself, have provided a rich opportunity to further explore
the dynamic history of this unique Canadian institution. I could not
have done it, however, without Michael Bliss's leadership, guidance,
and support. This essay, originally prepared during my postdoctoral
fellowship in 1999–2000, traces the origin of Connaught Laboratories
and the original Canadian foundation upon which it has grown.

Known as Connaught Laboratories during most of the 1920s through
to the 1940s, and as Connaught Medical Research Laboratories after
1946, the Labs remained a uniquely organized, non-commercial, and
self-sustaining part of the University of Toronto from 1914 until 1972,
when it was sold to the Canadian Development Corporation (CDC), a
federal Crown corporation, and privatized. By 1989 the CDC had
divested much of its interest in Connaught and Institut Mérieux of Lyon,
France, acquired a controlling stake in the company. By this time, Institut
Mérieux had formed an alliance with the Pasteur Institute.[5] Over the
next decade Connaught remained the Canadian component of what
became known as Pasteur Mérieux Connaught, which, in turn, was
owned by Rhône Poulenc, a French multinational chemical, agricultural,
and biotech company. In December 1999 Rhône Poulenc and the German pharmaceutical and chemical company Hoechst joined forces to
create a new pharmaceutical/biotech giant known as Aventis. In the
process, Connaught's identity changed in a significant way for the third
time since 1972. Pasteur Mérieux Connaught became known as Aventis
Pasteur, and its Canadian component became the 'Connaught Campus'

of Aventis Pasteur. However, within five years, Aventis was transformed into the even larger Sanofi-Aventis Group following the acquisition of Aventis by Sanofi-Synthélabo of Paris. The original Connaught identity thus shifted yet again to become the Canadian component of Sanofi Pasteur, the global vaccine business of Sanofi-Aventis.

While the Connaught name has been reduced to a subtitle, its identity as part of Aventis Pasteur, and now Sanofi Pasteur, clearly underscores the primacy of Louis Pasteur and the Pasteur Institute in the history of vaccines. The new names also serve to mark the important inspirational and practical role the Pasteur Institute played, especially through Dr John Gerald FitzGerald's (1882–1940) experience and network of contacts there, in the origin of Connaught and the unique place it held within the University of Toronto for fifty-eight years.[6] Indeed, FitzGerald had originally considered calling his new antitoxin laboratory the Pasteur Institute in the University of Toronto. No other university in the world had or has undertaken such an integrated and self-supporting public-health research, manufacturing, teaching, and public service–based biologicals distribution enterprise. Thus, the central question for this paper is, How and why did the University of Toronto assume responsibility for this unusual work in 1914? Moreover, the Pasteur Institute was created in 1888, quickly followed by the establishment of some forty similar private and state serum institutes in other parts of the world,[7] but not in Canada until the founding of Connaught. Why the delay?

## Connaught's Global Roots

The discovery of the Pasteur rabies treatment in 1885–6, and the subsequent founding of the Pasteur Institute in Paris in 1888, sparked a wave of institution building around the world focused, first, on preparing the new rabies treatment and, second, after the early 1890s, on producing the newly discovered diphtheria and tetanus antitoxins. These new public-health institutions were often based directly on the Pasteur Institute model; that is, a privately endowed, public dispensary of biological products, also focused on scientific research and teaching, and financially supported by the production and commercial distribution of biological health products.[8]

While the Pasteur Institute soon spawned a network of Pasteur Institutes around the world,[9] the Pasteur model also inspired a variety of other approaches to supplying the new biologicals. Initially, Pasteur had plenty of moral support from the French government to build his institute, but little of the financial kind. Elsewhere in Europe, particularly in Germany, the government played a much larger role in establishing and operating what became known as state serum institutes, most of which were also dependent upon varying levels of private philanthropy and public subscriptions to supplement the income they derived from the commercial sale of their products, especially to support research. Some institutes, particularly those that competed with one another in Germany, built close relationships with pharmaceutical companies to manufacture antitoxins and vaccines, while the institutes focused on testing, standardization, product development, research, and teaching. This was the case with the Paul Ehrlich Institute in Frankfurt and the nearby Hoechst firm.[10]

Encouraged by popular interest in the new life-saving products and the political and scientific rivalry between France and Germany, the Pasteur Institute and the Koch, Behring, and Ehrlich Institutes were established with minimal resistance from the public, the state, or the medical profession. The situation in Great Britain was quite different, as strong resistance from anti-vivisectionists, and thus political hesitation from the British government, frustrated the establishment of what became the Lister Institute of Preventive Medicine. There was also the specific desire among its founders to not form a centre similar to the Pasteur Institute. The dual goals for the British institute were to undertake scientific research into the causes, prevention, and treatment of diseases in man and animals, and also to supply biological products. But with minimal government funding or involvement, the Lister Institute was always hungry for endowments to pursue its research goals, and, as a production laboratory, was also expected to augment its income for research by the profits on its sales. The Lister Institute was therefore forced to take a market approach to distributing its products and compete with European commercial pharmaceutical companies. However, while it struggled for funding and public and political support, the scientific work of the Lister Institute ranked internationally with that of the other medical research institutes of the pre–First World War period, including the well-endowed Rockefeller Institute of New York.[11]

The impact of the Pasteur Institute and the other serum institutes it spawned was not felt in North America on a significant level until after 1895, when the New York City Department of Health, with much public and political fanfare, produced and administered the first supplies of diphtheria antitoxin on the continent.[12] Rabies was less of a problem in North America, and so there was little pressure to establish an official Pasteur Institute, or European-scale serum institutes, in the United States or Canada until the mid-1890s, when the effectiveness of diphtheria antitoxin had been established.

There was, however, a small and almost forgotten commercial enterprise established in December 1889 known as the New York Bacteriological and Pasteur Institute. Founded by Dr Paul Gibier, a former collaborator of Pasteur's, and with his agreement, the New York institute had no further links with Paris, however, and seems to have disappeared by 1917. During its existence, this small North American Pasteur Institute published a journal, *The Bulletin of the Pasteur Institute*, served as a rabies treatment centre for the United States and Canada, and was one of the first companies to produce and market the new antitoxins in North America. Indeed, in 1894–5, Gibier's institute was the source of serum for the first Canadian tests of diphtheria antitoxin in Toronto and Montreal.[13] There is also evidence of a Pasteur Institute in Chicago, which opened in July 1890, although little more is known about it.[14]

In North America, it was the increasing threat of such epidemic diseases as cholera that catalysed the establishment of public health boards at the state, provincial, and city levels from the 1830s on, albeit not always on a permanent, professional, or scientific basis. In New York City, the 1892 cholera epidemic prompted the city government to establish an independent diagnostic and bacteriological research laboratory under the leadership of Dr H.M. Biggs and Dr W.H. Park, the latter man becoming the North American authority on diphtheria antitoxin production. This expertise was quickly transferred around the United States, initially to Philadelphia, the Massachusetts State Board of Health, and the Hygienic Laboratory of the Marine Hospital Service (the forerunner of the U.S. Public Health Service) in Washington, DC.[15]

It was not long after Park's first diphtheria antitoxin was produced that several large pharmaceutical companies, such as Parke, Davis and Mulford Laboratories, began to produce the new biological wonder drugs on a large scale for the North American market, including Canada.[16] Park's New York City Health Department Laboratory was able to produce and distribute antitoxin and other biologicals as a free public service until the 1930s, despite the often strong opposition of doctors, politicians, and the pharmaceutical industry. Their resistance stemmed from a new encroachment of the state into the private business and profits of physicians and drug companies. Such opposition resulted in the Philadelphia Health Department abandoning biologicals production by 1904.[17] In 1903, when faced with similar commercial pressures, the Massachusetts State Board of Health responded aggressively to charges from the pharmaceutical industry of poor quality and primitive biological manufacturing conditions by arguing that, while not perfect, the serums produced by the state government were 'standard in everything but price. The state produces this at a cost of less than twenty-five cents a bottle. The druggists charge something like two dollars a bottle for what they sell.' Moreover, 'the difference between a public and a private laboratory is that the first finds its chief incentive in the service of science, while the second is of necessity primarily concerned with making money.'[18]

## Canadian Roots

The economic and state versus industry issues debated in Massachusetts do not seem to have been a major concern in Europe. However, in a reflection of long-standing cross-border trade and political concerns, these economic and commercial issues resonated among Canadian doctors, as well as the public, during the early years of the new century.

In 1905 diphtheria antitoxin was the focus of a lively discussion at a meeting of the Ontario Medical Association. Some Ontario doctors were still unconvinced of the serum's value, despite the experience of ten years, particularly, it was stressed, in the city of Chicago. In Ontario the antitoxin had been imported by the Provincial Board of Health from American pharmaceutical companies since 1894–5. Nevertheless, the diphtheria death rate in the province remained as high as 12 per cent. In reporting on the OMA meeting, the *Canada Lancet* stressed, 'This we think should not be the case; and we fear is due to the expense of the antitoxin placing it beyond the reach of some of the poorer patients. In such cases we think the municipality should supply it. We know of many instances where the doctor supplied it rather than see the patient die.'[19] A year later, in an editorial focused on 'Discovery and Commercialism,' the *Canada Lancet* found it remarkable that the discoverer of diphtheria antitoxin, Von Behring, received nothing for his discovery, yet commercial manufacturers had made millions out of it, while the public had been 'charged a very long price for the serum.' It was suggested that 'such a discovery as this should be placed under the highest authority in the government of the country. Why should manufacturers be allowed to grow rich from Behring's serum, and pay nothing for it?'[20]

This was a position that the editors of the *Canada Lancet* had taken since 1895, when the concern was less about price and more about quality control. An editorial noted how the Canadian medical profession, in light of recent experience with 'the fads of the German and French physicians,' was 'a little shy of the serum therapy.' 'Will the profession not be liable to the perpetration of fraud by those who may desire to speculate?' To ensure that 'we are procuring anti-toxine in the blood serum that we may demand,' the journal suggested 'that the Government take hold of this matter and employ salaried officials to carefully prepare and preserve the serum as it may be demanded. The test of the value of the serum now before us is by no means reliable.'[21]

In 1895 the *Canada Lancet* hoped that the federal government would assume this responsibility. However, despite strong lobbying, in particular by such Canadian public-health pioneers as Dr Edward Playter from as early as 1874, a Dominion Department of Health would not be established until 1919.[22] In 1866 the prime minister appointed Dr Frederick Montizambert as director general of public health. However, his mandate was primarily the quarantine of immigrants.[23] While several other federal departments had an interest in health matters, albeit primarily animal and plant health, it remained practically and politically impossible for Ottawa to make any focused effort towards producing a Canadian supply of anti-toxins or controlling the quality of the many drugs that were imported.

The only government in Canada with any chance of supplying anti-toxins at this time was that of Ontario, in particular its Provincial Board of Health. The board was established in 1882 and by the 1890s had assumed a progressive posture towards controlling infectious diseases. Smallpox was of particular importance, especially in the wake of the great 1885 epidemic in Quebec and Eastern Ontario, and the Provincial Board was able to secure a local supply of vaccine from a farm in Palmerston.[24] The board then set up, in 1890, the first of a network of provincial laboratories, which focused on bacteriological and chemical work. The Ontario laboratory predated New York City's and all but four other government laboratories in North America. However, the earlier U.S. city and state labs were largely focused on testing food and water, while investigating rabies outbreaks was among the first projects tackled by the Ontario laboratory.[25]

The Ontario Provincial Laboratory was as much a product of what Sandra McRae has called the 'scientific spirit' of medicine at the University of Toronto[26] as it was of any particular scientific or medical policy of the Ontario government. Echoing the close scientific, personal, and physical ties between the biology and medical faculties since the early 1880s, especially with respect to laboratory research, the origins of the Provincial Laboratory, and later Connaught, reflected the converging interests of key members of the Provincial Board of Health and professors of medicine and 'sanitary science' at the nearby provincial university. Practical laboratory demonstrations in sanitary science began in the medical faculty in 1889, while the first bacteriologist of the Provincial Laboratory was Dr J.J. McKenzie, a former assistant of Professor Ramsay Wright in the university's biology laboratory. Indeed, after first locating at Yonge and Queen Streets, the Provincial Laboratory shared space in the University of Toronto Biological Building, then in the new Medical Building after it opened in 1903, before settling into its own government facility at number 5 Queen's Park in 1911. Dr John A. Amyot succeeded McKenzie in 1900, and in 1910 was also appointed part-time professor in the newly created Department of Hygiene and Sanitary Science at the university. In 1904 the Medical Faculty had recommended that a Diploma in Public Health, or DPH, be established; however, with no facilities for courses, only didactic instruction in hygiene was given to undergraduate students between 1906 and 1910.[27]

The establishment of a department of hygiene at the University of Toronto coincided with several other important events in 1910 that were critical catalysts to Connaught's origin. Under circumstances not unlike those leading to the founding of the Pasteur Institute itself, in early 1910 the worst rabies epidemic in Ontario to date prompted strong lobbying from Canadian doctors, especially the Toronto Academy of Medicine, for the establishment of a Pasteur Institute in Toronto. While the medical men approached the Ontario cabinet for action, it is significant they asked that 'such an institute should be established in connection with the University.' As the Canada Lancet stressed, 'If such an institute was established it would be possible to obtain the serum, which cannot be exported from the United States.' Otherwise, victims of the 'mad dog scare' had to travel across the border to New York City for the Pasteur rabies treatment.[28] 'Needless to say, this incurred a much greater expense than most people can afford.' In 1910 the Provincial Board of Health found itself in a better position to respond. A sum of $1000 was quickly secured to provide for rabies treatments at two special clinics at Toronto General Hospital and the Hospital for Sick Children, the treatment being given by medical staff of the Provincial Board for a fee of $25 per case to cover the cost of vaccine specially imported from the New York City Health Department.[29]

In 1910 there were also increasingly vociferous calls, particularly from the Canadian Medical Association, for Ottawa to establish a national health department, an issue the CMA, and others, had pressed on and off in Ottawa over the previous decade.[30] There was also a proposal from the chief inspector of immigration, Dr P.H. Bryce, who had been the first secretary of the Ontario board of health, for a National Institution for Scientific Research, modelled after the Pasteur Institute. Among other duties, the Canadian institute would prepare serums, vaccines, and other health products for plants, animal, and man.[31] Neither proposal was successful, although the federal government did establish a Health Branch for the newly created Conservation Commission, to which Dr Charles Hodgett was appointed medical adviser. (Hodgett had succeeded Bryce as secretary of the Provincial Board of Health in Ontario in 1903.) This commission had no executive powers and served merely an advisory role for Canadian governments, with Sir Edmund Osler, brother of the famous Sir William Osler, presiding over its Public Health Committee.[32]

Hodgett's position as secretary of the Ontario board of health was given to Dr J.W.S. McCullough, a long-time member of the board, who was also appointed chief officer of health and deputy registrar-general for the province.[33] From these positions, McCullough implemented many of the public-health reforms he had often spoken about, including establishing full-time district health officers and compulsory smallpox vaccination, when the Ontario Public Health Act was passed in 1912.[34]

In 1910 McCullough, along with Hodgetts and Amyot, had been among the founders of the Canadian Public Health Association. The new association published the Toronto-based Public Health Journal as its official organ.[35] Canada's governor general, the Duke of Connaught, who had a close interest in public health, served as official patron of the CPHA and presided over its inaugural congress in Montreal in December 1911.[36] Among the conference's recommendations was a call for federal supervision of biological products.[37] This was a more politically acceptable resolution than had been proposed a few months earlier, when the federal government announced that it was about to establish a national laboratory in connection with a new federal department of health. The proposal, which originated with the Conservation Commission, suggested that a federal laboratory 'would provide a cheaper and purer supply of bacterins, antitoxins etc in Canada.' It would also enforce standards, provide means for experimentation with new medical discoveries, and also cover a wide field of educational work relating to health conservation. While the idea was greeted with great interest, the *Canadian Journal of Medicine and Surgery*, nevertheless, concluded, 'It would be a mistake, however, for the Canadian Government to organize and run a factory for the manufacture and sale of human biological products, in opposition to well-organized private concerns.'[38]

While the editors of the *Canadian Journal of Medicine and Surgery* felt confident in the stability, quantity, and quality of the antitoxins produced by American pharmaceutical companies – advertising revenues from which were supporting its publication – others were not so sure, especially about the long-term stability of the U.S. biologicals supply and, more important, about its price tag for those who needed their life-saving benefits the most. Dr John G. FitzGerald was one Canadian doctor increasingly uncomfortable with this situation in 1911, but he was not yet in a position to do anything about it.

## FitzGerald's Canadian Public Health Plan

Born on 8 December 1882 in the rural village of Drayton, Ontario, the eldest son of Alice and William FitzGerald, a pharmacist with Irish roots, the tall, slim, red-headed John Gerald FitzGerald sought early to rise above his obscure origins and become a doctor. He wasted little time, and in 1903 became the youngest yet to graduate from the University of Toronto Medical School, although he soon found himself frustrated by the suffering he encountered in practice. Yielding to what would become his characteristic restlessness, enthusiasm, and ambition – characteristics also of a manic-depressive condition that would underlie both his creative genius and the self-destructive tendencies that would surface later in his life, tragically leading to his suicide in 1940 – he signed up as ship surgeon on the *S.S. Philadelphia* in 1904. Whether or not he sensed his own psychiatric condition and hoped to be able to do something about it, FitzGerald turned his attention to psychiatry and the study of nervous and mental diseases and their prevention. He interned at the Buffalo State Hospital in 1904-5 and then worked at Sheppard Hospital in Baltimore and Johns Hopkins Hospital until late in 1906. He then returned to Toronto to become pathologist and clinical director at the Toronto Asylum for the Insane, also working as a demonstrator in the Department of Psychiatry at the University of Toronto during 1907-8. But, as one of his friends later wrote, 'the young man's restless mind could never be content with any activity savouring of routine.' Perhaps also growing frustrated with the limited individual results that he could achieve in psychiatry, despite his energy and campaigns for significant institutional reform, FitzGerald shifted his interests in 1908 towards pathology and the revolutionary subject of bacteriology while spending a year as a research student at Harvard University. He returned to Toronto in 1909, this time ready to lecture on bacteriology at the University of Toronto.[39]

Much as 1910 was an important year for public health in Canada, it was also significant for FitzGerald, both personally and professionally. He was married in April 1910 to Edna Leonard of London, the heiress of a foundry fortune, and shortly after their wedding they sailed for Europe. FitzGerald would spend his summer as a research student at the Pasteur Institutes in Paris and Brussels, establishing close friendships with Émile Roux, director of the Paris institute, as well as other European leaders in the field.

When FitzGerald returned to Toronto he was eager to apply what he had learned. In early 1911 he single-handedly set up a Laboratory of Serum Diagnosis in the University's Department of Pathology and Bacteriology, offering to the medical profession a variety of diagnostic testing services, as well as a supply of rabbit serum.[40] However, not long after announcing his new laboratory service, FitzGerald was offered a position as associate professor of bacteriology at the University of California in Berkeley.[41] By the summer of 1911, FitzGerald was back in Europe for more postgraduate study, this time based in the pathological anatomy department of the University of Freiburg in Germany. During both summers, FitzGerald also spent time at the Lister Institute, as well as at the New York City Department of Health and other city and state laboratories on the American east coast, likely before and/or after his trans-Atlantic voyages.[42]

FitzGerald was no doubt impressed and inspired by what was being done with biological products produced by these institutions. However, he was also aware of their limitations with respect to funding, research, and distribution, their relationship to universities and public health education, as well the prices of their products, whether within a commercial market or if bought and distributed as a free public service by government health departments. While in California, FitzGerald was able to assimilate his recent experience, but he was eager to apply it, preferably in Canada, and pick up where he had left off with his efforts to provide a diagnostic service and serum supply within the University of Toronto.

In the spring of 1913 FitzGerald got his chance when Amyot invited him to return to Toronto to assist with the production of the Pasteur

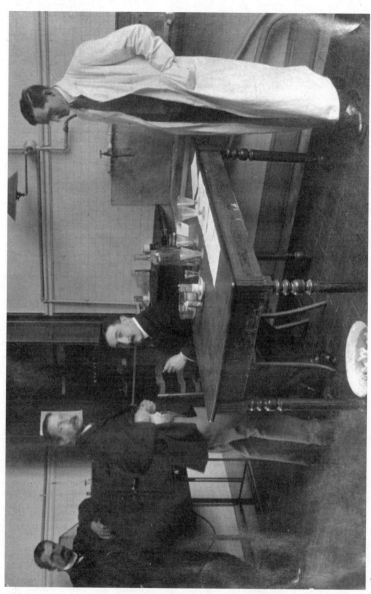

Dr John G. FitzGerald (in white lab coat) at the Pasteur Institute, Brussels, summer 1910. (James FitzGerald / SP-C Archives)

rabies treatment at the Ontario Provincial Laboratory and, if sufficient funds were raised to pay his $350 per month salary, to assume the position of part-time associate professor of hygiene at the University of Toronto.[43] Despite receiving a new endowment of $25,000 per year in 1913 to support medical research from 'some of Toronto's wealthy men,' the University of Toronto was actually in poor financial shape when FitzGerald returned. He was eager to carry out the plans that he had formulated while away, the success of which depended upon the support of the university, which was running a deficit.[44]

During the summer of 1913 FitzGerald focused his energies on working with Amyot and his assistant, William 'Billy' Fenton, to produce the first made-in-Canada supply of the Pasteur rabies treatment, FitzGerald taking advantage of his unique connections with the New York City Health Department for supplies, advice, and moral encouragement.[45] By August, while he and Fenton were preparing the rabies vaccine, FitzGerald began to ask his many contacts about the actual costs of producing antitoxins on a large scale. He discovered that, for example, the New York State Health Department, which gave antitoxin free upon the demand of any physician, was able to produce a purified diphtheria antitoxin, ready for filling, for between 5¢ and 6¢ per 1000 units.[46] FitzGerald saw no reason that he could not produce antitoxins for a similar price, with the facilities and support of the university, and make such biologicals available to the Provincial Board of Health at cost for free distribution to the public.

By the fall of 1913, enough money had been raised for FitzGerald to assume his part-time university appointment in the Department of Hygiene,[47] which by this time had graduated its first student to complete the full DPH course, Dr Robert D. Defries.[48] In 1911 the first DPH from the department had been granted to Dr H.V. Hill, who was given his diploma based only on his extensive public-health experience. Hill went on to help establish the Institute of Public Health at the University of Western Ontario in 1911,[49] leaving the Toronto Faculty of Medicine wondering whether or not it was worth investing in the necessary facilities and staff if many potential graduate students went down the road to London. In the fall of 1912, with the university ready to abandon a DPH course, Defries applied, which, together with pressure on the faculty from Amyot and McCullough, ensured that the course was given. FitzGerald was later appointed. McCullough had just implemented the new Ontario *Public Health Act*, an important part of which was the hiring of full-time district health officers across the province.

He needed qualified candidates quickly, all of whom would require a DPH. The demand for DPH graduates would also soon grow across the country, and Amyot, FitzGerald, McCullough, and Defries all saw an important national role for Toronto's fledgling Department of Hygiene, an educational role that was also important to the plan that FitzGerald was developing. In the fall of 1913 four candidates registered for the Toronto DPH course, which was taught by FitzGerald, with Defries assisting as demonstrator.[50]

During that fall, FitzGerald, without consulting with the board of governors, took advantage of an offer by Billy Fenton to help build a small stable and laboratory behind his house at 145 Barton Avenue, near Bathurst and Bloor Streets in what was then west Toronto. FitzGerald borrowed from his wife's inheritance to pay for the construction and necessary equipment, in addition to five horses, purchased for $5.00 each, and that would serve as the real antitoxin factories.[51] After spending just under $3000, by early December the modest wood-frame stable and laboratory covered with tin was ready and four of the horses, 'Crestfallen,' 'Surprise,' 'Fireman,' and 'J.H.C.' were given their first of many small but increasingly larger doses of diphtheria toxin.[52] By the end of March 1914, after producing the first batches of Canadian-made diphtheria antitoxin since January, which the Provincial Board of Health had already bought, FitzGerald formally approached the university's board of governors with what seemed to be a radical proposal.[53]

**Building a Public-Health Factory**

It has often been suggested that FitzGerald's proposal for the University of Toronto to assume responsibility for his antitoxin production enterprise was a 'revolutionary' one for the university to accept. While it clearly was unusual to expect a university to operate a biologicals factory, it is, however, evident that the University of Toronto, as the provincial university, was open to just such an idea. As a 1928 *Maclean's* magazine article on the Connaught story noted, 'Fortunately, the University of Toronto is not entirely ruled by precedent or manacled by convention.'[54] Indeed, by virtue of its 'scientific spirit' and the close personal relationships between the Faculty of Medicine and the Provincial Board of Health, the university had already been suggested as a home for a Canadian Pasteur Institute in 1910. FitzGerald was thus confident that he would have the support of the board of governors,

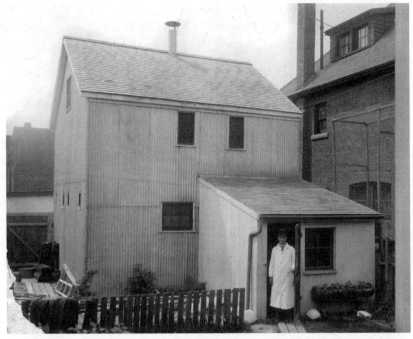

Barton Avenue Stable, backyard of 145 Barton Ave., Toronto, home of William Fenton (standing in doorway), 1913. The birthplace of Connaught Laboratories. (SP-C Archives)

especially of Sir Edmund Walker, chairman of the board, Sir Edmund Osler, and Sir Robert Borden, president of the university. The only limiting factor seemed to be whether or not the university could afford to fund FitzGerald's ambitious plans.

On 31 March 1914 FitzGerald wrote to Edmund Osler, detailing how much had been spent to date building the Barton Avenue stable and preparing antitoxin, how much had been earned already from the Provincial Board of Health, and how much was anticipated from sales to health departments in the City of Toronto and elsewhere across Ontario and Canada. He noted that at least $6000 was necessary for the university to take over the work, while 'an additional like amount should be available to meet the initial cost of a small place in the country at the earliest possible moment.' Under these circumstances, FitzGerald was confident that 'the work will be self-supporting within three to six months, probably less,' especially as the Provincial Board was prepared to undertake distribution at once. However, FitzGerald knew that he could not carry the work any further personally, but 'it can be done in the University, under University auspices only if funds are available.'[55]

Before taking the matter to the board, President Falconer let FitzGerald go ahead and make the necessary modifications in the Department of Hygiene, which then consisted of FitzGerald's office on the ground floor of the Medical Building's north wing, and a 'Museum of Hygiene' in the basement. However, since funds were tight at the university – it required $1,400,000 from the province but would still run an $85,000 deficit in 1914 and expected a $120,000 deficit in 1915 – Osler provided at least $500 of his own money to cover the immediate expenditures of converting the Museum of Hygiene into a laboratory.[56] On 23 April 1914 a special committee of the board of governors met to discuss FitzGerald's proposal. With Osler's personal and financial backing, and an expectation that the university would eventually provide funding, the committee recommended establishment of an 'Antitoxin Laboratory in the Department of Hygiene,' effective 1 May 1914.[57] There is some evidence, however, suggesting that FitzGerald had originally considered calling the laboratory the 'Pasteur Institute in the University of Toronto.'[58]

While the University of Toronto had agreed to assume official, and eventually, financial responsibility for the new Antitoxin Laboratory, it is clear that FitzGerald's enterprise would actually receive very little, if any, direct funding from the university. FitzGerald had desired to create a self-supporting organization, and much to the delight of the university bursar struggling with a deficit, he was never a financial burden. Even after FitzGerald was officially appointed director of the Antitoxin Laboratory, it was expected that his salary would be paid out of its operating expenses, the university being responsible only for his position as associate professor of hygiene.[59]

Over the first few months of the Antitoxin Laboratory's official existence, FitzGerald focused on expanding the modest facilities Amyot had managed to find in the basement and sub-basement of the Medical Building, converting the old Museum of Hygiene into a general laboratory, a bacteriological lab, and a room for sterilizing glassware, and adding space in the sub-basement for, among other things, processing blood plasma and packaging and storing finished products.[60] FitzGerald also worked on expanding the output and range of products, including typhoid vaccine, tetanus antitoxin, and anti-meningitis serum to meet demands from British Columbia and elsewhere, and developing a capacity for research and enlarged facilities for teaching. As he concluded in his first annual report as director of the Antitoxin Laboratory for the period ending 30 June 1914:

The value of the laboratory is thus greatly enhanced, since the Public Service aspect is made to go hand in hand with teaching and research, a combination possible only when the work is being done in connection with the University. It is the hope of those responsible for the Laboratory that it may in this way be possible to gradually develop in Canada, laboratories analogous in scope to those of the Lister Institute in London and the Pasteur Institute in Paris, Brussels and elsewhere.[61]

After a productive summer, the sudden onset of the First World War at first threatened to end FitzGerald's ambitious plans prematurely. However, the conflict quickly provided an opportunity for the fledgling laboratories to rapidly expand. In November 1914, surprised at the unexpected impact of wound infections, the British Expeditionary Force ordered that all wounded soldiers be given prophylactic doses of tetanus antitoxin as soon as possible, an order also given by the other armies on both sides of the front. A severe shortage of tetanus antitoxin ensued shortly, despite the efforts of serum labs in the United Kingdom, France, Germany, and the United States. As Defries described the situation to the university governors at the end of January 1915, 'not a fraction of the necessary amount was available,' since the entire output was spoken for in advance by the Allied Powers. Defries, who had quickly become FitzGerald's right-hand man, especially directing tetanus antitoxin production, outlined a plan whereby over the next five to six months, the Antitoxin Laboratory could produce enough serum for every Canadian soldier for 65¢ a dose, compared to $1.25 a dose, which was the lowest price at which the Canadian Red Cross could purchase it from the New York City Health Department. The proviso was that expanded stables and laboratories were needed as quickly as possible.[62]

President Falconer and the board of governors quickly approved the plan, Falconer telling Prime Minister Borden that it was a 'patriotic duty that we in Canada should manufacture tetanus antitoxin for our own expeditionary forces.' The board, however, was unable to provide the $3000–$4000 that was immediately needed, suggesting that it was up to FitzGerald to raise the money. Falconer had already approached a number of wealthy Toronto men for support, who suggested that the Dominion government should meet this war-related cost. McGill University had already received special grants for war work, so when Falconer asked Borden for a federal grant of $4500, he noted that no new precedent would be established.[63]

Shortly after Falconer had made his appeal to Ottawa, Colonel Albert E. Gooderham, a local distiller and member of the university board of governors, as well as chairman of the Ontario Red Cross Society, visited Falconer's office after a board meeting. He immediately wrote a cheque for $3000, on the condition that the money be used to provide facilities for the preparation of tetanus antitoxin so that a supply might be made available to the Canadian Red Cross. After thanking Gooderham, Falconer recognized that he had a potential problem should the Canadian government grant additional funds and then find that the Red Cross was given the entire output of antitoxin.[64] Although he considered withdrawing the university's request for a grant from Ottawa, by late February he decided to ask for $5000 instead of $4500 after he found out that the federal government was well supplied with antitoxin for the short term.[65]

The potential conflict was averted by early March after FitzGerald arranged to immediately supply the Red Cross with 5000 packages of antitoxin that he was able to purchase from the New York City Health Department at a special reduced price. In the meantime, Gooderham's $3000 gift would be used to equip the Antitoxin Laboratory for producing a Canadian supply by August. The federal grant would also be used to expand the laboratory facilities, but if the government needed a supply before August, FitzGerald would also use his connections to buy it from New York City at a similarly reduced price.[66] Once the federal grant was finally received in May, Falconer returned Gooderham's cheque as FitzGerald expected that the Antitoxin Laboratory would be able to produce enough antitoxin to meet the needs of both the Canadian military and the Red Cross by August.[67]

By this time, however, Gooderham had offered a much more valuable gift in support of FitzGerald's enterprise. Shortly Gooderham wrote his $3000 cheque, Falconer suggested that he visit FitzGerald to learn more about his plans, as they had never actually met one another. Gooderham immediately arranged to see FitzGerald in his office in the Medical Building, and after a ninety-minute discussion about his plans, FitzGerald showed Gooderham around, including a boiler room in the basement where he planned to stable the extra tetanus antitoxin horses. Gooderham did not think much of that idea and said to FitzGerald, 'I suppose for twelve or sixteen thousand dollars it would be possible to purchase a

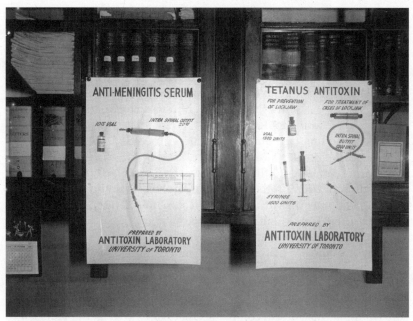

Essential First World War biologicals: Antimeningitis Serum, Tetanus Anti-toxin, Antitoxin Laboratory, University of Toronto, 1916. (SP-C Archives)

few acres of land on Yonge Street and build a stable and some laborato-ries there.' A few days later Gooderham asked that FitzGerald meet him at the offices of Stevens and Lee, architects, to review some preliminary sketches Gooderham had asked be done, on his own initiative, of the lab-oratory and stable buildings he was offering to build once a suitable site was found. To this end, in early April 1915, Gooderham once again gave FitzGerald a phone call, asking him to take a car trip, along with Gooder-ham's real estate agent, up north to York township. The agent had already heard about a possible site on the York-Vaughan town line at Dufferin Street in what was once the village of Fisherville. After making the twelve-mile drive along dirt roads, they found a long, derelict fifty-six-acre farm property that included a farm house, bank barn, and a dis-used chopping mill. FitzGerald saw no need to visit any other properties. Gooderham then asked his agent to track down the owners and find out their price, but told him, 'Don't let them know that I am interested in it.' Gooderham was anxious to complete the sale and proceed with erecting the new buildings, both to expedite the production of antitoxin and because he was planning to leave for England shortly, and, concerned about the war, he asked his son to carry out his wishes should he not be able to return.[68]

The war situation also prompted FitzGerald to enlist in May 1915. Fortunately, he did not have to go to the front, at least not yet, but was assigned to take charge of the Bacteriological Unit at the Camp Niagara training camp, a posting that enabled him to devote part of his time to directing the Antitoxin Laboratory.[69] While plans for the new farm building were finalized and construction proceeded, the stables of the old Ontario Veterinary College were offered, at no charge, by Dr King Smith, to accommodate the extra fourteen horses assigned to tetanus antitoxin production. In the meantime, diphtheria antitoxin production continued and the output distributed across the country, from St John's to Victoria, FitzGerald stressing in his second annual report that 'the support accorded the laboratory has greatly exceeded the most sanguine expectations, and its place in the scheme of public health activities is Canada made manifest.' His staff had grown from six to sixteen, five of whom worked exclusively in the new Tetanus Branch.[70] By the end of 1915, however, FitzGerald's unusual enterprise was being noticed by the American pharmaceutical companies that were no longer able to sell as many of their antitoxins and vaccines in Canada.

In early December 1915 it was evident that representatives of certain companies were spreading rumours, similarly to what had occurred earlier in American cities and states that distributed antitoxins as a public service, that the University of Toronto products were prepared by non-competent students, their stables and labs were not properly equipped, and their products were not as potent and caused more reactions than the commercial products. Dr E.J. Banzhoff, of the New York City Health Department, who had been in almost daily communication with FitzGerald since the beginning of the Antitoxin Laboratory, had frequently heard such rumours and rallied to FitzGerald's defence.[71] Calgary's medical officer of health, Dr C.S. Mahood, had been visited by one of these representatives and later wrote to Banzhoff, as well as a number of other health officers and hospitals in Canada that had been using the Antitoxin Laboratory products.[72] The Ottawa Board of Health had recently received its first supply and found that there were some reactions, but they were no worse than from any other source.[73] The experience of the Riverdale Isolation Hospital in Toronto was similar, its medical superintendent, Dr M.B. Whyte, stressing to his Calgary Hospital counterpart, Dr A. Fisher, 'I believe it is everyone's duty to support the project undertaken by the University of Toronto, whose aim is not to profit by the manufacture of Antitoxin but ultimately to have the cost borne by the Provincial Governments and Antitoxin distributed free of charge to the people. I believe this will shortly be done by the Ontario Government and we have Dr. FitzGerald and the University of Toronto to thank for the efforts put forth by them to obtain this end.'[74]

On 2 December 1915 Falconer received a letter from FitzGerald outlining the proposal from the Ontario board of health that McCullough had prepared, offering to distribute the products of the Antitoxin Laboratory for free across the province. As FitzGerald noted to Falconer, this would make the university laboratories the official source of public-health biological products in Ontario and practically eliminate commercial firms, at present, competing in Ontario. For FitzGerald personally, 'This marks the second step in the plan I had in mind when I first undertook this work and its culmination at this early date is a source of considerable gratification. I think we may look to the future with a reasonable certainty that the new stables and laboratories will have a definite place in the scheme of public health endeavors in Canada.'[75] Ontario's free distribution plan began on 1 February 1916, a month after FitzGerald purchased the cattle stock and remaining vaccine supply from Dr H.B. Coleman's Smallpox Vaccine Farm in Palmerston.[76] After its first year the cost of Ontario's free distribution program totalled $40,000, about a quarter of what an imported commercial supply would have cost.[77]

By the fall of 1916 the new farm property was largely occupied and its small staff focused on an expanded level of antitoxin production for the war effort and the home front. However, it was not yet ready to be officially handed over to the university until 25 October 1917, which happened to be Gooderham's wedding anniversary.[78] During the months leading up to the official opening of what was to be called the 'Connaught Antitoxin Laboratories and University Farm' – named after Gooderham's friend, patron of the Canadian Public Health Association, and former governor general, the Duke of Connaught – FitzGerald was focused on securing more autonomy for the laboratory. Specifically, he wanted the authority to engage or disengage staff as necessary, without reference to the board of governors.[79] He also wanted to secure the future of the 'Connaught Laboratories Research Fund,' to which all future surpluses from the sale of products were to be segregated from general university funds, and the income from which would support research in preventive medicine.[80] Finally, FitzGerald suggested to President Falconer that in order for Connaught to provide a truly national service – and since Ontario and Saskatchewan were now providing largely the financial support of labs through free distribution of products – he recommend an honorary advisory committee of the Connaught Laboratories be established. Representatives of each provincial government and the federal government would be appointed to this committee and would meet annually to consult with FitzGerald in regard to scientific problems in which Connaught could be of service. As FitzGerald stressed to Falconer, 'It is the belief of the Director, that, in this way, the Connaught Laboratories may come ultimately to occupy the position in Canada, that the Lister Institute does in Great Britain and the Pasteur Institute in France.'[81]

October 25, 1917, was a rainy day for an official opening ceremony. However, the spirits of the dignitaries and others in attendance on the covered stage set up next to the new laboratory building were lifted with the announcement from Premier Hearst that the Ontario government would contribute a $75,000 endowment in support of research at Connaught. It was also announced that Gooderham had also contributed another $25,000 for Connaught's research fund.[82] In all the press coverage of the official opening, however, there was no indication of any financial contribution from the University of Toronto itself. When asked why the university was involved in such an unusual manufacturing enterprise, Sir Edmund Walker, chairman of the board of governors, explained: 'Through the laboratories the university would extend the work it is carrying on as a great instrument of good for the entire community apart from the educational purpose, by way of direct service for the betterment of general conditions throughout the country.'[83]

## Conclusions

In creating Connaught, it is clear that FitzGerald had offered the University of Toronto a valuable opportunity to expand the 'scientific spirit' in medicine that it had nurtured since the 1880s to a new level of national and international public service, but without having to invest any of its own capital resources, limited as they were during this period. As a self-supporting and separate department of the university by 1919, for the most part, Connaught's unique arrangement would continue until 1972, when the University of Toronto decided to sell it to the Canadian Development Corporation, a federal Crown corporation. By this time, in the

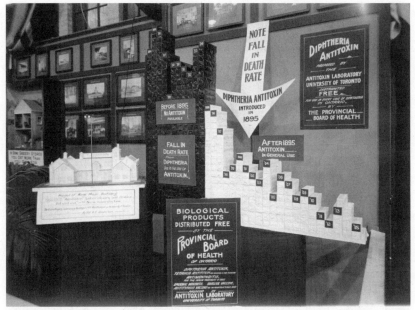

Ontario Department of Health Exhibit, Impact of Diphtheria Antitoxin on diphtheria death rates, 1895–1915. The exhibit highlights the free availability of diphtheria antitoxin from Antitoxin Laboratory, University of Toronto, and a model of the main building for expanded production then under construction at 'New University Farm,' 1916–17. (SP-C Archives)

wake of such prominent vaccine-related events as the 'Cutter incident' with the Salk vaccine in the United States in 1955, concerns about the risks of the live Sabin polio vaccine after 1962, coupled with the Thalidomide babies tragedy in Canada in the early 1960s, the university's newly restructured governing council was worried about the potential legal liabilities Connaught's work inherently flirted with. The council and others in the university were also worried about rapidly increasing government regulatory power over biological products, coupled with relentless pressure from commercial pharmaceutical companies who, among other complaints, resented Connaught's tax-free status. There were passionate arguments in support of Connaught's continued relationship with the university, particularly from Dr James K.W. Ferguson, Connaught's director since 1955. However, the university's new generation of leaders, less familiar with Connaught's many contributions and unique mission, and faced with a rapidly expanding student body and shrinking provincial funding, were increasingly desirous of the capital that Connaught's research fund had accumulated, as well the financial windfall its sale would bring.[84]

Despite Connaught's transformation into a profit-driven corporation after 1972 and, eventually, into the Canadian component of the global Sanofi Pasteur organization, Dr FitzGerald's original mission has remained largely intact: that is, to develop, manufacture, improve, and distribute, through provincial health departments, essential public-health products at a price that is within the reach of everyone. Well before FitzGerald had crystallized his vision for what became Connaught Laboratories, several distinctive Canadian elements provided him with fertile ground, in particular: the problem of expensive U.S. imports of antitoxins and vaccines; persistent and growing public-health challenges (diphtheria, rabies), strong interest in public health and the power of bacteriology to meet and prevent such challenges among key medical, scientific, and political leaders at the University of Toronto and in the Ontario government; and the emergence of national interest in public health, reflected in such organizations as the Canadian Public Health Association. FitzGerald's personal background, his international exposure to European and American approaches to public health and the provision of biological products, and his extraordinary drive focused and expedited the evolution and application of an emerging and quite distinctive Canadian approach to preventing disease and protecting national, as well as international, health. The essential role Connaught played in the development of insulin, as told by Michael Bliss, as well as of polio vaccines, as I have documented, for example, in addition to many other important biological products (i.e., heparin, diphtheria toxoid, pertussis and smallpox vaccines, various combined vaccines), clearly depended upon this distinctive Canadian approach to public health, an approach Connaught simultaneously reflected, reinforced, and furthered from its modest beginning in a backyard stable.

NOTES

The author, Christopher J. Rutty, PhD, is the owner of Health Heritage Research Services, Toronto (http://www.healthheritageresearch.com; contact: hhrs@healthheritageresearch.com). The original version of this paper was presented during the Colloquium series, Institute for the History and

Philosophy of Science and Technology, University of Toronto, on 26 January 2000, and supported by a Hannah Institute for the History of Medicine / Associated Medical Services Postdoctoral Fellowship.

1 'Some of the work of the Department of Hygiene of the University of Toronto,' *Canadian Journal of Medicine and Surgery* 42 (October 1917): 93.
2 On the history of Connaught see R.D. Defries, *The First Forty Years, 1914–1955: Connaught Medical Research Laboratories, University of Toronto* (Toronto: University of Toronto Press, 1968); Paul Bator, with A.J. Rhodes, *Within Reach of Everyone: A History of the University of Toronto School of Hygiene and the Connaught Laboratories*, vol. 1, *1927–1955* (Ottawa: Canadian Public Health Association, 1990); Paul Bator, *Within Reach of Everyone: A History of the University of Toronto School of Hygiene and Connaught Laboratories Limited*, vol. 2, *1955–1975, With an Update to the 1990s* (Ottawa: Canadian Public Health Association, 1995); Pierrick Malissard, 'Quand les Universitaires se font entrepreneurs: Les Laboratoires Connaught et l'Institut de Microbiologie et d'Hygiene de l'Université de Montréal, 1914–1972,' PhD thesis, Department of History, Université du Québec a Montréal, 1999; Christopher J. Rutty, 'Robert Davies Defries (1889–1975),' in L.N. Magner, ed., *Doctors, Nurses and Medical Practitioners: A Bio-Bibliographical Sourcebook* (Westport, CT: Greenwood Press, 1997), 62–9; Craig Defries, 'Now Is the Time: The Early Years of Dr. Robert Davies Defries, Associate Director of the University of Toronto's Connaught Laboratories and the School of Hygiene and the Decisive Intervention Taken by That Organization in the Ontario and Toronto Public Health Lobby's Efforts to Control Diphtheria,' MSW thesis, School of Social Work, Carleton University, 1993.

On Connaught's diphtheria toxoid work, see Jane Lewis, 'The Prevention of Diphtheria in Canada and Britain, 1914–1945,' *Journal of Social History* 20, 1 (1986): 163–76; C.E. Dolman, 'Landmarks and Pioneers in the Control of Diphtheria: The Donald T. Fraser Memorial Lecture, 1973,' *Canadian Journal of Public Health* 64 (July 1973): 317–36; on insulin: Michael Bliss, *The Discovery of Insulin* (Toronto: McClelland and Stewart, 1982); C. Sinding, 'Making the Unit of Insulin: Standards, Clinical Work, and Industry,' *Bulletin of the History of Medicine* 76 (2002): 231–70; on heparin: James Marcum, 'The Development of Heparin in Toronto,' *Journal of the History Medicine and Allied Sciences* 52 (July 1997): 310–37; on penicillin: Ronald Hare, *The Birth of Penicillin and the Disarming of Microbes* (London: George Allen and Unwin Ltd, 1970); on polio vaccines: Christopher J. Rutty, 'Do Something! Do Anything! Poliomyelitis in Canada, 1927–1962,' PhD thesis, Department of History, University of Toronto, 1995; Christopher J. Rutty, Luis Barreto, Rob Van Exan, and Shawn Gilchrist, 'Conquering the Crippler: Canada and the Eradication of Polio,'

*Canadian Journal of Public Health*, 96 (March–April 2005), special insert, I-1–I-2; and on smallpox: Luis Barreto and Christopher J. Rutty, 'The Speckled Monster: Canada, Smallpox and Its Eradication,' *Canadian Journal of Public Health* 93 (July–August 2002), special insert, I-1–I-20.

3 See note 2; see also R.D. Defries, 'The Connaught Medical Research Laboratories, 1914–1948,' *Canadian Journal of Public Health* 39 (August 1948): 330–44; R.D. Defries, 'The Connaught Medical Research Laboratories during the Second World War, 1939–1945,' *Canadian Journal of Public Health* 40 (August 1949): 348–60; and J. Callwood, 'The Miracle Factory That Began in a Stable,' *Maclean's*, 1 October 1955.

4 Christopher J. Rutty, 'The Canadian Polio Experience: A Personal Journey Through the Past,' *Ars Medica* 1, 2 (Spring 2005): 60–73.

5 Martine Spence, 'European Investment Abroad: A Case Study of Acquisition of Connaught Biosciences Inc. by Rhône-Poulence S.A.,' MBA paper, Concordia University, Montreal, April 1991.

6 For biographical background on J.G. FitzGerald see especially Bator and Rhodes, *Within Reach of Everyone*; Rutty, 'Robert Davies Defries'; C. Defries, 'Now Is the Time'; and Hare, *The Birth of Penicillin* (see note 2). See also James FitzGerald, 'Sins of the Fathers,' *Toronto Life*, February 2002, 66–72.

7 Harriette Chick, Margaret Hume, and Marjorie MacFarlane, *War on Disease: A History of the Lister Institute* (London: André Deutsch Ltd, 1971), 22.

8 G.L. Geison, 'Pasteur, Roux, and Rabies: Scientific versus Clinical Mentalities,' *Journal of the History of Medicine and Allied Sciences* 45 (1990): 341–65; G.L. Geison, *The Private Science of Louis Pasteur* (Princeton: Princeton University Press, 1995); B. Latour, *The Pasteurization of France*, trans. A. Sheridan and J. Law (Cambridge, MA: Harvard University Press, 1988); A.M. Moulin, 'The Pasteur Institutes between the Two World Wars: The Transformation of the International Sanitary Order,' in P. Weindling, ed., *International Health Organisations and Movements, 1918–1939* (Cambridge: Cambridge University Press, 1995), 244–65; P. Weindling, 'Scientific Elites and Laboratory Organization in fin de siècle Paris and Berlin: The Pasteur Institute and Robert Koch's Institute for Infectious Diseases Compared,' in A. Cunningham and P. Williams, eds, *The Laboratory Revolution in Medicine* (Cambridge, New York: Cambridge University Press, 1992), 170–88; Ilana Löwy, 'On Hybridizations, Networks and New Disciplines: The Pasteur Institute and the Development of Microbiology in France,' *Studies in the History and Philosophy of Science* 25 (1994): 655–88.

9 See, for example, Nancy Stepan, *Beginnings of Brazilian Science: Oswaldo Cruz, Medical Research and Policy, 1890–1920* (New York: Science History Publications, 1976).

10 Jonathan Liebenau, 'Paul Erlich as a Commercial Scientist and Research Administrator,' *Medical History* 34 (1990): 65–78; Paul Weindling, 'From Medical Research to Clinical Practice: Serum Therapy for Diphtheria in the 1890s,' in John V. Pickstone, ed., *Medical Innovations in Historical Perspective* (London: Macmillan, 1992), 72–83.

11 Chick, Hume, and MacFarlane, *War on Disease*.

12 Elizabeth Fee and Evelynn M. Hammonds, 'Science, Politics, and the Art of Persuasion: Promoting the New Scientific Medicine in New York City,' in David Rosner, ed., *Hives of Sickness: Public Health and Epidemics in New York City* (New Brunswick, NJ: Rutgers University Press, 1995), 155–96.

13 Mallisard, 'Quand les universitaires se font entrepreneurs,' 59–60.

14 Genevieve Schiffmann and Jaroslav Nemec, *Medical Research Institutions Named after Medical Men* (Bethesda: National Library of Medicine, 1969), 49.

15 See, for example, Fee and Hammonds, 'Science, Politics and the Art of Persuasion'; Jonathan M. Liebenau, 'Public Health and the Production and Use of Diphtheria Antitoxin in Philadelphia,' *Bulletin of the History of Medicine* 61 (1987): 216–36; Barbara Gutmann Rosenkrantz, *Public Health and the State: Changing Views in Massachusetts* (Cambridge, MA: Harvard University Press, 1972); and Victoria A. Harden, *Inventing the NIH: Federal Biomedical Research Policy, 1887–1937* (Baltimore: Johns Hopkins University Press, 1986).

16 Jonathan Liebenau, *Medical Science and Medical Industry: The Formation of the American Pharmaceutical Industry* (Baltimore: Johns Hopkins University Press, 1987), 48–56.

17 Liebenau, 'Public Health and the Production and Use of Diphtheria Antitoxin in Philadelphia,' 236.

18 Rosenkrantz, *Public Health and the State*, 124–7.

19 Editorial, 'The Value of Diphtheria Antitoxin,' *Canada Lancet* 38, 9 (May 1905): 836–7.

20 Editorial, 'Discovery and Commercialism,' *Canada Lancet* 39, 5 (January 1906): 463–4.

21 Editorial, 'Treatment of Diphtheria with Anti-toxine,' *Canada Lancet* 27 (February 1895): 189–90.

22 R.D. Defries, 'Dr. Edward Playter: A Vision Fulfilled,' *Canadian Journal of Public Health* 50 (September 1959): 368–77.

23 Editorial, 'Inaguration 1911, Canadian Public Health Association Congress: The Vote of Thanks – Dr. Montizambert,' *Public Health Journal* 3, 1 (January 1912): 8–10; see http://www.cdnmedhall.org/laureates.

24 J.T. Phair, 'Public Health in Ontario,' in R.D. Defries, ed., *The Development of Public Health in Canada* (Toronto: Canadian Public Health Association, 1940), 67–85; W.B. Spaulding, 'The Ontario Vaccine Farm, 1885–1916,'

*Canadian Bulletin of Medical History* 6 (1989): 45–56; Baretto and Rutty, 'The Speckled Monster.'

25 J.W.S. McCullough, 'A Review of 10 Years Work of the Provincial Board of Health of Ontario, 1910–1920,' in *Annual Report of the Provincial Board of Health, 1920* (Toronto, 1921); Fee and Hammonds, 'Science, Politics and the Art of Persuasion,' 185.

26 Sandra McRae, 'The Scientific Spirit in Medicine at the University of Toronto, 1880–1910,' PhD thesis, University of Toronto, 1987.

27 Phair, 'Public Health in Ontario,' 75–7; R.D. Defries, 'Postgraduate Teaching in Public Health in the University of Toronto,' *Canadian Journal of Public Health* 48 (July 1957): 285–94; R.D. Defries, 'Brief Historical Account of the Development of Graduate Teaching in Public Health at the University of Toronto,' 1924, Sanofi Pasteur–Connaught Campus Archives (hereafter SP-CA), 83-001-10.

28 Miscellaneous, 'A Pasteur Institute,' *Canada Lancet* 43, 7 (March 1910): 554.

29 Editorial, 'The Rabies Outbreak,' *Canadian Journal of Medicine and Surgery* 27, 4 (April 1910): 222–6; Editorial, 'Rabies in Canada,' *Dominion Medical Monthly* 35, 3 (March 1910): 128; R.D. Defries and N.E. McKinnon, 'The Rabies Problem and the Use of Rabies Vaccine (Semple) in Canada,' *University of Toronto Medical Bulletin* 9 (1929): 8.

30 Editorial, 'A Secretary of Public Health,' *Dominion Medical Monthly* 35, 6 (June 1910): 246–8; Editorial, 'A National Department of Health,' *Canada Lancet* 43, 11 (July 1910): 806–7.

31 P.H. Bryce, 'A Dominion Health Service,' *Canadian Therapist and Sanitary Engineer* 1, 8 (August 1910): 393–4.

32 Editorial, 'Dr. Charles Hodgetts Joins the Federal Service,' *Canadian Journal of Medicine and Surgery* 28, 6 (June 1910): 383; Phair, 'Public Health in Ontario,' 71–2.

33 News, 'Dr. J.W.S. McCullough Succeeds Dr. Hodgetts,' *Canadian Journal of Medicine and Surgery* 28, 3 (September 1990): 184–5.

34 Phair, 'Public Health in Ontario,' 72; J.W.S. McCullough, 'Relation of the Medical Profession to the Public,' *Canada Lancet* 41, 2 (October 1907): 108–20.

35 Bator with Rhodes, *Within Reach of Everyone*, 1: 9–10; Editorial, 'The Conference of Public Health Men,' *Dominion Medical Monthly* 35, 5 (Nov. 1910): 192–93.

36 Editorial, 'The Canadian Public Health Association Congress,' *Public Health Journal / State Medicine and Sanitary Review* 2, 11 (November 1911): 503–7; Editorial, 'Inauguration 1911, Canadian Public Health Association Congress,' *Public Health Journal State Medicine and Sanitary Review* 3, 1 (January 1912): 3–10.

37  C.B. Higgins, 'Biological Products,' *Public Health Journal* 3, 1 (January 1912): 28–31.
38  Editorial, 'A National Laboratory at Ottawa,' *Canadian Journal of Medicine and Surgery* 30, 3 (August 1911): 111–13.
39  For more biographical details of FitzGerald's life, see note 6 above, especially FitzGerald, 'Sins of the Fathers,' and C.B. Farrar, 'I Remember J.G. FitzGerald,' *American Journal of Psychiatry* 120 (July 1963): 49–52. Examples of Dr FitzGerald's efforts towards institutional reform in psychiatry include J.G. FItzGerald, 'The Modern Methods of Treating the Insane,' *Canada Lancet* 40, 10 (June 1907): 906–9, and 'A Brief Resume of the Development of Clinical Psychiatry,' *Canada Lancet* 41, 2 (October 1907): 102–8.
40  Memo, 'Laboratory of Serum Diagnosis' (ca. 1911), University of Toronto Archives (hereafter UTA), A67-0007, box 13, File 'FitzGerald 1911.'
41  (President, University of Toronto) to J.G. FitzGerald, 25 February 1911, UTA, A67-0007, box 13.
42  FitzGerald, 'Sins of the Fathers.'
43  F.A. Mouré to J.G. FitzGerald, 11 July 1913, J.G. FitzGerald papers held by James FitzGerald.
44  Editorial, 'Medical Research at University of Toronto,' *Dominion Medical Monthly* 39, 6 (December 1912): 208; News, 'Medical Research at the University of Toronto,' *Canadian Journal of Medicine and Surgery* 33, 2 (February 1913): 149–50; News, 'The University of Toronto,' *Dominion Medical Monthly* 42, 5 (May 1914): 186. For more on the financial health of the University of Toronto during this period, see Marianne P.F. Stevens, 'Dollars and Change: The Effect of Rockefeller Foundation Funding on Canadian Medical Education at the University of Toronto, McGill University, and Dalhousie University,' PhD thesis, Institute for the History and Philosophy of Science and Technology, University of Toronto, 2000.
45  F.S. Fielder to J.G. FitzGerald, 5 August 1913; Fielder to FitzGerald, 12 September 1913, SP-CA 83-006-06.
46  W.S. Magill to FitzGerald, 8 August 1913, ibid.
47  Receipt, Bursar of the University of Toronto, 24 October 1913, FitzGerald papers.
48  Rutty, 'Robert Davies Defries (1889–1975),' 62–9.
49  Murray L. Barr, *A Century of Medicine at Western* (London: University of Western Ontario, 1977), 205–10.
50  Defries, 'Postgraduate Teaching in Public Health in the University of Toronto,' 285–7.
51  Defries, *First Forty Years*, 5.
52  Horse Records, SP-CA, 83-006-06; FitzGerald, 'Statement, Preparation of Diphtheria Antitoxin and Rabies Vaccine in Department of Hygiene,

University of Toronto, to April 1, 1914,' attached to FitzGerald to Edmund Osler, 31 March 1914, UTA, 67-0007, box 28.

53  FitzGerald to Osler, ibid.

54  Frederick Edwards, 'A Peacetime Munitions Plant,' *Maclean's*, 15 January 1928, 4.

55  FitzGerald to Osler, 31 March 1914, UTA, A67-0007, box 28.

56  R. Falconer to E. Osler, 1 April 1914, and Osler to Falconer, 3 April 1914, UTA, A67-0007, box 31; E. Osler to FitzGerald, 3 April 1914, and FitzGerald to Falconer, 8 April 1914, UTA, A67-0007, box 28.

57  Minutes, UTA, A83-0036, box 19.

58  Memo of Account attached to FitzGerald to Falconer, 12 May 1914, UTA, A67-0007, box 28.

59  Mouré to FitzGerald, 19 June 1914, FitzGerald papers.

60  Defries, *First Forty Years*, 10.

61  Annual Report of Director Antitoxin Laboratory, Year ending 30 June 1914, SP-CA, 83-005-03. Also published in *University of Toronto President's Annual Reports*.

62  R.D. Defries to J.W. Flavelle, 29 January 1915, UTA, A67-0007, box 35.

63  Falconer to R.B. Borden, 30 January 1915; Borden to Falconer, 2 February 1915; Falconer to Osler, 8 February 1915; Osler to Falconer, 9 February 1915, UTA, A67-0007, box 35.

64  Falconer to A.E. Gooderham, 16 February 1915, UTA, A67-0007, box 34.

65  Falconer to Minister of Militia, 23 February 1915, UTA, A67-0007, box 35.

66  Falconer to Gooderham, 3 March 1915, UTA, A67-0007, box 34.

67  Falconer to Lt.-Colonel Winter, 5 May 1915, UTA, A67-0007, box 35. See also FitzGerald memo, 27 May 1915, UTA, A67-0007, box 37; and J.G. FitzGerald, Historical Memo, October 1935, SP-CA, 83-001-09.

68  FitzGerald, Historical Memo, ibid.

69  FitzGerald to Falconer, 3 May 1915, UTA, A67-0007, box 34.

70  Annual Report of Antitoxin Laboratory, 30 June 1915, SP-CA, 83-005-03.

71  E.J. Banzhoff to C.S. Mahood, 9 December 1915, SP-CA, 83-006-06.

72  Ibid.

73  R.P. Hardman to A. Fisher, 4 December 1915, and R.P. Hardman to FitzGerald, 4 December 1915, SP-CA, 83-006-06.

74  M.B. Whyte to A. Fisher, 12 December 1915, ibid.

75  FitzGerald to Falconer, 2 December 1915, UTA, A67-0007, box 38a.

76  Falconer to FitzGerald, 23 December 1915, ibid.

77  'Provincial Supply of Antitoxin,' *Canada Lancet* 50, 7 (March 1917): 333–4.

78  Defries, *First Forty Years*, 29.

79  FitzGerald to Falconer, 5 September 1917, UTA, A67-0007, box 47a.

80  FitzGerald to Falconer, 10 September 1917, ibid.

81  FitzGerald to Falconer, 10 September 1917, ibid.

82  'Opening of the Connaught Laboratories at the University Farm, University of Toronto,' *Public Health Journal* 8, 11 (November 1917).

83  'Splendid Gift to University,' *Mail & Empire*, 26 October 1917.

84  Bator, *Within Reach of Everyone*, 2: 128–9; Malissard, 'Quand les universitaires se font entrepreneurs,' 293–302.

# 11 Defining Disability, Limiting Liability: The Care of Thalidomide Victims in Canada

BARBARA CLOW

In the early 1960s, thousands of children around the world were born with serious physical deformities after their mothers had ingested thalidomide. Horrified by the ravaged bodies of newborns, the public, the medical profession, and the state sought an explanation for the tragedy as well as an appropriate response to the suffering of the babies and their families. Diverse programs of investigation, remediation, and compensation gradually took shape in many countries. But officials struggling to assess the impact of thalidomide faced formidable obstacles because exposure to the drug was exceedingly difficult to document. Consequently, they tackled the problem from both ends, trying to track down those affected by the drug while following the trail of pills and syrups. Searching for the victims of thalidomide, doctors and other investigators emphasized the most visible physical defects, namely, compromised limb development or phocomelia. In the process, phocomelia became emblematic of thalidomide exposure for both the public and the medical profession.

In Canada, as elsewhere, the government took a rather different view of phocomelia. Arguing that this type of birth defect could and did develop spontaneously, independent of thalidomide use, federal and provincial officials were reluctant to accept limb deformities as sufficient proof of exposure. They consequently demanded more reliable evidence, such as hospital or pharmacy records, patient files, and/or the testimony of prescribing physicians. As one might expect, evidence of this kind could be an exceedingly elusive commodity. By defining phocomelia as a naturally occurring congenital malformation and demanding medical confirmation of drug use, the state successfully limited its liability for the suffering caused by thalidomide.

Although many infants born in Canada during the early 1960s exhibited the 'classic' signs of thalidomide exposure, they were judged ineligible for aid without acceptable evidence that their mothers had taken the deforming drug.

Before considering the issues of disability and liability, I want to spend a little time discussing the events that led up to the establishment of special 'habilitation' programs for the Canadian victims of thalidomide. The story begins with the manufacturing and marketing of the drug, and the gradual recognition of its teratogenic properties. Once we are acquainted with the broad outlines of the thalidomide tragedy, we will look more closely at the relationship between ideas about congenital malformations and decisions about access to state-sponsored programs of care.

## Manufacturing and Marketing

Thalidomide first appeared in West Germany in 1957, under the trade name Contergan. It was synthesized in 1953 by Chemie Grünenthal and then tested in animal and human subjects before being released for general consumption. These early experiments suggested that Contergan was not only an effective sleeping aid, but also an exceptionally safe one. In contrast to other sedatives popular in the 1950s, such as barbiturates, thalidomide could be ingested in large quantities without causing death.[1] The manufacturer and the government consequently felt confident that the drug could be sold without a prescription. By 1959 thalidomide was not only the most popular sleeping pill in West Germany, it was also an ingredient in a dozen other medicines sold over the counter for the treatment of colds, flu, headaches, neuralgia, and asthma.[2]

As Contergan was sweeping the West German market, Chemie Grünenthal also licensed pharmaceutical firms in other countries to manufacture and/or distribute thalidomide. By the early 1960s the drug was available in forty-six countries around the world: 'eleven European, seven African, seventeen Asian, and eleven North and South American.'[3] In Canada, two manufacturers cornered the thalidomide market: the Cincinnati-based firm Richardson-Merrell and Montreal pharmaceutical company Frank W. Horner Ltd. In September 1960 Richardson-Merrell submitted a New Drug Application to the United States Food and Drug Administration, and the following month sent a similar application to the Canadian Food and Drug

Directorate. While U.S. officials, notably Frances Kelsey, refused to approve the drug for sale because they were dissatisfied with the details of toxicity studies, Canadian regulators apparently felt that the safety of thalidomide had been well established by European experience and five hundred pages of documentation submitted by the American company.[4] On 1 April 1961 Richardson-Merrell's brand of thalidomide, Kevadon, went on sale in Canada. Six months later, Frank W. Horner joined the competition with its product, Talimol. Both products were available only by prescription, despite Richardson-Merrell's appeal for broader distribution 'in view of the established safety of this product.'[5] Permission was refused on the grounds that sedatives and tranquillizers, no matter how harmless, should not be made freely available to the public.

Although pharmaceutical manufacturers harped on the safety of thalidomide, as early as 1956, doctors conducting clinical trials in Hamburg noticed dizziness and loss of balance among elderly patients treated with Contergan. Moreover, as sales of thalidomide sky-rocketed, so too did reports of other disturbing side-effects, including severe constipation, hangover, loss of memory, hypotension, petechial hemorrhages, trembling, incoordination, numbness, and even partial paralysis.[6] Officials at Chemie Grünenthal insisted that these noxious side-effects developed only with overdosing or extended treatment, and they claimed that symptoms subsided with the cessation of thalidomide therapy.[7] At best, these reassurances were half-truths, proffered in the interests of preserving a marketing strategy predicated on the drug's safety. Manufacturers continued to insist that the drug was harmless, even in the face of mounting evidence linking it with severe birth defects. In 1960, as pharmaceutical preparations containing thalidomide flooded world markets, doctors began to notice a disturbing increase in phocomelia, an unusual anomaly involving the absence or shortening of the arms and/or legs due to the malformation of the long bones, with associated deformities in the hands, feet, fingers, and/or toes. Increasing pressure from the public, the medical profession, and the state finally convinced Chemie Grünenthal to recall the drug on 27 November 1961. Distillers (Biochemicals) Ltd in Great Britain followed suit the same day and the Swedish manufacturer, Astra, withdrew its product two weeks later.[8]

Meanwhile, Canadians continued to enjoy access to thalidomide until the spring of 1962. Although federal regulators learned about the possible connection between the drug and congenital malformations in

December 1961, they were lulled into a false sense of security by the fact that Kevadon and Talimol were available only by prescription. Government officials were satisfied that warning letters issued to physicians by the manufacturers would, 'in effect, withdraw it from the market insofar as pregnant women are concerned.'[9] Through the winter, both Richardson-Merrell and Horner kept in regular contact with the Food and Drug Directorate, assuring the government that evidence implicating thalidomide as the cause of birth defects was 'inconclusive.' But late in February 1962 a damning report on thalidomide appeared in *The Lancet*, and three days later the government finally removed the drug from the Canadian market 'pending clarification.' For months afterwards, officials in the Food and Drug Directorate worked to trace and retrieve supplies of thalidomide lurking on the shelves of pharmacies and in medicine cabinets or squirrelled away in doctors' desk drawers. Although these efforts probably saved some children from exposure, more than four million tablets had made their way into Canadian homes and hospitals during eleven months of legitimate sales, while at least another million pills had been distributed as samples. By 1962 countless infants and their families had already suffered the devastation wrought by thalidomide.[10]

## Managing a Tragedy

As the medical profession, the public, and the parents of deformed babies struggled to come to terms with the tragic impact of thalidomide, the Canadian government swung into action. The minister of national health and welfare, Waldo Monteith, commissioned a review of new-drug approval procedures and an investigation of the damage caused by thalidomide. At the same time, he invited the provinces to help develop 'habilitation' strategies for the victims and their families.[11] Through the fall of 1962, with the aid of an advisory committee of experts, a comprehensive program of care evolved. Hospital and diagnostic services were already freely available through a publicly funded insurance plan introduced in 1957. Provincial and federal governments agreed to share the remaining costs of managing thalidomide deformities, including such items as doctors' fees, surgery, drugs, prosthetic devices, psychological assessment and support, special education or vocational training, custodial care, and even income supplements.[12] Federal authorities earmarked $200,000, in addition to standard health grants, for the support of these programs, making close to half a million dollars available to help thalidomide victims and their families.[13]

## Disability and Liability

With the general outlines of a treatment plan in place, federal and provincial administrators faced the unenviable task of determining who would be eligible for care at the expense of Canadian taxpayers: in other words, which deformed babies were really thalidomide babies. Given the extraordinary nature of the birth defects associated with the drug, we might expect that the issue of eligibility would have been easily resolved. Although estimates of the incidence of phocomelia before the introduction of thalidomide are hardly reliable, ranging from one in four million to one in five thousand, they were nonetheless uniformly low.[14] Indeed, the rarity of phocomelia and the sudden epidemic of new cases had first alerted doctors to the dangers of the drug. According to one West German expert in congenital malformations, before 1961 'he had seen more babies with two heads than with phocomelia.'[15] Moreover, any lingering doubts about the cause of these unusual limb deformities should have been dispelled when rates dropped dramatically after governments banned the drug.

Although the attention paid to abnormal limb development undoubtedly helped to expose the teratogenic properties of thalidomide, there were, in fact, a great many drawbacks associated with singling out this malformation. On the one hand, prenatal exposure to thalidomide induced a wide variety of anomalies, ranging from facial hemangiomas and paralysis, which presented few health risks, through disabling deformities of the limbs, eyes, and ears, to life-threatening abnormalities of the gastro-intestinal, genito-urinary, and cardio-vascular systems. Consequently, infants born with normal limbs and defective hearts or ears might still be victims of the drug.[16] On the other hand, thalidomide was clearly not the only cause of limb malformations. Genetic anomalies and a variety of environmental hazards could produce deformities that resembled phocomelia.[17] As Jean Webb, head of the Child and Maternal Health Division at National Health and Welfare, observed, 'The question of what constitutes a thalidomide induced anomaly is a very thorny one.'[18]

Doctors advising the federal government recognized these difficulties: 'It is impossible,' they observed, 'to determine with certainty which children born during the period in question have deformities due to thalidomide.'[19] As a result, medical experts urged the authorities to provide care for every *potential* victim of thalidomide; any infant born with suspicious deformities whose mother *could have* ingested the drug.[20] But the state, unwilling or unable to commit itself to this extent, set out instead to *count* the babies damaged by thalidomide. Federal officials combed through death certificates, birth registries, and hospital records for evidence of congenital malformations, contacting physicians and parents for more information about specific infants.[21] Despite the salience of many different birth defects, these epidemiological studies consistently targeted abnormalities of the limbs. Questionnaires demanded detailed descriptions of the arms and legs of babies, consigning discussion of all other anomalies to one or two lines. Similarly, a hospital survey initiated in August 1962 asked only for information about bone and joint or multiple malformations, actively discouraging reportage of eight other categories of defect.[22] From these investigations, Canadian officials concluded that although thalidomide created an 'unusual pattern of congenital malformation,' similar anomalies could and did appear spontaneously.[23] In other words, phocomelia was suggestive of, rather than definitive, regarding exposure to thalidomide. Not only was this view at odds with the beliefs of many clinicians and researchers, both in Canada and abroad, it also exposed a fundamental contradiction in the government's investigations of the tragedy: having set out to find thalidomide victims by searching for phocomelic babies, the authorities proceeded to deny that the babies they found were necessarily victims of thalidomide.

In the months and years following the thalidomide tragedy, physicians continued to diagnose exposure, quite literally, at a glance. For example, a specialist at Toronto's Hospital for Sick Children was shocked to discover that one of his patients was not classified as a victim of thalidomide. 'It was ... a surprise to me,' he wrote, 'to know that [this girl] was not officially registered as a thalidomide child, as it never really occurred to me that she could be anything else. Her deformities are absolutely typical, and she was born at the time during which thalidomide was available.'[24] Although this child was eventually accepted into Ontario's habilitation program, the provincial authorities made their decision grudgingly. 'This type of deformity was well recognized prior to the introduction of ... thalidomide,' wrote one official. 'However, in spite of the lack of confirmation by her physician that [the mother] had received thalidomide during her early pregnancy, it is possible that she may have obtained the drug in some other way and we are adding this child to those benefitting under the Thalidomide Programme.'[25] Cases such as this one not only confirmed official reluctance to rely on phocomelia as proof of thalidomide exposure, it also indicated the type of evidence preferred by administrators: professional testimony.

As with the emphasis on phocomelia, the demand for documentation of exposure was fraught with problems. Although some doctors readily admitted prescribing thalidomide for their patients, others were less willing to cooperate with investigators. In British Columbia, for example, medical health officers approached practitioners in person because they recognized that 'many physicians would be loath to submit information in writing because of future possibilities of legal litigation.'[26] Moreover, some doctors were defensive or openly hostile when questioned about their use of the drug. One physician, responding to an official inquiry, wrote, 'I *of course* have no cases who receive[d] this drug.'[27] Despite the government's confidence, professional testimony was an uncertain source of information about thalidomide exposure. Case files and hospital logs did not necessarily provide more reliable or accessible evidence. In this era, many practitioners liberally distributed samples of drugs without keeping any records. As a result, they might simply not know which medicines they had dispensed to their patients. One doctor admitted, 'I *might* have given ... patient a small sample of thalidomide with the occasion of some house call. However I doubt it very much.'[28] In the same way, some hospitals routinely administered sleeping pills, including Kevadon and Talimol, for in-patients without entering the information on every medical chart.[29] One woman who had been hospitalized and medicated during her pregnancy believed she had been given thalidomide, but neither her own doctor nor hospital staff could or would confirm her fears.[30] Finally, a significant proportion of mothers who had ingested thalidomide did not obtain the pills from a doctor or hospital, but rather from family, from friends, or at work.[31] In such cases, it was virtually impossible to document exposure.

The demand for professional evidence of thalidomide use, in combination with the government's stunning conclusions about phocomelia, dramatically reduced the numbers of children who qualified for federal and provincial aid. Among thousands of deformed babies born in Canada between 1960 and 1963, only 115 met the strict criteria of eligibility established by the government, and more than 40 of these children had died as a result of severe congenital malformations long before the habilitation programs became available.[32] Consequently, though the government had set aside hundreds of thousands of dollars to care for the victims of thalidomide, only a tiny fraction of this money was expended for drugs, surgery, prosthetic devices, and support. Between 1963 and 1971, for example, Ontario's habilitation program served fewer than twenty children at a total cost of less than $34,000.[33]

## Conclusion

Federal officials insisted these guidelines for access to the programs were 'not intended as a restrictive definition beyond which the provinces could not go in accepting children for rehabilitation assistance.'[34] Although provincial authorities sometimes exercised their discretionary powers, accepting children who did not qualify for care according to the federal definition, they made few exceptions. Many deformed children were simply denied assistance, usually because their parents could not substantiate thalidomide exposure.[35] Moreover, despite the alleged flexibility of the Canadian government, parents and doctors inquiring about thalidomide programs were told in no uncertain terms that 'assistance is limited to babies with congenital malformations where the drug thalidomide was taken by the mother during her pregnancy.'[36] By redefining the significance of phocomelia, federal authorities sought to create two categories of birth defects: naturally occuring or 'normal' abnormalities, for which they had no responsibility, and iatrogenic or 'abnormal' abnormalities, for which they might have some responsibility. By insisting on documented evidence of thalidomide exposure, the government limited the number of children who would fall into the second category of congenital malformation, curtailing its liability. As the thalidomide babies have grown into adults, initiating claims for compensation against the federal government, this definition of eligibility has persisted, becoming even less flexible and less inclusive.

NOTES

1 Richard E. McFadyen, 'Thalidomide in America: A Brush with Tragedy,' *Clio Medica* 11 (1976): 79.
2 Henning Sjöström and Robert Nilsson, *Thalidomide and the Power of the Drug Companies* (Middlesex, UK: Penguin, 1972), 38–9.

3 Yoichiro Yamakawa, 'The Legal Settlement of Thalidomide Cases in Japan,' in T. Soda, ed., *Drug-Induced Suffering's Medical, Pharmaceutical, and Legal Aspects* (Amsterdam: Excerpta Medica, 1980), 365; Sjöström and Nilsson, *Thalidomide*, 39–40, 147; The Insight Team of the *Sunday Times*, London, *Suffer the Children: The Story of Thalidomide* (New York: The Viking Press, 1979), 29, also 1, 45; Ethel Roskies, *Abnormality and Normality: The Mothering of Thalidomide Children* (Ithaca: Cornell University Press, 1972), 1–2.

4 McFadyen, 'Thalidomide in America,' 80; Canada, Department of National Health and Welfare, Health Protection Branch (HPB), 'Chronology Re Thalidomide,' 17 August 1962.

5 Jean F. Webb, 'Canadian Thalidomide Experience,' *Canadian Medical Association Journal* 89 (1963), 987–92; Sjöström and Nilsson, *Thalidomide*, 136–46.

6 Insight Team, *Suffer the Children*, 30–2; Sjöström and Nilsson, *Thalidomide*, 46–59.

7 'Chronology re Thalidomide,' 5.

8 Sjöström and Nilsson, *Thalidomide*, 94–104.

9 'Chronology re Thalidomide,' 9.

10 June Callwood, 'The Unfolding Tragedy of Drug-Deformed Babies,' *Maclean's*, 19 May 1962, 13; HPB, 'Survey of Effects of Thalidomide,' Charles B. Walker, Officer-in-Charge, Biostatistics Section, 18 June 1962.

11 'Chronology re Thalidomide,' 16–17.

12 HPB, 'Memorandum: Aid for Thalidomide Babies,' John E. Osborne, Director, Research and Statistics, to G.D.W. Cameron, Deputy Minister of Health (MOH), August 1962. See also Roskies, *Abnormality*, 3–7.

13 HPB, 'Chronology re Thalidomide,' 16–17.

14 Sjöström and Nilsson, *Thalidomide*, 95; HPB, 'Review – Thalidomide and Congenital Anomaly,' Child and Maternal Welfare Division, 14 June 1962.

15 Insight Team, *Suffer the Children*, 96.

16 HPB, 'A Definition of the Syndrome Associated with Thalidomide' and 'Thalidomide Syndrome,' August 1962.

17 HPB, F. Clarke Fraser, Department of Genetics, McGill University, to Jean Webb [see note 18], 4 July 1962. According to Fraser, half of infants born with phocomelia in Liverpool had no known history of thalidomide exposure, but two mothers had taken Doriden, the generic drug glutethimide.

18 HPB, Jean F. Webb, Chief, Child and Maternal Health Division, National Health and Welfare, to E.S. Hillman, MD, Montreal Children's Hospital, 30 October 1962.

19 HPB, 'Recommendations of Sub-Committee on Prosthetic Problems to Expert Committee on Rehabilitation of Congenital Malformations Associated with Thalidomide Based on Trip to United States Centres,' 7 November 1962.

20 HPB, 'A Definition of the Syndrome Associated with Thalidomide,' August 1962; Memorandum, John E. Osborne, Director, Research and Statistics, to G.D.W. Cameron, Deputy MOH, National Health and Welfare, August 1962; 'Management of Affected Children of Mothers Who Had Taken Thalidomide during Pregnancy,' J.C. Rathburn, Professor and Head, Department of Paediatrics, Faculty of Medicine, University of Western Ontario, 5 October 1962.

21 HPB, G.D.W. Cameron, Deputy MOH, National Health and Welfare, to M.E. Lydall, Administrator, Grace Hospital, Ottawa, 25 June 1962, HPB; Memorandum, 'The Thalidomide Problem,' Gordon H. Josie, Consultant, Planning and Evaluation, to Jean Webb, 3 August 1962; 'Plan for Study of Congenital Deformity Associated with Maternal Thalidomide Intake,' 23 August 1962; 'Pilot Study on the Use of Thalidomide during Pregnancy in the Ottawa Area,' ca. August 1962.

22 HPB, Form letter, Hospital survey, ca. August 1962.

23 HPB, Webb to unknown, 26 May 1965; Webb, 'Canadian Experience,' 6; Osborne, 'Aid,' 4; Rathburn, 'Management,' 1.

24 Archives of Ontario (AO), J.H. to James S. Band, Deputy Minister, Department of Social and Family Services, Ontario, 10 February 1969, RG 10-187-1-36; see also RG 10-187-1-19, 10-187-1-21, and 10-187-1-11.

25 AO, J. Ellis Moore, Director, Maternal and Child Health Services, Special Health Services Branch, to C.K. Stuart, Med. Consultant, Social and Family Services, 30 December 1968, and Moore to Stuart, 28 April 1969, RG 10-187-1-36.

26 HPB, J.A. Taylor, Deputy MOH, BC, to G.D.W. Cameron, Deputy MOH, National Health and Welfare, 7 August 1962. See also HPB, Memorandum, Re Study of Thalidomide in Pregnancy, Webb to K.C. Charron, Director of Health Services Directorate, National Health and Welfare, 30 July 1962.

27 HPB, Unknown physician to T.K. Scobie, Secretary, Academy of Medicine, Ottawa, 10 July 1962 [emphasis added].

28 AO, Initial report, P.S., n.d., RG 10-187-2-17, Correspondence, General – 1962–7. See also HPB, interviews with Drs Hurtig and Dooley, 3 August 1962.

29 Roskies, *Abnormality*, 30–1.

30 AO, Case 11, RG 10-187-1-11, 1967–77.

31 Roskies, *Abnormality*, 30–1. According to Roskies, of 20 women whose children were treated at the Rehabilitation Institute of Montreal for thalidomide-related deformities, only 12 had received the drug from a doctor. Similarly, close to a third of women whose children were registered in Ontario's habilitation program had obtained the drug from sources other than a prescribing physician. See AO, RG 10-187-1-1 to 10-187-1-36.

32 Information on congenital malformations was not uniformly or consistently gathered in Canada before the thalidomide tragedy. Estimates of the incidence

of birth defects resulted in educated guesses, such as the rate of 10.4 to 11.3 per 1000 live births in Ontario. HPB, Simi Memorandum, Departmental Secretary to K.C. Charron, Director, Health Services Directorate, National Health and Welfare, 'Replies to Questions in the House of Commons, September 27, 1962.' See also HPB, Webb to Jim Carney, Story editor, *Close-Up*, CBC, Toronto, 4 December 1962.

33  AO, Recapitulation of Expenses, 1963–1871, RG 10-187-2-6; J.E. Moore to H. Sharp, Executive Assistant, Public Health Division, 1 August 1972, RG 10-187-2-19.

34  HPB, Webb to E.S. Hillman, MD, Montreal Children's Hospital, 30 October 1962.

35  AO, M.R.Warren, Director, Fort William and District Health Unit, to Martin, Director, Public Health Administration Branch, Department of Health, 30 August 1962; and Warren to Matthew Dymond, MOH, Ontario, 29 April 1963, RG 10-107-0-663, Drug Thalidomide, D10-5, 1962-4.

36  HPB, Webb to Professor A.M. Linden, Osgoode Hall Law School, Toronto, 5 September 1963. See also HPB, Murray A. McBride, MP, to John Munro, Minister of National Health and Welfare, 23 January 1969, and Memorandum, Philip Banister, MD, to Unknown, 10 February 1969.

# 12 'Comfort, Security, Dignity': Home Care for Canada's Aging Veterans, 1977–2004

JAMES STRUTHERS

In recent years the cost of caring for an aging society has risen to the top of Canada's social-policy agenda. Ballooning health budgets, over-crowded emergency rooms, lengthy waiting lists for institutional care, and the patchwork nature of home care are regular staples of media coverage of Canada's health-care landscape. These same issues also loom large in Roy Romanow's 2002 royal commission report on the future of Canada's health-care system.[1] Although the causes of a per-ceived crisis in health care are complex, the relationship between an aging population and rising health-care expenditure is an ongoing and often 'alarmist' feature of current policy and media debate. Increas-ingly, it has also driven discussions around the need for a national home-care strategy as a more cost-effective alternative to the poten-tially crippling burden of institutional care, over the next three decades, for Canada's burgeoning population of seniors.[2]

A quarter of a century ago Veterans Affairs Canada (VAC) con-fronted similar pressures as it faced the demographic and economic consequences of its aging population of First and Second World War veterans and veterans of the Korean War. Through a gradual series of regulatory changes in veterans' benefits stretching from 1928 to 1966, all those serving overseas in time of war had gained the right to insti-tutional long-term bed care, if needed, in a VAC facility.[3] Yet by the late 1960s, faced with growing difficulties attracting high-quality doctors and nurses to work in what were fast becoming 'rest homes with obso-lescent facilities,' populated mostly by frail and indigent First World War veterans, the department was increasingly anxious to get out of the business of directly administering nursing home care. Over the next two decades ten of VAC's eleven institutions, with a total capacity of almost seven thousand beds, would be turned over to the provinces in exchange for agreements guaranteeing a designated number of 'contract beds,' financed by Ottawa, for Canadian veterans requiring long-term care in provincial health facilities.[4]

Although by the beginning of the 1980s VAC was, for the most part, no longer running hospitals or, more accurately, long-term-care facilities itself, it still faced a substantial and ill-defined financial commitment for providing care, if required, to the massive cohort of surviving Second World War veterans with overseas service, a group numbering more than 317,000, half of whom would reach age sixty-five by 1985. Out of the imperatives of this moral and fiscal obligation emerged a significant social-policy experiment: Canada's first and to date only national home-care initiative, the Veterans Independence Program (VIP). Launched in April 1981 as the Aging Veterans Program, the VIP (it was renamed in 1986) has become one of Canada's least known but most successful examples of community-based home care as an alternative to institutionalizing the elderly.

Through the VIP, VAC anticipated the needs of an aging population and developed a coherent, effective, and highly popular model for the delivery of community-based home care, albeit for a select clientele, from one end of the country to the other, long before debates around the need for a national home-care strategy emerged in force during the 1990s. The VIP was also one of the first government programs to embrace gerontological perspectives on alternatives to institutionalization as well as to acknowledge, however cautiously, the rights of care-givers. Now that Canada as a whole over the next three decades faces similar challenges posed by a rapidly aging population, the policy example provided by the VIP deserves a wider audience.

As early as 1957 some VAC officials had begun to lobby for a 'Charter for Aged Veterans' through which the department could take the lead in Canadian gerontological research. Its doctors, nurses, psychiatrists, and hospitals constituted the 'core of a professional staff that could ... point to a better understanding and thoroughly practical approach to the Ageing citizen problem.' A new 'charter,' built upon VAC's experience in the field, could serve as an 'inspiration to the whole field of Gerontology throughout the country.'[5] Although prescient, such recommendations fell upon deaf ears for the next quarter-century.

The significant exception was Deer Lodge Centre in Winnipeg. At this veterans' facility, from the mid-1960s onwards, Dr Jack MacDonell, widely acknowledged as one of the founders of geriatric medicine and gerontology in Canada, pioneered the concept of multidisciplinary team-based approaches to the care of the elderly, day hospital clinics, respite care for caregivers, and community-based home care as a lower-cost and more humane alternative to the unnecessary institutionalization of aging veterans.[6] As a young physician in 1960, MacDonell had visited the United Kingdom to train with Ferguson Anderson, Marjorie Warrens, and Lionel Cosins, giants of British geriatrics in the post–Second World War era.[7] Anderson's core principle for geriatric medicine was that 'older people are happier and healthier in their own homes if they are fit enough to be there and so desire.' Problems as simple as bad feet, poor diet, severe constipation, or impacted ear wax – conditions all easily treatable at home – commonly led to misdiagnosis and unnecessary institutionalization of the elderly. Careful home assessments could reveal the roots of such conditions and determine the capacity of family members to provide care.[8]

Before joining VAC in 1967 as chief geriatrician at Deer Lodge, MacDonell experimented with these ideas at Municipal Hospital, a Winnipeg tuberculosis and polio treatment facility which, by the early 1960s, had evolved into a mostly chronic-care institution for the aged. Upon moving to Deer Lodge he launched an even more ambitious program to de-institutionalize as many as possible of its aging veterans.[9] Multidisciplinary teams were sent out to examine the physical layout of the veteran's home and, as MacDonell later recalled, ask pertinent questions: 'Is it on one or two floors? How were the kitchen facilities? How far is the bathroom? If they were not convenient, we would see what we could do to make the patient more mobile and able to cope. If that wasn't within the realm of possibility, we would ask "how can we alter the physical set-up in the home in order to make it compatible with day care?"'[10] A wheelchair pool was created for families so that veterans could be moved about more easily. Victorian Order of Nurses (VON) nurses were sent into veterans' homes to assist wives with bathing and health care for their husbands. With the help of the local branch of the Canadian Legion, MacDonell also established a system of social transportation to get veterans to and from his Day Hospital at Deer Lodge, the first of its kind in Canada. If a wife complained that she couldn't cope,

invariably we'd pick him up in an ambulance, and 'whish' he was back in the hospital. Well then, word got around that 'Hey, they really believe in what they're doing. They really will help us.' So the program was a success.

But if we hadn't said, 'Yes, that's fine, we'll pick him up,' and create some trust in the system, it wouldn't have gone far … Medicine was provided. Prostheses were provided. Canes and crutches were provided. So before home care started, we had a program. It wasn't called home care. But that's the kind of support that, through the Day Hospital, we were able to provide. And maybe that's where the Veterans Independence Program got the idea.[11]

Winnipeg, a city of vibrant ethnic neighbourhoods and strong community activism, was fertile ground in the 1960s for such innovative experiments in home care. In 1957 the Age and Opportunity Centre, one of Canada's first attempts to coordinate area planning and research on the needs of the elderly, was launched by the city's social planning council. It soon became a focal point for attracting to Winnipeg leaders in community-based care such as Betty Havens and Evelyn Shapiro, both of whom would subsequently become key advisers to VAC and to Manitoba's own long-term care system, the first in Canada to make home care, after 1974, its principal point of access.[12] As Havens recalled: 'Sometimes you get a critical mass of people who have similar philosophies or ideologies or concerns and because they are in the same place they can move things forward with great strides … And because these ideas worked here, in a sense you were selling Veterans Affairs and others a product you could show them, not just that you talked about.'[13]

By the late 1970s, the department was willing to listen to such ideas as a result of aggressive lobbying from the Canadian Legion and the War Amps of Canada over waiting lists, in the hundreds, for veterans wishing access to long-term-care beds in VAC facilities. Despite a recent $11 million renovation and expansion of Sunnybrook Hospital in Toronto, the Legion noted in 1975, 'its 400 beds are filled, there's an overflow of nearly 200 in a nearby building and a long waiting list. Most of the patients are First World War veterans. Others are from the Boer War. As yet, few WWII vets have checked in.' The solution, the Legion argued, was for Ottawa to build more beds, and quickly.[14]

These demands, combined with the spectre of 330,000 Second World War veterans who would be turning sixty-five by 1985, deeply alarmed department officials. VAC would either have to reverse its decade-long policy of decentralizing institutional care to the provinces, entice them into building more long-term beds than they currently needed, or find other, less costly policy alternatives for meeting Canada's acknowledged obligations to its aging veterans.[15]

Beginning in early 1977, the department began exploring alternative policy options. Two years later, a small working group, led by VAC's program medical adviser Dr Blair Mitchell, completed their report.[16] The most important ideas shaping the group's work came from Manitoba, in particular Deer Lodge, where the task force travelled to get a first-hand look at MacDonell's Day Hospital. There they encountered in action the home-care principles of Sir Ferguson Anderson. Through a four-day conference on 'Alternatives to Long Term Care' hosted by the University of Manitoba, officials also met with Betty Havens and Evelyn Shapiro.[17] The end result, a lengthy memorandum to cabinet entitled 'The Aging Veteran and DVA,'[18] completed in December 1979, made a strong case for the advantages of the home-care option. Many veterans, who only needed a place to live, had been attracted to the department's institutional-care facilities by the cheap $120 monthly cost, unchanged since 1949, rather than through medical necessity. The department's current policy of simply 'warehousing' these and other veterans in hospitals, the memorandum argued, was

> expensive and not cost-effective; to a large degree it almost totally ignores the severe plight of many aged veterans and their spouses. A very significant number of veterans are in (expensive) hospital beds, not because they need to be but because we're unable to do the things that need to be done to keep them in the community ... It is clear to everyone that the unnecessary institutionalization of old people contributes to their deterioration and hastens the process of senility.[19]

The alternative was a new 'Aging Veterans Program' (AVP) to provide a 'more effective and less costly way' of meeting this need through programs designed to 'embrace support services delivered at the patient's home.' Apart from the delivery of professional and health-related services in the veteran's own residence, the AVP would also provide home modifications necessary to support independent living, social transportation to get veterans to and from out-patient or day hospital facilities, and, in a major innovation, housekeeping and groundskeeping services, where necessary. The goal was to 'make certain that [veterans] live, as long as is possible, in their own homes, in as happy and as healthy a state as can be.' Wherever possible, VAC would not provide services directly, but rather would 'selectively top up' provincial home-care coverage for eligible veterans, where it was available. In this way the department hoped to 'disengage gradually and as opportunity affords, from our present direct provision of care at the nursing home level ... leaving the actual operation of health systems to provincial jurisdictions.' Such a retreat 'would likely be more acceptable if offset by ... more use of community facilities and home-delivered services.' Since Canada's veterans were aging significantly faster than the general population, the department simply could not wait for provinces to act on their own to meet their needs.[20]

The first clients eligible for the proposed AVP were to be all aging veterans with overseas service who, either due to war injury or economic need, might require assistance in remaining in their own homes, a group estimated at 27,000 clients over the next five years. The price tag was $153 million. Once the proposal went to Treasury Board in the summer of 1980, however, it was scaled back to a far more modest 'pilot project,' targeted at a maximum of 3500 veterans who could relate their need for home-care services directly to a war-related 'pensioned condition.' Money for the new program, fixed at $21 million spread out over the next five years, was to be found from within VAC's existing budget.[21] The AVP's key goal was 'to contain the increasing adverse effects of aging in Canada's veteran population more effectively and at reduced cost.' A second objective, which would grow in importance as time went on, was 'to maintain the self-sufficiency of [the veteran's] spouse.' Since she was most often his primary caregiver, 'her health status is of concern to the department.' The new program would also spread Canada's support for aging veterans more equitably across the country. Compared to the department's 2400 chronic-care beds located in large cities where less than half of all veterans actually lived, AVP services would be made available everywhere.[22]

The AVP was announced in Parliament in early November 1980 and began operations in April 1981.[23] Despite its restrictive eligibility conditions and small start-up population, senior department officials argued that the pilot project was a 'foot in the door,' which they hoped could be 'expand[ed] quickly to include all needy veterans and civilians with qualifying service at such future time as the fiscal climate might permit.'[24]

Of all the support provided through the AVP, assistance with housekeeping and groundskeeping was the most trailblazing, since no provincial home-care program then (or now) offered equivalent stand-alone services. Their inclusion reflected the core belief of the department's key gerontological advisers that preserving the dignity of the elderly was essential to their ability and willingness to live independently. As Darragh Mogan, the key official behind VAC's home-care initiative, put it:

> People can be sick as all hell, but if their dignity in the community is maintained, in other words if they maintain themselves more or less to the standard of the community, they'll do a heck of a lot to stay home. If the surroundings and environment begin to fall apart, they will too. They'll give up ... Hence, the groundskeeping, housekeeping elements which are by far the most popular components of the program, even now.[25]

Four issues, present at the AVP's inception, would remain contentious over the next twenty-five years. The first was how to prove whether home care actually saved money that would otherwise be spent on hospital beds. Without such evidence, the AVP, like other community-based home-care programs at the provincial and local level, could be viewed by budget-conscious treasury and finance officials as an 'add-on' rather than a substitute cost for existing health-care spending, which simply generated new clients for an already over-burdened system.

A related issue was determining the intended core clientele for the program. Within the pension-based hierarchy of VAC, those who had suffered a war-related disability, although 'not [the] veterans in greatest need ... historically had the political "first call"' on any new program.[26] Initial eligibility for the AVP reflected this priority. Until 1984 only veterans with pensionable disabilities could apply. When few did in the program's early years, VAC district counsellors were instructed to 'beat the bushes' in order to find them.[27] The greatest need for the program, however, existed among the much larger category of low-income War Veterans Allowance (WVA) recipients. These were the men actually taking up most of the domiciliary care beds in VAC-sponsored facilities because of economic and social rather than medical necessity. If the cost-saving potential of home care was to be demonstrated, this was the group that had to be targeted. If limited only to pensioned veterans, the AVP could never prove it could save money.[28]

The third issue was use of the AVP as a 'gateway' into eligibility for the full package of VAC health-treatment benefits. Since veterans in institutions were already entitled to such care, in order to make the AVP an attractive substitute the department stipulated that qualifying for any one component of its home-care program would confer eligibility for the full range of treatment benefits such as eyeglasses, hearing aids, dental care, and drugs. Only a full assessment by a VAC medical team could qualify a veteran to receive any of these items. However, district counsellors soon discovered in marketing the AVP to veterans that 'in many cases what people wanted [was] not [AVP] but treatment benefits. It was a gateway ... It didn't take very long to figure it out: "I don't really need somebody to do my housekeeping but I sure would like somebody to pay for my glasses, my dental, and all the other benefits that follow."'[29]

A final issue was the status of veterans' wives or other family members who provided them with care. From the beginning the architects of the program recognized 'the vital role of spouses in maintaining the well-being of entitled veterans.'[30] Relieving some of their burden through contributions for home support or respite care was therefore in the department's long-term interest. However, this acknowledgment did not lead officials to include wives within the circle of eligibility for the AVP beyond the limited provision that veterans' widows could continue to receive housekeeping and groundskeeping contributions for a maximum of thirty days after their husband's death. 'A "family member" is a "family member." Society expects families to have ties and responsibilities and to accept these,' VAC minister Bennett Campbell argued in 1983 in making the case against extending AVP benefits to caregivers.[31]

Despite a slow start, within a year the AVP pilot project had met its initial target of reaching 3000 disabled veterans and was proving increasingly popular. As a result, VAC began planning for a major extension of the program to the much wider group of low-income clients receiving the WVA who, from the beginning, had been seen as the key clientele for its services. The timing was right. Since half of the veteran population would reach age sixty-five within two years, increasing numbers would become eligible for the combination of Old Age Security (OAS) and the Guaranteed Income Supplement (GIS). As a result, VAC expenditures on the income-tested WVA for those below sixty-five were projected to shrink from $437 million in 1983–4 to only $110 million by 1991, a saving of more than $300 million for the department. 'Less than one-third of this amount will accommodate health care needs of aging veterans,' officials argued.[32] Simply combining the administration of the WVA with the much vaster OAS-GIS infrastructure within National Health and Welfare would free up the resources needed to finance the cost of expanding the AVP. Building a larger home-care service across the country would also pay dividends for Canadian society as a whole. By the year 2000, VAC officials pointed out that

Canada will be faced with the reality of the 'grey wave' resulting from the aging of the 'baby boom' era children. Significant gaps in services, program know-how, and geriatric research must be filled. The Department is in the unique position to develop and provide creative responses for veterans that could have wide acceptance in the community in time to be of service to the future mass of elderly Canadians.[33]

Expanding home care would also be popular not only among veterans, but with their children, 'who traditionally are supportive of the Government for the care given to their parents.' By contrast, failure to act would be viewed by veterans and their families as evidence of a 'lack of government commitment to fulfilling responsibilities identified in the Veterans Charter.'[34] Since all those who served overseas were eligible to apply for access to domiciliary or nursing-home care paid for by VAC, they should also all be eligible to apply for the AVP, and the sooner this was made possible the better. Measures 'delayed too long ... might "miss the boat" in terms of answering the need' of Canada's rapidly aging Second World War veteran cohort.[35]

Although there was no hard data from the pilot project to say exactly how much Ottawa might save from this 'more humane approach to care,'[36] officials simply compared the difference between the $4400 average annual price per person for the AVP and the $36,000 yearly cost of operating a nursing-home bed. From this perspective, they argued, an expanded AVP would allow Ottawa to meet its acknowledged obligations to aging overseas service veterans at 'one-eighth the cost of institutionalization.' Put differently, by spending an additional $57 million annually, the department could either keep 14,000 veterans living 'in their own communities, most in their own homes' or, for the same money, assist 'only 1,280 veterans ... in new Type 1 and Type 2 institutional beds.'[37] The choice seemed clear. 'The cost of the traditional response to the plight of old people who can no longer survive at home on their own – that is of warehousing them in institutions – will go right off the clock in a few years,' VAC deputy minister Bruce Brittain warned the Trudeau cabinet in defending his department's home-care proposal. 'Costs, however, can be contained by the program ... we have submitted today.'[38]

Enticed by the anticipated savings to be generated from harmonizing the delivery of WVA with OAS-GIS, the federal government agreed in February 1984 to a modest and phased-in extension of the AVP over a four-year period to 'all high risk veterans groups.' Between 1984 and

1986 all veterans aged sixty-five or over receiving WVA, and not just
disability pensioners, would become eligible to apply for AVP home-
care services. Over the following two years, pensioned and non-
pensioned veterans unable to qualify for WVA because they were
already receiving OAS would also become eligible if they needed assistance in living at home. When this AVP extension was completed by
1988–9, the department estimated that the program would have a caseload of 11,105 veterans and, measured in constant dollars, would cost
an additional $40.6 million annually.[39]

These estimates of modest program growth soon evaporated once a
new Progressive Conservative government led by Brian Mulroney took
office in September 1984. During the election, capitalizing on the deep
unhappiness of the Canadian Legion and War Amps over the relocation
of VAC headquarters from Ottawa to Charlottetown, the Tories targeted
veterans as an important constituency by promising to sharply reduce
the processing time and significantly expand the range of veterans' benefits. To make good on this pledge, Mulroney appointed a high-profile
cabinet minister from the Diefenbaker era, George Hees, as his new minister of veterans affairs. The seventy-four-year-old Hees, a Member of
Parliament since 1950, was a decorated Second World War veteran who
had been wounded during overseas service. He became one of Canada's
most popular and successful advocates of veterans' needs. 'All Canadians are special but veterans are very special,' Hees proclaimed upon taking up his new cabinet position. 'They went overseas and took a chance
on getting their heads blown off so their country could remain free. For
that reason I want all veterans and their submissions treated with the
very greatest of generosity, courtesy, and efficiency ... I want the benefit
of the doubt to be given to the veteran.'[40] As one department official
recalled, 'There was just a major difference in approach ... The bottom
line was "be generous." And people were very generous. That permeated the organization very rapidly.'[41]

Hees's first initiative was to insist that the name of the Aging Veterans Program be changed to the Veterans Independence Program, or
'VIP.' Hees liked the acronym VIP because the initials captured perfectly the message he had been publicizing since taking over the
department. 'The new name reflects the Government's philosophy that
veterans are very special Canadians.'[42] The program soon proved to be
extraordinarily popular with veterans as well, to an extent unantici-
pated by VAC. Because of its extension to a much wider category of
veterans and heavy promotion by both department counsellors and

veterans' organizations, reflecting Hees's clear signal that his staff should embrace a 'climate of generosity' towards veterans, the VIP's caseload grew by 70 per cent a year between 1984 and 1989 during a time when other national social programs were experiencing 'clawbacks.' By the latter year 40,000 veterans were accessing VIP services, compared to the caseload of 11,000 originally forecast for that date in 1983.[43] The department's new focus on preventive health and social services for aging veterans also brought about a transformation in VAC's personnel. By 1987 52 per cent of counsellors in district offices had university degrees. Another 25 per cent had either completed or were enrolled in community-college certificate or in-housing training courses in gerontology.[44] Women were also emerging as a rapidly growing presence within all levels of the department. By the end of the 1980s VAC was no longer an organization administered by (male) veterans for (male) veterans.

Despite this explosive caseload growth, by 1987 the department still had no solid evidence that the VIP was actually saving Ottawa money.[45] Was home care provided through the VIP an add-on or a substitute cost for long-term-care beds in the community, senior officials asked? Without more research there was no way of knowing. To answer these questions in 1987 VAC commissioned a well-known independent consulting firm, Price Waterhouse, to explore whether the VIP was actually delivering the goods in terms of both saving money on bed care and increasing the self-sufficiency of veterans. Before beginning their work the consultants flagged a number of methodological problems facing their study. First, there was no control group with whom VIP clients could be compared, so there was no way of knowing what would have been their fate in the absence of the program. Second, since the VIP topped up provincial home-care services, wherever possible, it was difficult to separate out its effects from those of other programs. Third, cost-effectiveness was only one rationale for the VIP. The other was improving veterans' health and self-sufficiency. This objective could be met whether or not they were actually in danger of institutionalization. Finally, given the insufficient supply of long-term-care beds within many if not most communities, it would be hard to demonstrate whether or not the VIP delayed or prevented institutionalization. Without a true choice, how could one know whether home care was the preferred option?[46]

These reservations notwithstanding, the Price Waterhouse consultants undertook their study, which was completed by the summer of 1989.

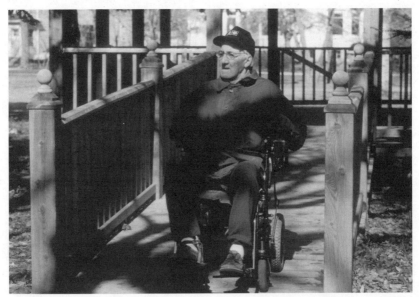

VIP provides home modifications for disabled veterans. (Courtesy Veterans Affairs Canada)

The study provided the first thorough portrait of the VIP caseload. The typical client, in 1988, was a married male between sixty-five and seventy-five years old living with his spouse and family or friends. Most owned their own home. Three-quarters were pensioners. One-half had been admitted to hospital at some point over the past three years. Seventy-five per cent rated their own health as 'fair' or 'poor' and 80 per cent were suffering from at least one chronic ailment. Two-thirds could be left unattended in their own homes, 7 per cent could not be left by themselves, and 21 per cent could only be left alone for up to three hours. Only 35 per cent of their caregivers were rated as being in excellent or good health, and one-quarter were in poor heath. This was a key finding, the report noted, since 'caregiver health status has implications for the amount and type of services needed by veterans to enable them to remain in their own homes.' Most clients were receiving housekeeping or groundskeeping services through the VIP that were supplied by independent providers, friends, or family members, the last method being by far the most preferred.[47]

The study's most important finding was the high level of client satisfaction with the VIP. Over 90 per cent of both veterans and their caregivers reported that they were 'moderately' or 'extremely' satisfied with the services they were receiving. Three-quarters of the veterans and over half of their counsellors, caregivers, or nurses said that the VIP had made a moderate or great deal of difference in their life satisfaction, mostly because of reduced worry, which was the most common factor cited by veterans for why the program had improved their health. The 'vast majority' of clients reported difficulties in managing at home before receiving the VIP. Without it, almost half said they would have difficulty doing yard work or snow shovelling, 36 per cent said general home maintenance would be a problem, and 20 per cent singled out difficulty climbing stairs or getting in and out of the bath. One-quarter were extremely limited in their ability to perform activities of daily living. Eighty-six per cent said the VIP had made a moderate or large difference in their ability to manage in their own home. In short, in terms of meeting one of its principal goals, improving the self-sufficiency of veterans, the program was clearly a great success.

The VIP was also having a major impact on veterans' caregivers, 88 per cent of whom reported that the VIP had made a 'moderate' or 'great deal' of difference in reducing their burdens. Fifty-six per cent said it had improved their own health. This too was a key finding. 'When the health of the caregiver is good,' the consultants noted, 'it can be expected that they will take on a variety of care activities on behalf of the veteran. If their health is poor, many of [these activities] ... will likely be transferred to the formal service system.' Put differently, keeping the veteran's wife healthy would reduce the long-term costs of veterans' benefits to the state.[48]

But did the VIP reduce significantly the demand for institutional beds? On this key point, the Price Waterhouse study was less conclusive. Most VIP clients, it observed, 'were not at high risk of institutionalization.'[49] Since the most common services provided through the program were groundskeeping and housekeeping rather than personal or direct patient care, this finding should not have been all that surprising. Nonetheless, it did create problems for underscoring the VIP's cost effectiveness. No part of the report was more troublesome than its attempt to estimate how much money the VIP had actually saved. Depending on the assumptions used, estimates of cost-savings could 'vary from $6 million to $214 million.' Such a huge range was not very helpful in making a convincing case for the cost effectiveness of the

VIP. The consultants' best estimate was that the program most likely saved Ottawa $33 million a year. However, this was a conclusion that 'should be treated with caution.'[50]

VAC agreed. These assumptions were 'so soft [they are] an easy target for criticism,' senior officials argued. Unfortunately, this was exactly 'the area that the Department must have a handle on to support the VIP to senior levels of government,' particularly in light of newly revised forecasts that within seven years the program's caseload could peak at 120,000 clients. As a result, VAC decided to underscore the high level of client satisfaction with the VIP revealed by the Price Waterhouse study and to focus on quality-of-life arguments for supporting the program. 'It should be dealt with in a way that expresses the psychological, emotional, and social importance of seniors remaining in their homes or community.'[51]

During Hees's remaining years as VAC minister questions of cost-saving receded into the background as the range and scope of veterans' benefits expanded dramatically. In the 1984 election campaign the Progressive Conservatives had promised to extend eligibility for the WVA to those who had volunteered for active duty during the Second World War and were assigned to serve in Canada for a period of at least a year, a group known as Canada Service Only (CSO) veterans.[52] After four years of failing to deliver on this promise and in response to unrelenting pressure from the Canadian Legion to make good on it before the upcoming 1988 election, the Mulroney government, largely through Hees's efforts, agreed to a scaled-down compromise. All 327,000 CSO veterans, a group slightly larger than the 317,000 veterans who had 'theatre of war' service overseas, would now be eligible to apply for the VIP, even though they enjoyed no guarantee of a long-term-care bed. If approved, they would also 'gateway' into the full range of veterans' health treatment benefits, one of the principal objectives the Legion pursued on their behalf.[53] This decision, in combination with the ongoing aging of the veterans' population, provided a further boost to the already exponential growth rate of the VIP. Between 1988 and 1992 the program's caseload more than doubled from 40,400 to 87,900. Program expenditures rose from $54 million to $168 million.[54]

At the same time, disturbing new warnings emerged from a 1988 VAC study which predicted that, notwithstanding the VIP's widespread popularity and rapid growth, the department would soon be facing a major shortage of long-term-care beds as its client population became older and frailer. In 1988, male veterans, at an average age of sixty-eight, constituted one-third of the total Canadian male population over age sixty-five and half of all disabled elderly men. Since 1984, because of the VIP, the department had frozen its total number of departmental and contract beds on the assumption that its home-care program would cut the demand for long-term care by approximately 1200 beds. By 1988 the department had 1100 beds in its four remaining institutions, and another 3000 reserved 'on contract' for veterans in provincial or non-profit facilities. Taken together, their cost absorbed almost half of its total health-care budget.

By 1991 more than 7000 veterans would need institutional care, the report predicted. Ten years later, when demand peaked, the total need was forecast at 11,000 beds caring for 7 per cent of the eligible veteran population, almost half of whom would need the most expensive Type 3 category of chronic care. The price tag ranged from $520 million in capital and $220 million in operating costs if VAC built and ran the facilities itself, to $200 million in capital and $45 million in operating costs if it worked through the provinces. These 'conservative' assumptions, the authors of the report argued, were 'startling, if not alarming.' Nonetheless, failure to act would be viewed as a '"breaking of faith" on the part of the government and a denial of earlier promises and assurances that veterans would be fully compensated for their sacrifices on behalf of Canada.' Coming up with an answer to the looming bed shortage, the authors concluded, constituted 'the single most important component of Veterans' Affairs planning for the veteran population in its twilight years.'[55]

The most puzzling aspect of the study was its downplaying of the VIP's role as the answer to the ballooning costs of long-term care. For the past decade VAC officials had argued that the department was ahead of the field in developing an innovative community-based home-care strategy as an alternative to building costly institutional beds, a strategy that by the late 1980s was extraordinarily popular among veterans. Now, this new study warned that, despite the VIP, more long-term beds were needed – and lots of them. What had gone wrong?

The VIP had saved money through the freeze on new contract beds throughout the 1980s. At the same time, the numbers of veterans on waiting lists for access to long-term institutional care had risen from 330 in 1983 to 821 by 1987. No matter how well the VIP had responded to maintaining veterans' self-sufficiency in the home, it apparently had not succeeded in reducing waiting lists or the previously estimated needs for additional long-term-care beds. Instead, what had occurred was

> an easing of the demand for lower levels of institutional care. Patients who have been quietly suffering at home without assistance are now able to enjoy an improved quality of life and independent functioning. As well, stresses on the primary care giver, often the spouse ... are eased to make their lives more tolerable ... However, demand for an already scarce supply of long-term institutional beds continues as the individual who can now safely be cared for at home is replaced in the queue by someone whose health care needs cannot be effectively provided at home.

The VIP, in other words, would 'not eliminate pressures for veterans' long-term care beds.' There was an 'urgent need' to build more of them. In the meantime, 'waiting lists will continue to grow at an increasing rate and utilization of home care services will be extensive.'[56] This was not an argument that advocates of the VIP within the department wanted to hear.

By the early 1990s the fiscal pressures on VAC also intensified in response to a rapidly deteriorating economic climate and growing pressure from the Finance Department and Treasury Board for fiscal restraint and across-the-board cuts. Even veterans would not be immune from these demands for sacrifice. The 'era of generosity' had come to an end. The department's organizational culture of 'courtesy, generosity, and speed ... which has been inculcated in our staff and has, in the past, characterized Canada's relationship with its veterans ... must [be] turn[ed] around to reflect fiscal reality,' VAC's new minister, Kim Campbell, warned.[57]

Over the first half of the 1990s this tougher fiscal environment provoked a series of clashes between veterans' organizations and the department. In 1990, in a largely symbolic cut, the department eliminated heavy housekeeping – the seasonal cleaning of walls and ceilings, chimneys, drapes, and carpets – from the list of VIP home-care services. Representing an estimated $8 to $10 million annual saving within a $1.5 billion VAC budget, this did not seem like a drastic change.[58] Instead, the decision – undertaken without first consulting veterans' organizations – provoked a firestorm of criticism from the War Amps, the Legion, and opposition MPs precisely because of its symbolism. As Liberal VAC critic Fred Mifflin put it, 'Something is being taken away from veterans for the first time since the Great Depression. We should not be taking something away from veterans, we should be racking our brains trying to find something to give them.'[59] War Amps president Cliff Chadderton, wielding the image of frail amputees 'tottering back and forth on step ladders' in their efforts to clean walls and chimneys so that they could keep up their homes, was particularly devastating in his attack on the department's decision, even entering into negotiations with CTV's flagship W5 news program for a feature on the topic on the eve of the 1993 federal election.[60] Not surprisingly, a compromise was eventually reached, leading to the reinstatement of heavy housekeeping for all war pensioners' with 100 per cent disability status.[61]

This blow-up, one of the most acrimonious in the department's post–Second World War history, underscored the difficulties of attempting to take away services from veterans.[62] It also highlighted the challenge of balancing entitlement and need within the VIP. Disabled veterans, who had appreciated assistance coping with the more difficult seasonal tasks of independent living when they were in their sixties, were hardly willing to forego these same services once they and their spouses were ten years older. It was a lesson that would not be soon forgotten.

Similar tensions emerged over VAC's decision, after 1990, to begin enforcing the pensioned condition, or the direct linkage between war-related injury and the need for VIP benefits, far more vigorously on the one-third of the program's caseload receiving a disability pension. At this point the political imperatives of fiscal restraint increasingly clashed with the growing frailty of Canadian veterans. District counsellors and health officials in the field could reach no consensus on how the pensioned condition should be interpreted, resulting in wide variations in departmental practice across Canada. Should hearing loss or flat feet be used to establish VIP eligibility for housekeeping or groundskeeping services? Should arthritis, respiratory illness, or heart problems, not easily traceable to war, be used as criteria for establishing a pensioned condition?[63] Here is where the needs and rights of veterans collided, mediated through the lens of old age. As even senior VAC officials conceded, the attempt in the 1990s to vigorously enforce the pensioned conditioned on a frailer clientele was 'absurd.'[64]

The result was a growing movement within VAC, as the century drew to a close, away from an entitlement-driven pension regime and towards a new philosophy of client-centred services, focused increasingly on the entire family context surrounding the frail veteran and his caregiver. As one official put it, 'Our idea was "let's get to the need, and let's find a way that we can link the health problem to the pension process."'[65] This new approach was made fiscally easier as the VIP caseload peaked at 87,900 in 1993, significantly below the earlier forecast of 120,000, and began to decline gradually for the first time in its history in response to the accelerating mortality of the veteran population. By 2000 the program's caseload had dropped by over 20 per cent to 68,900, the average age of veterans reached eighty-two, and the percentage deemed 'at risk' more than doubled from 20 per cent to 42 per cent. In response, senior VAC officials soon were asking why there should be any criteria for linking the VIP to a war-related disability.[66]

A similar focus on need rather than entitlement emerged around the growth of waiting lists for long-term-care beds, the issue that had prompted the creation of the VIP in the first place. This time debate raged over the category of those Overseas Service Veterans (OSVs) who had no war-related injury, whose needs up to this point were almost completely unknown by either veterans' organizations or VAC. Between 1997 and 2002 dire predictions of acute shortages of long-term-care beds for this group dominated discussions between department officials, veterans' organizations, and the Senate Subcommittee on Veterans Affairs. OSVs, who numbered somewhere between 150,000 and 180,000, were described by the National Council of Veterans' Associations (NCVA) as the 'phantom group' because they did not qualify for disability pensions, income-tested WVA, or the VIP, and therefore had had little to no contact with VAC since 1945. Their single entitlement, by virtue of their overseas service during the war, was the right to a department-funded, priority-access bed in a long-term-care facility.[67] In his 1996 report the auditor general drew attention to how little VAC knew about the anticipated needs of OSVs or the extent to which they might claim their right to a long-term-care bed now that they had reached the age of seventy-five and were beginning to experience greater health risks. The department 'could face significant unplanned costs' from this group, he warned.[68]

Privately, VAC officials were also concerned that over the next three to eight years OSVs might generate a demand for thousands more beds, compared to the 4000 currently in use.[69] In 1999 the Senate Subcommittee on Veterans Affairs released its influential report *Raising the Bar: Creating a New Standard in Veterans Health Care*, which also flagged the issue, arguing there was 'a very real concern that a substantial percentage of the 160,000 overseas veterans entitled to a priority access bed will invoke this right.'[70] At presentations before the Senate subcommittee each year between 1997 and 2002 Cliff Chadderton, chairman of the NCVA, raised the same alarm:

> Five years ago we brought to your attention the issue of the phantom veteran. We know he exists, but we have no record of him. However, he served in World War II. He is back in Canada now. There is no doubt that if he continues to live he will require a long term care bed ... We do not really know how many there are ... We told this committee four years ago that there is a crisis hanging over our heads. It is not here now because we are able to find ways and means of finding beds for veterans or of giving them the veterans' independence program so that they can remain in their own homes. However, we pointed out that situation will not continue. The crisis will only get worse.

VAC would require anywhere from 6000 to 10,000 more beds during this 'crisis period,' Chadderton predicted.[71]

In a hard-hitting, three-part series on veterans' hospitals between 1999 and 2000 the *Legion* magazine also zeroed in on the problem of three-year waiting lists for admission to veterans' facilities in Victoria, Ottawa, and Halifax. 'It is up to VAC to provide the veterans beds when they are needed, whether that means building new facilities, building additions, or contracting beds in other facilities.' In a blunt editorial, the magazine argued, 'We have been too comfortable with the view long put forward by VAC that the Canadian veterans are treated better than veterans anywhere else in the world ... VAC should tackle the remaining problems of outdated facilities. It should also address the situation in Victoria, Ottawa and Halifax where the facilities are modern but the waiting lists are intolerably long – up to three years. There's a simple solution: more beds.'[72] After two decades arguing that home care was the better alternative, it now seemed that the department was back where it started.

Or was it? Senior officials remained sceptical that spending anywhere from $250 million to $500 million building more beds was the answer, especially for a group such as the 'phantom' OSVs whose needs were so uncertain. As one senior official put it, 'We know that people don't want to be in institutions, so why would you put a whole lot of money into building beds that people may not want in the long run anyway?'[73] Instead, the department devised, as an alternative, an innovative pilot project targeted at the OSV client group to test their need and desire for institutional care. Beginning in 1999, 139 OSV veterans on waiting lists for VAC beds at facilities in Victoria, Ottawa, and Halifax, although not entitled to VIP home-care services or health-treatment benefits because they lacked either a pensionable disability or the required low-income qualification, were nevertheless 'deemed eligible' for both until a long-term-care bed became available.[74] As VAC's deputy minister at that time explained, 'Although we didn't have the legislative authority ... we did certainly have the moral authority in terms of the intent of the legislation and it was something ... we really did want to have a look at to see what kind of difference it would make. The other reality is that it was a quarter to a fifth of the cost to provide veterans services in their own homes than in a facility.'[75] Through the pilot project, OSVs gained access to home patient care, personal care, housekeeping, groundskeeping, ambulatory health care, social transportation, and home adaptation services, plus the full range of VAC health-treatment benefits at an estimated annual average cost of $10,400 per client.[76]

The OSV pilot project became the department's response to the auditor general's and veterans organizations' concerns about the needs of the so-called 'phantom group.' It also provided a concrete example of how the new client-centred service approach could be used creatively to address the unmet needs of clients in a cost-effective manner. The VIP benefits and services these veterans received improved their health care as well as their lifestyle while they were on waiting lists by allowing them to stay closer to their families for longer periods and at the same time reduced pressure on and provided respite for their caregivers. Cliff Chadderton, chairman of the NCVA, remained deeply sceptical, calling the project a 'stop-gap, band-aid measure ... It will not correct the situation at all. What is the solution? ... The federal government will have to go to the provinces and say ... "We would like to dedicate ... more beds."'[77]

His critique, however, was soon eclipsed by the key finding of the project. The OSV clients on the waiting lists did not want a bed. Although quite frail and very ill, if given a choice they wanted to stay at home. Over 92 per cent of those who participated in the project, when actually offered a bed at a nearby veteran's facility, turned it down in favour of continued support at home through the VIP.[78] Thus, it was now clear that there was more to waiting lists than met the eye. Within a year the OSV pilot project was expanded to all OSVs on priority-access waiting lists across Canada, with identical results. After receiving the VIP and treatment benefits, 90 per cent chose to remain at home even when a bed became available, resulting in major savings for the department. The average client on the pilot project spent approximately $3600 in VIP services and $3000 in treatment benefits annually, compared to the $50,000 yearly cost of a priority-access bed.[79] Figures like these finally drove home to Finance Department and Treasury Board officials the cost-effectiveness of the VIP. 'Everybody was a doubting Thomas,' the department's former director of health services recalled. 'But the central agencies knew what they saw. They saw files. They knew how sick these people were and they were still willing to stay home.'[80] After two decades of pioneering Canada's most extensive model of community-based home care, those running the VIP now had convincing evidence that even Type 2 and Type 3 clients, whose need for expensive institutional care was immediate and irrefutable, when given a real choice backed by a strong network of home-care sources, preferred to 'age in place' rather than within a long-term-care facility.

In this sense, the OSV pilot project finally provided VAC with strong arguments to counter the sheer power of waiting lists to drive the agenda towards purchasing or building more beds. 'People love beds ... They love institutions. They love it for everybody else, but they don't love it for themselves,' officials wryly observed. 'So if anyone wants to review the impact of the Veterans Independence Program, they have to look at that pilot project.'[81] In June 2003, as a result of the VIP's success, eligibility for the program was extended to all OSVs who demonstrated a need for it.[82] More questions remained, however. How long could access to the VIP and treatment benefits delay institutionalization? To what extent was the decision to remain at home attributable to the resources made available through VIP as opposed to other factors? And what was the impact on caregivers? In assessing the 'cost' advantage of the VIP, department officials acknowledged, it always had to be remembered that 'for most recipients, the care and support provided by family members (most often the spouse) comes at no cost to the state.'[83]

The needs and rights of spousal caregivers of veterans re-emerged forcefully onto the VAC policy horizon during the same period as the debate over waiting lists was unfolding. Along with better access to beds, the demand that wives receive lifetime eligibility for VIP services in their own right, following the death of their husbands, became the other key demand of veterans' organizations from 1997 onwards. The

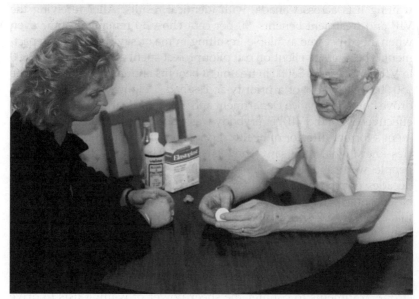

VIP provides home health care for aging veterans. (Courtesy Veterans Affairs Canada)

rising mortality of Second World War veterans as the century drew to a close sharply underscored their growing concern for the fate of their partners. 'Certainly in the mind of the veteran, [the VIP] was taking care of both of them, allowing both … to live in the house,' Legion Service Director Jim Rycroft told the Senate Subcommittee on Veterans Affairs in 2001. 'We are trying to honour the veterans' wishes to take care of the surviving spouse.'[84] As veterans themselves put it during focus-group sessions with the department, 'Spouses … suffered with us and should be compensated. If I pass away, my wife is out in the cold.' Similar demands were echoed by their wives. 'We are the caregivers of veterans. They will give you service as long as the veteran is living. If he dies, what will happen to me? Will all those benefits be cut off?'[85]

Before 1990 spouses only continued to receive VIP housekeeping and groundskeeping services for up to thirty days following their husband's death. Beginning in 1990 these benefits were extended on compassionate grounds for up to twelve months. However, the wife's entitlement remained tied directly to recognition of her husband's wartime service, not her own contributions as his caregiver. Department regulations were 'very explicit as to who our clients are ... Housekeeping and groundskeeping ... are the only two aspects of the VIP which also indirectly benefit the spouse while being provided to the veteran,' senior officials argued. As a result, these were the only two VIP services that could be continued for the widow, albeit for a limited period. 'Eligibility to a spouse is not being recognized; eligibility still resides through the veteran.'[86]

By the end of the 1990s, this constrained recognition of the key role of veterans' caregivers in allowing a frailer population of veterans to remain at home became the target of growing criticism both inside and outside the department. Within VAC's Gerontological Advisory Council, established in 1997, academics and veterans made common cause around the rights and contributions of caregivers.[87] Reflecting an explosion of research across North America in the 1990s on the significance of informal caregiving, including an innovative 'Care for the Caregiver' program co-sponsored by VAC itself,[88] gerontologists on the council argued that the department's historic focus on the *veteran's* benefits provided a poor fit with its new service philosophy of taking the entire context of family caregiving into account.[89] 'Attempts to support caregivers with policies developed to support care recipients are cumbersome,' a departmental study in 2001 pointed out. 'As VAC moves towards a focus on the veteran family unit, it should be prepared to provide direct benefits to informal caregivers,' including not only lifetime eligibility for the VIP but the provision of full health-treatment benefits, where necessary. The familialist ideology surrounding the VIP since its origins in 1981, which normalized the family's responsibility for care, had masked or muted the rights and needs of caregivers whose unpaid labour was essential to the low cost and continued success of the program. A new policy of 'equal support for caregiving contributions of equal value' was required.[90]

All such arguments in favour of granting benefits to caregivers, including lifetime eligibility for VIP services, were rejected by Ottawa on the grounds that such a change implied a dramatic redefinition of who the 'true' clients of VAC really were. As Canada moved closer to the sixtieth anniversary celebrations of V-E Day and the 'Year of the Veteran,' however, these defences collapsed in the face of a swelling tide of public commemoration honouring the contributions of veterans and their spousal caregivers.

In the spring of 2003 Veterans Affairs Minister Rey Pagtakhan announced that his department would soon bring forward policy changes to address the key needs identified by Canadian veterans' organizations, the most of important of which was providing lifetime continuation of VIP housekeeping and groundskeeping services to the surviving spouses of veterans. Pagtakhan's speech clearly displayed the hierarchy of arguments underpinning this historic shift in the department's mandate. This policy change, he argued, 'offer[ed] Canada an opportunity to further express our nation's unending gratitude to our Veterans. These changes *also* recognize the value of lifelong caregiving that has been provided to Veterans with disabilities by their spouses.' The same commemorative rationale was reflected in Legion president Allan Parks's expression of thanks to the Chrétien government for ensuring that, through this recognition of their wives, 'the sacrifices of Canadian Veterans will not be forgotten.'[91]

At first limited only to wives whose husbands died after 12 May 2003, lifetime eligibility to VIP housekeeping and groundskeeping services was made retroactive, by December 2004, to all spouses widowed since the program's inception in 1981 after a storm of public and parliamentary criticism at the niggardliness of the original decision to disentitle 27,000 other veterans' wives who had lost continued access to VIP services because their husbands died prior to May 12, 2003.[92]

Ottawa's belated policy reversal would add another $200 million to the cost of the program over the next five years. Nonetheless, 'it was simply the right thing to do,' Paul Martin's new VAC minister Albini Guarnieri acknowledged in justifying the change. 'We felt they were essentially unpaid partners of Veterans Affairs who were helping us care for our veterans. They deserved our support in their declining years.' Guarnieri also added her voice to the significance of commemoration in shaping this decision. 'The Year of the Veteran will be a national history lesson, a national show of gratitude for our veterans and an opportunity to renew our commitment to remembrance and pass that tradition on to a new generation.' The VIP was also a 'model for the rest of Canada,' she argued, which the provinces should follow. 'The challenge for all levels of government is to promote the kind of healthy independent living that allows seniors to live in the community longer, to be in a caring family environment longer, and to be in an institutional environment as a very last resort.'[93]

Guarnieri's juxtaposition of veterans' special entitlement with the relevance of the VIP model to debates around the need for a national home-care program reveals the contradictory legacy of the program. The VIP's rapid growth and enduring popularity among veterans' families is evidence of both the attractiveness and need for community-based home-care strategies that provide a broad continuum of support for aging in place. The most widely used elements of the VIP, self-managed housekeeping and groundskeeping services, although not high profile nor generally available within provincial home-care programs, have arguably played a key role in bringing veterans and their partners into care plans designed to avoid a caregiving crisis.

At the same time, veterans and their widows have such a choice because they are privileged clients of the Canadian welfare state in recognition of their sacrifices in time of war. The right of all OSVs to a federally funded long-term care bed was the VIP's original policy driver. This was not an entitlement veterans' organizations would let Ottawa forget. As one VAC study pointed out, 'Because many veterans believed they had a right to services ... [they] were more "open" about what they needed ... Services such as the VIP are acceptable to them because VIP is a service that they have earned.'[94]

This is a sentiment American political sociologist Theda Skocpol, in her study of the GI Bill of Rights, has termed 'legion populism.'[95] But as the American example illustrates, legion populism does not always translate well into claims that are easily winnable by a wider public. Today American veterans enjoy a range of publicly funded medical and hospital services that Canadians take for granted, but that have not led to a successful campaign, south of the border, for universal, publicly funded health insurance. A similar challenge confronts those arguing for the addition of something like the VIP home-care model to our national package of health-care entitlements. For this to occur, VIP-like services must first be seen as essential and affordable, not just for 'very special Canadians,' but for everyone who requires them in order to age in comfort, security, and dignity in old age.

## NOTES

I wish to thank Veterans Affairs Canada for their generous cooperation and support of this research project, and Peter Neary as well as Norah Keating for their helpful comments.

1 Canada, Commission on the Future of Health Care in Canada, Final Report, *Building on Values: The Future of Health Care in Canada*, November 2002. See also Patricia M. Baranek, Raisa Deber, and A. Paul Williams, *Almost Home: Reforming Home and Community Care in Ontario* (Toronto: University of Toronto Press, 2004).

2 Morris L. Barer, Robert G. Evans, and Clyde Hertzman, 'Avalanche or
Glacier? Health Care and the Demographic Rhetoric,' *Canadian Journal on
Aging* 14, 2 (1995): 193–224; Ellen Gee and Gloria Gutman, eds, *The Oversell-
ing of Population Aging: Apocalyptic Demography, Intergenerational Challenges
and Social Policy* (Toronto: Oxford University Press, 2000). Marcus Hollander,
*Final Report of the Study on the Comparative Cost Analysis of Home Care
and Residential Care Services* (Victoria: National Evaluation of the Cost-
Effectiveness of Home Care, 2001) provides the most thorough Canadian
analysis of the cost advantages of home care over residential care.
3 Veterans Affairs Canada (VAC), Charlottetown, Research Directorate,
'Chronology of Regulatory Changes Affecting Eligibility of Overseas Service Only Veterans for Institutional Care,' app. E (n.d.), 1–5; provided by
David Pedlar, Director of Research, VAC.
4 VAC, Veterans Affairs Canada–Canadian Forces Advisory Council Reference Paper, *The Origins and Evolution of Veterans' Benefits in Canada, 1914–
2004*, 'J. Consolidation and Adaptation,' March 2004; http://www.vac-acc
.gc.ca/general/sub.cfm?source=councils/vaccfac/reference; accessed
22 September 2005.
5 VAC, VIP Records, file 2740–1, vol. 7, D.F. Ferguson to J.A. Coulombe, 'New
Formula for the Aged Veterans,' 25 February 1985, enclosing copy of memo
by Dr E.B. Convery, Adviser in Geriatrics, to Senior Treatment Medical Officers, 'An Example for the Country: A Service to the Ageing,' 19 November
1957. Coulombe, the Assistant Deputy Minister for VAC, penned in the mar-
gin 'Most interesting – it took nearly 25 years to initiate this program.'
6 MacDonell received the Order of Canada in 1976 in recognition of his contribution to Canadian geriatrics. He was also one of the founders of the
Canadian Association on Gerontology in 1971. For biographical information see Dr Jack A. MacDonell at http://www.umanitoba.ca/honours/
index; accessed 22 September 2005. For MacDonell's work at Deer Lodge
Centre see http://www.deerlodge.mb.ca/about_dlc/history.asp, 'Deer
Lodge Centre History'; accessed 4 February 2004.
7 Jack and Asa MacDonell, joint interview by author, Toronto, 2 January 2004.
Asa MacDonell, wife of Jack, was also a physician and a former administrator at Deer Lodge Centre. Her work was instrumental in the creation of the
geriatric Day Hospital at Deer Lodge.
8 On the pioneering work of Ferguson Anderson, Marjorie Warrens, and
Lionel Cosins in Britain, see Pat Thane, *Old Age in English History: Past Experience, Present Issues* (New York: Oxford University Press, 2000), 443–53.
9 MacDonell interview, 2 January 2004.
10 Ibid.

11 Ibid.
12 Betty Havens, telephone interview by author, Winnipeg, 27 October 2003; Evelyn Shapiro, interview by author, Winnipeg, 22 October 2003; Signe Hansen, interview by author, Winnipeg, 23 October 2003.
13 Havens interview, 27 October 2003.
14 'A Veterans' Hospital That Looks More Like a University Residence,' *Legion* magazine, September 1975; 'More than Just Shelter,' *Legion* magazine, editorial, October 1976; 'Summing It All Up – A Comprehensive Brief,' *Legion* magazine editorial, July 1977.
15 VAC, VIP Records, file 2730–5, 'The Aging Veteran and D.V.A.,' November 1978.
16 VAC, VIP Records, file 2860-1, Darragh Mogan, 'The Veterans Independence Program: A Second Legacy to the People of Canada,' 29 April 2002, 1–3. Stu Tubbs, Darragh Mogan, Duncan Conrad, and Signe Hansen were the other members of the VAC task force on alternatives to institutional care; VAC, VIP Records, file 2730-5, W.B. Brittain, Deputy Minister of Veterans Affairs to P.A. McDougall, Deputy Minister of National Health and Welfare, 'The Aging Veteran and DVA: A Policy Proposal,' 27 December 1979.
17 Darragh Mogan, former director-general of health services, VAC, interview by author, Charlottetown, 11 July 2003; MacDonell interview, 2 January 2004; 'The Aging Veteran and DVA.'
18 In 1984 the 'applied title' of the department changed from the Department of Veterans Affairs (DVA) to Veterans Affairs Canada (VAC).
19 VAC, VIP Records, file 2730-5, W.B. Brittain, 'Memorandum to the Minister,' 20 December 1979.
20 VAC, VIP Records, file 270-5, 'Aging Veteran Program, Part 1, Proposal,' 5 June 1980; file 2730-0, memo from A. Garman, 'Aging Veterans Policy,' 24 September 1980; file 190-A6, draft form letter to physicians re the AVP, n.d. but ca. February 1981; file 2730-5, discussion paper 'The Aging Veteran and DVA,' 30 June 1980, reference discussion paper VA-1-80-DP; file 2730-5, vol. 2, 'Revised Assessment Report, The Aging Veteran and DVA,' 2 July 1980; file 2730-5, 'The Aging Veteran and DVA,' 30 June 1980. No provincial home-care programs were available in the four Atlantic provinces, nor in large parts of rural and small-town Canada.
21 VAC, VIP Records, file 2740-1, vol. 1, G.I. Hurley, memo, 'Extension of the Aging Veterans Program,' 23 March 1981; file 2730-5, 'The Aging Veteran and DVA.'
22 VAC, VIP Records, file 2730-5, 'The Aging Veteran and DVA.'
23 VAC, VIP Records, file 2730-1, 'News Release Communique, 7 November 1980 on "The Aging Veterans Program"'; file 195-1, 'Aging Veterans Program,

minutes of meeting of steering committee, Winnipeg Manitoba, 6–7 November 1980.' Services eligible for support included groundskeeping, housekeeping, home modifications, friendly visiting, meals-on-wheels, home nursing, physiotherapy, occupational therapy, attendance at day hospitals, and day care, all subject to yearly ceilings. When these were no longer sufficient, the veteran would be 'assisted in obtaining admission to an appropriate institution in the community of his choice.' For those disabled pensioners who qualified, the AVP would provide up to $45 a day for adult residential nursing home care, $4300 per year for home care, $500 per year for ambulatory care, and $2500 per year for home modifications.

24  VAC, VIP Records, file 195, A-2, 'Meeting on the AVP, Montreal, 17 November 1980'; file 2730-0, 'Program Description,' n.d. but ca. July/August 1980.
25  Mogan interview, 11 July 2003.
26  VAC, VIP Records, file 2740-1, vol. 4, Darragh Mogan to Lyse Blanchard, MSSD, 17 November 1983; Jacques Boisvert, former chief of treatment benefits, VAC, interview by author, Charlottetown, 8 July 2003.
27  Duncan Conrad, former director of health benefits, VAC, interview by author, Charlottetown, 9 July 2003.
28  VAC, VIP Records, file 2740-1, vol. 1, James Smith, ADM, to Bruce Brittain, DM, memo on 'Extension of the Aging Veterans Program,' 23 March 1981; file 2740-1, vol. 1, James Smith to Bruce Brittain, memo on 'AVP – Extension,' 10 November 1981.
29  Don Wilson, former chief of treatment benefits, VAC, interview by author, Charlottetown, 10 July 2003.
30  VAC, VIP Records, file 2730-0, memo from Jacques Boisvert, chief of treatment benefits, to RD's/DR, 'Aging Veterans Program,' 27 October 1982.
31  VAC, VIP Records, file 2740-3, Bennett Campbell, Minister of Veterans Affairs, 'AVP Presentation – War Amps of Canada,' Winnipeg, 23 March 1983.
32  VAC, VIP Records, file 2740-5, vol. 1, Bruce Brittain to Bennett Campbell, 13 July 1983; file 2740-5, vol. 2, memorandum to cabinet, 'Aging Veterans Program / War Veterans Allowances and Civilian War Allowances Program,' 24 November 1983.
33  VAC, VIP Records, file 2740-5, 'Aging Veterans Program / War Veterans Allowances.'
34  VAC, VIP Records, file 2740-5, vol. 2, 'Discussion Paper, Aging Veterans Program Extension,' 24 November 1983.
35  VAC, VIP Records, file 2745-9 BF, 'Interim Review Report Extended AVP,' May 1982.
36  VAC, VIP Records, file 2740-1, vol. 4, Marjory Boyce, VAC gerontologist, to James Smith, ADM, 'Cost-Savings AVP: Possible Extrapolation from

Manitoba/Canada Home Care Study,' 28 November 1983; file 2740-5, 'Discussion Paper, Aging Veterans Program Extension,' 24 November 1983.
37 'Discussion Paper,' 24 November 1983; file 2740-5, vol. 2, 'Introductions, J.C. Smith, ADM VS,' 30 November 1983.
38 'Discussion Paper,' 24 November 1983.
39 VAC, VIP Records, file 2745-1, 'Aging Veterans Program Extension Work Plan,' n.d. but ca. March 1984; file 2740-5, 'Discussion Paper.'
40 'Veteran Performer,' *Legion* magazine, February 1985, 5–6, 16.
41 Boisvert interview, 8 July 2003.
42 VAC, VIP Records, file 2740-1, vol. 8, press release, 'More Progress at Veterans Affairs,' 16 January 1986; file 2860-1, vol. 4, 'Speech Notes for Minister, Newfoundland and Labrador Command of the Royal Canadian Legion Convention, 8 June 1987.'
43 VAC, VIP Records, file 2860-1, vol. 6, memo, 'Veterans Independence Program Submission Report for Treasury Board,' Departmental Statistical Unit, Economic and Program Support Division Programs Branch, August 1990.
44 VAC, VIP Records, file 2755-2-1, memo, 'Changes to Decision-Making Authority for the Veterans Independence Program,' 23 June 1987.
45 VAC, VIP Records, file 2860-1, vol. 4, Byron Lindsay, Planning & Development Officer, to Darragh Mogan, memo, 'Caring for the Elderly (Disabled) Veteran,' 29 January 1987.
46 VAC, VIP Records, file 765-8, 'Request for Proposals for an Evaluation Study of Veterans Affairs Veterans Independence Program,' December 1987.
47 VAC, VIP Records, file 765-8, Price Waterhouse Management Consultants, 'Final Report Evaluation of the Veterans Independence Program,' 20 June 1989, 40.
48 Ibid., 40–1.
49 Ibid., 47.
50 Ibid., 58, 64.
51 VAC, VIP Records, file 765-8, Derek Sullivan, A/Director Program Administration to Darragh Mogan, 'Veterans Independence Program Evaluation,' 22 November 1989; file 765-8, Derek Sullivan to Darragh Mogan, 'Veterans Independence Program Evaluation,' 18 October 1989; file 765-8, Derek Sullivan to Darragh Mogan, 'Veterans Independence Program, (VIP) Evaluation,' 10 July 1989; file 765-8, Darragh Mogan memo, 'Quick Notes on Evaluation/Audit,' 11 July 1989; file 765-8, R.A. Hollinger, Project Director, VIP Project, memo, 'VIP Evaluation Report,' 10 July 1989.
52 'An Unfulfilled Promise,' *Legion* magazine editorial, September 1987. Gaining WVA eligibility for CSO veterans had been an objective of the Canadian Legion since 1974.

53 VAC, VIP Records, file 2865-9, memo, 'CSO Expansion,' 31 March 1988; file 2865-9, memorandum to cabinet, George Hees, 13 April 1988, 'Issue: Whether to accede to pressure from veterans' organizations to make those who served in the armed forces in World War II only in Canada eligible for War Veterans Allowance (WVA) at age 65'; VAC, Health Services Director-ate Resource Library, no. 320, Veterans Affairs Canada, 'Care for the Aging Veteran: 1990–2020, a Discussion Paper,' 15 April 1988, 83, 19.

54 VAC, VIP Records, file 765-8, vol. 10, 'Veterans Independence Program Component File': table, 'VIP Clients & Actual Expenditures, Main Esti-mates,' part III.

55 VAC, Health Services Directorate Resource Library, 'Care for the Aging Veteran: 1990–2020,' i–vi, 64, 1.

56 Ibid., 5, 32, 38, 51, 40, 38, 92.

57 VAC, VIP Records, file 2860-1, vol. 9, Kim Campbell, Minister of Defence and Veterans Affairs, to Gilles Loiselle, President of the Treasury Board, 7 January 1993.

58 VAC, VIP Records, file 2860-11-2, vol. 1, 'Fact Sheet: Changes in Veterans Affairs Programs: Budget 1990, 27 February 1990; Canada, House of Com-mons *Debates*, 8 March 1990, speech by Veterans Affairs Minister Gerald Merrithew, 9028. The elimination of heavy housekeeping services in the VIP was expected to affect 19,000 veterans, at an average annual cost of $500 per veteran.

59 'Budget Blues for Veterans,' *Legion* magazine, April 1990, 2; Canada, House of Commons *Debates*, 5 March 1990, speech by Fred Mifflin, 8788.

60 VAC, VIP Records, file 2860-11-2, vol. 7, Cliff Chadderton to J.D. Nicholson, (ADM) Veterans Affairs, 'Re: Heavy Housekeeping,' 6 July 1993; vol. 6, memo, 'Briefing Notes: 1990 Budget Cuts,' 18 January 1993.

61 VAC, VIP Records, file 2860-11-2, vol. 7, memo, Serge Rainville, ADM Veter-ans Affairs, to Nancy Hughes Anthony, DM, Veterans Affairs, 'Heavy Housekeeping, Summary of Meeting, 28 July 1993.'

62 VAC, VIP Records, file 2860-11-2, vol. 6, 'Briefing Notes: 1990 Budget Cuts,' 18 January 1993. As VAC officials acknowledged in hindsight, 'Of all the cutbacks and savings announced [in the 1990 budget] only ours actually removed money or other benefits from individuals. The media had some-thing of a field day, and veterans were outraged at being the only Canadi-ans asked, as individuals, to do their part in reducing the deficit.'

63 VAC, VIP Records, file 2860-20-1, vol. 2, Brian MacGregor memo, 'Pension-Related VIP, (1981–1983),' draft, December 1993, 2; Brian MacGregor, memo, 'Pension-Related VIP, draft July 1993,' 2–3; file 2345-8-1, Projects Directorate, 'VIP Services Study,' March 1991; file 2860-20-1, vol. 1, Treva

McNally to Duncan Conrad, memo, 'Summary of Regional Input on Pensioners Eligibility for VIP,' 5 June 1989; Wilson interview, 10 July 2003. By 1993 approximately one-third of the VIP caseload, 32,000 veterans, were disability pensioners.

64 VAC, VIP Records, file 2345-8-1, Projects Directorate, 'VIP Services Study,' March 1991, viii; Mogan interview, 11 July 2003.

65 VAC, VIP Records, file 2770-11, vol. 12, 'Making the Transition to Being a Client-Centred Agency – Changes in Roles & Functions,' enclosed in memo, 'National Project Sites,' 14 October 1997; 'Client-Centred Service Initiative,' from the desk of Dennis Wallace, ADM, Veterans Services, *Carillon*, January 1997; 'Coming Your Way Soon from VAC,' *Legion* magazine, September/October 1997; Conrad interview, 9 July 2003.

66 VAC, Statistics Directorate, Corporate Planning Division, 'Clients and Expenditures Forecasts, 2002–2003, Forecast Cycle,' October 2001, 'Clients by Program,' 15, and 'Expenditures by Program,' 17; Conrad interview, 9 July 2003. As VAC's Gerontological Advisory Council recently put it, 'As veterans age, the distinctions used to determine eligibility for programs and services are no longer relevant. Given the long-term impact of military services on health, all older veterans should have the right to access services to help them maintain their health as they age.' VAC, 'Keeping the Promise: The Future of Health Benefits for Canada's War Veterans,' Report of the Gerontological Advisory Council to Veterans Affairs Canada, November 2006, http://www.vac-acc.gc.ca/providers/sub.cfm?source=councils/gac/report_gac, 25; accessed 20 March 2007.

67 Canada, Senate, *Raising the Bar: Creating a New Standard in Veterans Health Care. The State of Health Care for War Veterans and Service Men and Women*, Report of the Subcommittee on Veterans Affairs of the Standing Senate Committee on Social Affairs, Science, and Technology, February 1999, Excerpt C, Standards of Care for the Independent Veteran, recommendation 49; Canada, Senate, 'Proceedings of the Subcommittee on Veterans Affairs,' Issue 1 – Evidence, 17 October 2000, testimony of Cliff Chadderton, Chairman, National Council of Veterans Associations.

68 Canada, Senate, 'The State of Health Care for War Veterans and Service Men and Women. First Report: Long-Term Care, Standards of Care, and Federal-Provincial Relations,' Report of the Subcommittee on Veterans Affairs of the Standing Senate Committee on Social Affairs, Science, and Technology, March 1998, 4.

69 VAC, VIP Records, file 5270-3-1, vol. 4, John Walker, Director Residential Services, to Darragh Mogan, 10 October 1999, enclosing OSV Wait List Pilot Evaluation Framework, Exposure Draft, 6 August 1999, 5.

70 *Raising the Bar,* Excerpt C: Standards of Care for the Independent Veteran, (A) The Veterans Independence Program.
71 Senate, Canada, 'Proceedings of the Sub-Committee on Veterans Affairs,' Issue no. 2, Evidence, evening meeting, 28 November 2001, testimony of Cliff Chadderton, 6, 10.
72 Tom MacGregor, 'A Pattern of Inaction,' *Legion* magazine, March/April 2000, 38; 'A Need for Action,' editorial, *Legion* magazine, March/April 2000, 4.
73 Verna Bruce, Associate Deputy Minister, VAC, interview by author, Charlottetown, 16 July 2003.
74 VAC, VIP Records, file 5270-3-1, vol. 3, memorandum, Verna Bruce to J.D. Nicholson, DM, 'Waiting List Pilot Project,' draft, 16 February 1999; Overseas Veteran Pilot Project, draft, 1 March 1999.
75 Larry Murray, former deputy minister, VAC, telephone interview by author, Ottawa, 4 September 2003.
76 VAC, VIP Records, file 5270-3-1, vol. 3, J.D. Nicholson, DM, memorandum to Minister, 'Subject: Waiting List Pilot Project,' June 1999; vol. 4, John Walker to Darragh Mogan, 'OSV Project – Victoria,' 10 April 1999, enclosing 'OSV Wait List Pilot Evaluation Framework,' draft, 6 August 1999. As Walker pointed out, the pilot project model was the 'least cost option ... for meeting the needs of OSVs.'
77 Canada, Senate, 'Proceedings of the Subcommittee on Veterans Affairs,' Issue 1 – Evidence, 17 October 2000, testimony of Cliff Chadderton.
78 VAC, VIP Records, file 5270-3-1, vol. 4, memo, Brian Ferguson, ADM, to Larry Murray, DM, 'Evaluation of the Overseas Service Veterans (OSV) at Home Pilot,' n.d.
79 David Pedlar and John Walker, 'Brief Report: The Overseas Service Veteran At Home Pilot: How Choice of Care May Affect Use of Nursing Home Beds and Waiting Lists,' *Canadian Journal on Aging* 23, 4 (May 2004): 367–9; VAC, VIP Records, file 5270-3-1, vol. 4, Brian Ferguson to Larry Murray, 'Evaluation of the Overseas Service Veterans (OSV) At Home Pilot,' n.d.
80 Mogan interview, 11 July 2003.
81 Judy Lougheed, Director Health Services, VAC, interview by author, 18 July 2003; John Walker, Director Residential Services, VAC, interview by author, 12 August 2003.
82 VAC, Veterans Affairs Canada–Canadian Forces Advisory Council, Reference paper, *The Origins and Evolution of Veterans' Benefits in Canada, 1914–2004,* March 2004, 27.
83 Mogan, 'The Veterans Independence Program,' 12.

84 Canada, Senate, 'Proceedings of the Subcommitee on Veterans Affairs,' Issue 1 – Evidence for 24 October 2001, testimony of Jim Rycroft, Director, Service Bureau, Canadian Legion, 5.

85 VAC, 'Review of Veterans' Care Needs Focus Groups,' prepared for Veterans Affairs Canada by Pollara, May 1997, 4, 18.

86 VAC, VIP Records, file 2345-8-2, Duncan Conrad to Darragh Mogan, memo, 'Extension of All VIP to Surviving Spouses,' 12 January 1990, enclosing memo, 'Extension of All Home Care Elements to Surviving Spouses'; 'Extension of Veterans Independence Program Benefits for All Home Care Elements for a Period of Up to One Year to Surviving Spouses,' November 1989; file 2860-11-2, vol. 4, Peggy Ogden, 'Record of Discussion/Decision, Issue: Continuation of VIP Housekeeping and Grounds Maintenance Services to Spouses of Deceased VIP Clients,' 11 June 1990.

87 VAC, Gerontological Advisory Council, minutes of meeting, Charlottetown, 15 October 1997, 5. Leading Canadian gerontologists appointed to the GAC included Victor Marshall, Neena Chappell, Evelyn Shapiro, and Norah Keating.

88 For a good Canadian example, see C.T. Baines, P.M. Evans, and S.M. Neysmith, eds, Women's Caring: Feminist Perspectives on Social Welfare (Toronto: McClelland and Stewart, 1991). On VAC's own 'Care for the Caregiver' training initiative, launched in cooperation with Nova Scotia's Centre on Aging at Mount Saint Vincent University, see VAC, VIP Records, file 5200–12-2, B/F, 'Care for the Caregiver Pilot Project Final Report,' September 1994 and http://www.vac-acc.gc.ca/providers/sub.cfm?source= caregivrmanual; accessed 22 September 2005.

89 VAC, GAC, minutes of meeting, Charlottetown, 25 June 1998, 4; GAC, minutes of meeting, Halifax, 2 May 2000, 10, 12–13; GAC, minutes of meeting, Edmonton, 26 October 2000, 3.

90 VAC, Norah Keating, Jacquie Eales, and Janet Fast, 'The Differential Impact of Veterans Affairs Canada Policies on the Economic Well-Being of Informal Caregivers,' Final Report to Veterans Affairs Canada, 28 February 2001, 1–2. See also VAC, 'Keeping the Promise: The Future of Health Benefits for Canada's War Veterans,' Report of the Gerontological Advisory Council to Veterans Affairs Canada,' November 2006, http://www.vac-acc.gc.ca/ providers/sub.cfm?source=councils/gac/report_gac, 24–6.

91 VAC, news release, 'Veterans Affairs Canada Announces Intent to Address the Most Urgent Needs of Canada's Veterans,' 12 May 2003.

92 The decision unfolded awkwardly in two stages, in response to continued public pressure. See Canada, Senate, 'Proceedings of the Subcommittee on Veterans Affairs,' testimony of Rey Pagtakhan, 29 October 2003; 'War

Widows in Battle for Benefits, *National Post*, 24 March 2004; 'Proceedings of the Subcommittee on Veterans Affairs,' testimony of Albini Guarnieri, 8 December 2004. Only widows whose husbands had been receiving VIP housekeeping or groundskeeping benefits at the time of their death were eligible for lifetime continuation of these same services.

93 Canada, Senate, 'Proceedings of the Subcommittee on Veterans Affairs,' testimony of Albini Guarnieri, 8 December 2004; 'Rules Changed that Restricted Help for Spouses of Some Vets,' *Peterborough Examiner*, 8 December 2004.

94 'Review of Veterans' Care Needs Focus Groups,' 38.

95 Theda Skocpol, 'Delivering for Young Families: The Resonance of the GI Bill,' *American Prospect* 28, 7 (September 1996).

# Medical Science and Practice

# 13 Wondrous Transformations: Endocrinology after Insulin

ALISON LI

> Hence it happens that the average layman's conception of the ductless glands centers embarrassingly around the organs of sex and their weird counterparts – 'monkey glands,' so much so that his newspaper acquaintance with 'goats' glands' and 'Black Oxen' forbids their association in his mind with such refined diseases as goiter and diabetes.
>
> Hans Lisser, 1925[1]

In 1922 the medical world greeted the discovery of insulin. The impact on diabetics and those caring for them was life-changing, but the discovery was also to have a huge impact on the field of endocrinology. Endocrinologist Hans Lisser, in a lively account of the first forty years of the Endocrine Society, called the discovery of insulin 'epoch-making' in 'stimulating vast productive research' on the endocrine organs.[2] He continued: 'This conquest, accordingly, receiving as it did world-wide recognition and acclaim, spurred intensive researches into other endocrine maladies, so that today innumerable patients are benefited by the newer, potent adrenal, ovarian and testicular hormones, none of which were available before the advent of insulin.'[3]

That same year, the American literary scene welcomed a new romantic novel by Gertrude Atherton. *The Black Oxen* told the story of a mysteriously beautiful woman who suddenly appears in New York society. She bears an uncanny resemblance to a well-known beauty of several decades before, and all society is abuzz with questions about her identity. This Countess Zattiany gains numerous admirers yet remains maddeningly aloof and enigmatic. Only one suitor, a persistent newspaperman, manages to win her heart and to slowly, painstakingly, piece together her story. Her mystery: she is indeed the beauty from many decades before, and is in fact more than sixty years old. Her secret? She has availed herself of the services of a well-known Viennese doctor and with his glandular therapy has become a most formidable creature: a woman with the radiant beauty and physical and mental vigour of a twenty-eight year old, paired with the daunting intellect and experience of a sixty year old. When the Countess Zattiany finally reveals her secret to the public and agrees to meet with a circle of her girlhood friends, the greying society matrons present responses ranging from admiration to bitter envy to outright horror that the countess has dared to tamper with nature.[4]

The novel was an instant hit and was later made into a film. Popular responses mirrored those of the matrons in the novel. The novel was roundly condemned from pulpits as dangerous and unnatural. At the same time, the author, Gertrude Atherton, was besieged with hundreds of letters from women pleading with her to tell them whether the scientific miracle depicted in the book was simply a fiction or was based on fact. Atherton was the author of a long string of successful popular novels, and in her day was sometimes mentioned in the same breath as her contemporary, Edith Wharton. Newspaper writers made suggestive references to the youthful vigour of the sixty-four-year-old Atherton and hinted at a resemblance between the author and her heroine, but the novelist herself remained coy. Atherton conscientiously replied to all inquiries by referring the writers to Dr Harry Benjamin, the New York disciple of the famous Viennese scientist Eugen Steinach, who was renowned for offering sex-gland operations for rejuvenation.

In the early twentieth century, endocrinology held the promise that perhaps genetics does for today's society, that of understanding and controlling the essential processes of life. Hormones were considered the key to sex, aging, growth, and behaviour, and their manipulation was touted as the potential source not only of new therapies for hormonal disorders but also of solutions to broader social problems. The field drew intense interest from scientists, clinicians, the pharmaceutical industry, and government.[5] At the same time, there was a more controversial side to the study of the glands of internal secretion, as shown in the sensation surrounding the Voronoff 'monkey gland' transplants for rejuvenation. Of particular concern to the medical establishment was the proliferation of commercial glandular products of doubtful value. Leading researchers warned patients and general practitioners against over-enthusiasm and credulity.

The insulin discovery and the public response over *Black Oxen* are contrasting faces of endocrinology in the early 1920s. Both stories evoke images of miraculous transformations. In one, children on the edge of death were brought back to life; in the other, aged men and women were restored to youth. Michael Bliss describes the clinical effects of insulin as Lazarus-like, 'the closest approach to the resurrection of the body that our secular society can achieve.'[6] Glandular rejuvenation evoked perhaps a more dangerous tale, the Faustian myth.[7] The first treatment was embraced by medical scientists as legitimating their work in the glands. The second was viewed warily by many of endocrinology's early leaders as bringing disrepute to their endeavours.

This paper is an exploration of the hopes and anxieties of the early leaders of endocrinology in the United States, focusing on the impact of the discovery of insulin on the development of the field. In retrospect, endocrinologists celebrate the insulin discovery as a key achievement in therapeutics, and one that lent a much-needed legitimacy to the nascent field of endocrinology. Insulin was a clear and distinct victory; it had a definite physiological action and served to treat a life-threatening disease. As Hans Lisser's plaint in the epigraph suggests, though, the clinical efficacy of insulin was only part of its appeal as 'good advertising' for endocrinology. To endocrinologists such as Lisser, the clearly reliable hormone therapies such as thyroxin and insulin treated 'refined' diseases such as goitre and diabetes. In contrast, the therapies that were more commonly associated with the glands in the public eye were the ones that strayed into sensational territory, the term 'rejuvenation' serving as a euphemism for shoring up the flagging libidos of aged men or feeding the vanity of stout matrons.

## Endocrinology as a Science

The scientific study of the endocrine glands emerged from the medical practice of organotherapy in the 1890s with Charles-Édouard Brown-Séquard's suggestion that potent substances – 'internal secretions' – could be derived from animal tissue and used to treat diseases that resulted from their deficiency. This idea arose from the French physiologist and neurologist's rejuvenation studies involving the grafting of testicular tissue. The first recognized success of this new form of therapy was British pathologist George Redmayne Murray's use of subcutaneous injections of thyroid juice to treat patients with myxoedema in 1891. This initiated a wave of enthusiasm for testing animal extracts in medical therapy. Laboratory scientists introduced a new rigour to the study of these extracts by measuring the immediate physiological effects using standard experimental techniques. In Britain, a collaborative effort of clinician George Oliver and physiologist Edward Schäfer led to the discovery in 1894 of the specific physiological effects of adrenal extract in raising blood pressure, accelerating the heartbeat, and contracting skeletal muscle. Schäfer articulated a new 'theory of internal secretions' in 1895, defining the materials secreted by glands into the bloodstream as the object of study.

Historians Diana Long Hall and Thomas Glick argue that endocrinology is a field rather than a discipline in that it is not unified by common techniques and concepts. Rather, it has drawn on the work of researchers from many disciplines, being successively dominated by morphological sciences (anatomy and histology), physiology, biochemistry, and molecular biology, and, throughout, tied to practical clinical and social concerns.[8] Until 1900, most of the work in this field was conducted in Britain, France, Germany, and Italy. In Britain, physiologists took the lead in research. After 1910, scientists in the United States began to make important contributions, particularly after chemists began to be involved.[9] One such contribution was the production of crystalline thyroid hormone by Edward Kendall in 1914–15. Surgeons also began to appreciate the significance of the endocrine organs to their work; in this period, they recognized syndromes associated with hormonal excess and performed surgery to relieve the symptoms of over-secretion. Richard Welbourn gives 'pride of place' to American surgeon Harvey Cushing, who founded the first school of neurosurgery and contributed more than anyone else during this period to the surgery of the endocrine glands, particularly the pituitary. Important developments involved the cooperation of physicians, surgeons, and laboratory scientists at such places as the Mayo Clinic.[10]

The early success with thyroid extract and adrenal extract in the 1890s led to much enthusiasm for organotherapy. As Bliss describes in this volume, for William Osler, the introduction of thyroid extract as therapy for myxoedema was one 'glorious instance' of the hope held out by medical science and a sign of the greater things to come from glandular treatments. Endocrinologist Hans Lisser later recalled:

This auspicious beginning, soon followed by equally marvelous transformations of cretinous children, accomplished so simply, conveniently and cheaply by the mere ingestion of thyroid tablets, naturally led to the hope and expectation that shortly similar extracts from the other ductless glands would become available for comparable miracles when the pituitary, parathyroids, pancreas, adrenals, ovaries, or testicles were functioning insufficiently. But, alas, these ardent wishes were to be denied fulfillment for almost half a century.[11]

Thyroid extract (and after 1914, thyroxin) clearly treated thyroid deficiency. The impact of adrenal extract was more mixed. Adrenal extract had clear physiological effects and was a great boon to medicine and surgery, yet did not neatly fit the model of hormone extracts as treatments for hormone deficiencies, as adrenaline did not serve to treat a well-defined adrenal insufficiency, Addison's disease. For two decades following the successes of the 1890s, despite much enthusiastic interest on the part of physicians, laboratory scientists, and the public, the study of the glands failed to generate another clear therapeutic agent.

### *The Black Oxen* and the Steinach Treatment

In this same period, new champions arose to follow in the footsteps of Brown-Séquard in attempting to produce rejuvenation using the glands. Like him, these were often respected scientists working within the framework of the science of their day. In his fine study of sex, glands, and hormones, Chandak Sengoopta traces the development of the science and therapeutics of the sex hormones. He provides an excellent analysis of the work of Steinach and Benjamin, and of Atherton's connection with their rejuvenation therapy, arguing that rejuvenation was much more than a passing fashion, and that it revolutionized the image of endocrine science.[12]

Sengoopta argues against a simplistic view of rejuvenation treatments as irresponsible quackery. He traces the three very different theoretical and therapeutic approaches offered by Eugen Steinach, an experimental physiologist, Elie Metchinikoff, a biologist, and Serge Voronoff, a surgeon. Voronoff's work in transplanting the testicles of apes into men is now often derided as 'monkey-gland' charlatanism. Sengoopta convincingly argues that each of these scientists developed therapies based on what they considered to be the sound biological principles of the time, though their work may have been flawed or based on hasty wish-fulfilment.[13] Moreover, Sengoopta demonstrates that rejuvenation was framed not only as a medical issue but one with broader social and political significance, tied to regenerating a tired civilization devastated by the Great War.[14] Julia Rechter and Julie Prebel outline the connections between 1920s endocrinology and eugenics. Rechter finds that in the mainstream press of the time, calls were made to use hormone therapies as a form of positive eugenics to help in the understanding and the repair of social deviants such as the feeble-minded, the criminal, and the insane.[15] Gertrude Atherton herself openly suggested that Germany use the Steinach operation to create new supermen leaders to restore the nation to its previous glory.[16]

Gertrude Atherton's successful novel of 1922 was followed by a popular film two years later. In the *New York Herald Tribune*, in March 1924, New Yorkers were told, 'Women Here Made Younger, Like Heroine in 'Black Oxen,' By Rejuvenation Treatment.'[17] Dr Harry Benjamin's rejuvenating treatment for women was a lesser known and less widely performed version of the Steinach treatment for men.[18] In the case of men, Steinach had developed a surgical technique of ligating the vas deferens, a procedure we know as the vasectomy. His theory was that, by preventing the work of the tissue that produced sperm, this procedure stimulated the work of a competing tissue, the one that produced the sex hormone of the testes. He argued that the renewed output of male sex hormone resulted in a striking increase in mental and physical vigour among, first, his test animals and, later, his human patients. In women, no surgery was performed. Instead, X-rays were used to irradiate the ovaries over the course of several discreet office visits. The irradiation generally made fertility impossible, but since this treatment was undertaken by menopausal women, this was not considered to be a problem. As in the case of the male Steinach treatment, the procedure was thought to stimulate the renewed production of the female sex hormones by the ovaries. Later in the decade, when the harmful effects of X-rays became better known, irradiation was replaced by diathermy, the passing of an electrical current through the body. In about 20 per cent of the cases, Benjamin supplemented the treatment with an extract of goat glands.

In the 1924 article Dr Benjamin reported on a number of successful cases he had treated, one of which was that of a sixty-four-year-old educator who 'for several years had complained of an increasing lack of mental activity,' concentration, and imagination. According to Atherton's biographer Emily Leider, this anonymous patient is unquestionably the novelist herself.[19] Only a decade after the publication of *The Black Oxen* did Atherton go public with the information that she herself had taken two 'reactivation treatments.' Atherton cited the fact that she had an eighteen-year-old protagonist in her latest novel as clear evidence that she had no problem capturing the viewpoint of a young girl despite her own seventy-eight years.[20]

In her autobiography of 1932, Atherton described her adventures with rejuvenation, or, as she and Benjamin preferred to call it, reactivation. A decade before, she explained, she had been dispirited, tired, and frustratingly at a loss for a subject for her next novel. She had gone to interview Benjamin in the hopes of using rejuvenation as the centre of a new story. However, Benjamin quickly convinced her to try rejuvenation for herself, and within a day or two she found herself back in his office to begin a course of eight treatments, spread over several weeks, which she described as 'painless and rather boring.' For a month, her 'brain was torpid' and she slept sixteen hours a day. She found that she could neither read nor keep up a conversation. She continued:

> And then, one day – it was about a week after the finish of the treatments – I had the abrupt sensation of a black cloud lifting from my brain, hovering for a moment, rolling away. Torpor vanished. My brain seemed sparkling with light. I was standing in the middle of the room when this miracle happened and I almost flung myself at my desk. I wrote steadily for four hours … It all gushed out like a geyser that had been 'capped' down in the cellars of my mind, battling for release.'[21]

### Endocrinology in the 1920s – Quackery and Professionalization

In her fine PhD thesis, Julia Rechter traces the popular perceptions of endocrinology in 1920s America, arguing that the hormones were depicted as the 'glands of destiny,' holding out vast possibilities not only of personal transformation that affected every aspect of mind, body, and personality, but of societal reform as well. Rechter demonstrates that even scientific professionals, though more cautions, concurred with the popular view on three points: (1) that endocrinology was an important experimental science, (2) that hormones fundamentally shaped physiology and character, and (3) that there was the possibility that, one day, scientists would be able to improve bodies and minds.[22]

Attention-grabbing stories such as *The Black Oxen* or newspaper reports of monkey-gland transplants proved to be a source of great anxiety to leaders of endocrinology. In 1967 Hans Lisser, an early president of the Association for the Study of Internal Secretions (later the Endocrine Society), portrayed the early years of the organization in colourful terms:

Its birth and infancy were troubled and at times sickly and distraught, fraught with difficulties, and even opposition. It survived and prospered eventually, but for many years it was hazardous to forecast whether this dashing and intrepid pioneering into a fertile, but suspect, field of medicine would fail or triumph. Indeed, on several occasions in those earlier years, some feared it might still all come undone. Hostility toward its earlier meetings was of such a nature that it might have been safer and wiser to have met in secret – for clinical endocrinology at that time was in disrepute. Meetings were poorly attended, audiences were hard to attract, programs were sparse and speakers were few ... Conditions were such that any younger clinician, not yet firmly established and despite an unblemished reputation, who dared to embark on a career in this field was looked upon askance, considered naïve and gullible or – perhaps worse – suspected of straying into the realm of quackery, and heading for the 'endocrine gold fields.' As phrased by Walter Cannon, 'He was threatened with ridicule and scorn because of the wild surmises and fantastic claims of brethren whose imagination outran both fact and reason.'[23]

Were Lisser's recollections of the 1920s accurate? On 6 June 1921, at the fifth annual meeting of the association, Harvey Cushing presented a presidential address that Lisser later recalled as a 'scalding ridicule of the endocrinology of the time ... [a] withering denunciation of pseudoendocrinology and quack endocrinologists.' In his magisterial biography of Harvey Cushing, Michael Bliss reveals that Cushing, the father of American neurosurgery and a leader in pituitary research, served as president of the Association for the Study of Internal Secretions from 1920 to 1921 under the most unusual circumstances. According to Bliss, Cushing was elected as president without his knowledge at a meeting that he did not attend, and he agreed to serve only out of a sense of duty and in order to help to suppress quackery. Cushing regarded the field of endocrinology as mostly 'poppy-cock' and was said to have called it 'endocriminology,' wary of the potions that often passed as glandular therapy. More fundamentally, he felt there was no clinical rationale for grouping together the treatment of various disorders of the ductless glands. According to Bliss, Cushing's castigation of glandular charlatans would have been understood by many in the audience at the presidential address to be an attack on the founder of the organization, Henry Harrower, a California mail-order businessman who sold glandular extracts.[24]

Using spirited metaphorical language, Cushing exclaimed:

We find ourselves embarked on the fogbound and poorly charted sea of endocrinology. It is easy to lose our bearings for we have, most of us, little knowledge of seafaring and only a vague idea of our destination. Our motives are varied. Some unquestionably follow the lure of discovery; some are earnest colonizers; some have the spirit of missionaries and would spread the gospel; some are attracted merely by the prospect of gain and are running full sale before the trade wind ... In the enthusiasm 'to embark *glandward* ho!' ... many of us have lost our bearings in the therapeutic haze eagerly fostered by the many pharmaceutical establishments.[25]

Early editors of *Endocrinology* also engaged in regular, fraught ruminations on the status of the field. In a 1921 editorial entitled 'What Is Endocrinology?' editor Roy Hoskins spoke of the special responsibility of association members to cease to entertain what he called 'pseudo-endocrinology,' 'lest a long suffering medical profession in disgust with the rank growth of weeds in our fertile field in reformatory zeal uproot wheat and tares alike.' He noted that there was no reliable evidence of the value of the pancreas as a source of hormone. In very few cases had it been proved that endocrine organs actually contribute a substance to the blood stream. The basic model of endocrine action was even in question. Hoskins was uncertain whether the endocrine organs operated by addition or subtraction; perhaps they functioned by taking something out of the blood. He concluded cautiously that the value of endocrine gland substances would, in the end, have to be a matter of empirical observation rather than speculation: 'That enlightened empiricism may lead to further valuable therapeutic deductions is not improbable. Such results are to be expected, however, not from promiscuous dosing with hit-or-miss mixtures, but from carefully controlled experiments carefully analyzed.'[26]

Endocrinologist Victor Medvei argues in his massive history of endocrinology that clinicians in the United States were 'less discouraged' to show an open interest in endocrinology than were those in Britain. Medvei recalls being present at a medical meeting in London even much later, in the 1950s, where 'a distinguished member got up and warned against attempts of the "Westendocrinologists" (referring to London's Harley Street of medical specialists in the West End of the city) who were suggesting untried diversions when a satisfactory surgical treatment was available!'[27]

Julia Rechter rightly argues that professional scientists were often neither clearly critics nor enthusiasts for the hormone craze. Often they were a mix of both. Moreover, the easy stereotypes of the cautious scientist versus the over-enthusiastic clinician do not adequately describe the complexity of positions held. Both groups expressed a mix of caution and zeal.[28]

### The Insulin Discovery

Despite the popular focus on the sensational aspects of endocrinology, especially the sex hormones, the endocrine researchers themselves were interested in a far wider panoply of endocrine glands and products. In a 1922 article entitled 'Invitations to Research in Endocrinology,' W.B. Cannon, the Harvard physiologist, suggested the vast scope available for future exploration, explaining that the endocrine organs play such an essential role in so many fundamental processes, from growth to the development of the nervous system, reproduction, metabolism, and the mobilizing of forces for an organism undergoing physical struggle. 'There is no more interesting field for research in medicine or biology at present than that of internal secretion.'[29] In articles such as this, leading endocrine scientists made broad surveys of research on the thyroid, the parathyroids, the adrenals, the pituitary, the thymus, as well as the sex glands. They spoke of promising new knowledge about the physiological function of these glands and their implications for therapeutics. The sorts of therapeutics described usually lacked the glamour (or even the luridness) of the gland treatments that appeared in the popular press, but they were treatments that relieved the very real human suffering that clinicians saw in their offices.

One other endocrine organ had attracted considerable attention from researchers: the pancreas. Since 1889, researchers in several countries had made attempts to isolate an active principle of the pancreas after Oskar Minkowski and Joseph von Mering discovered the link between the pancreas and diabetes, but two decades later there was still no convincing evidence that an effective extract had been made.

Michael Bliss's definitive study of the discovery of insulin illuminates one of the pivotal events in the history of endocrinology. From the summer of 1921 through the winter of 1922, Frederick Banting, assisted by Charles Best, worked at the University of Toronto attempting to make extracts of beef pancreas and injecting them into depancreatized dogs to determine whether the extracts could correct the symptoms of the pancreatic deficiency. They were supervised and supported by the noted carbohydrate physiologist J.J.R. Macleod, who made a laboratory available to them and gave them key advice. Also on the team was J.B. Collip, a biochemist from the University of Alberta. Collip's laboratory expertise allowed him to produce a purified extract in January of 1922 that was used successfully in a clinical trial. The Toronto team named their product insulin and collaborated with the Connaught Laboratories in Toronto and Eli Lilly and Company in the United States to manufacture the product.

Before the advent of insulin, a diagnosis of diabetes mellitus had been a death sentence. Very quickly after its discovery, insulin was hailed as a modern medical miracle, bringing back diabetics from the brink of death and allowing them to go on to live long, relatively healthy lives. The following year, 1923, the Nobel Prize was awarded to J.J.R. Macleod and Frederick Banting. Banting shared his award money with Best, while Macleod shared his with Collip.

**The Impact of Insulin on Endocrinology**

Historians and endocrinologists alike cite the insulin discovery as a signal achievement in the history of endocrinology. Victor Medvei called the discovery of insulin 'the most spectacular event in the field of endocrinology in the first half of this century, apart from the clinical use of cortisone, and perhaps the use of iodized salt for the prevention of goiter, because of the great number of people to benefit from it.'[30] Commentators note the special impact of the discovery in boosting the development of endocrine science. Medvei comments: 'The significance of the success of insulin in the treatment of a disease which was neither uncommon nor easy to control, proved to be a great fillip to the extension of hormone research.'[31] Hans Lisser explains that before this 'epoch-making' discovery, there was little that clinicians could offer to their 'beseeching patients' in terms of endocrine therapies. This lack was reflected at an institutional level since the Association for the Study of Internal Secretions depended on the support of clinicians for its survival. Lisser remembers: 'Accordingly, there was more or less disappointment expressed by our members, not only by complaint but too often by resignation. This made the financing of the early years exceedingly difficult. It was necessary to make continual appeals to the friends of our most interested members in order to fill our annually depleted ranks and keep the Association alive.'[32] Historian Nicolas

Rasmussen adds that the discovery 'vividly confirmed the medical and commercial potential of endocrinology, and raised the competitive tempo of the field.'[33]

The summer of 1922, Harvey Cushing, who had only a year before warned of embarking on 'the fogbound and poorly charted sea of endocrinology,' wrote to the Toronto insulin team congratulating them on their success, calling it 'perfectly stunning.'[34]

## The Leaders Respond

Through 1922, Frederick Banting and a dozen or so American clinicians, including leading diabetologists Elliott Joslin and Frederick Allen, performed clinical trials of insulin. They struggled with issues of dosage and diet, learning about insulin and its effects. On the whole, they were amazed by the marvellous transformations they witnessed. Michael Bliss notes that metaphors of salvation and resurrection were a feature common to writers and patients.[35]

In May Lewellys F. Barker addressed the sixth annual session of the association, discussing his concerns about inappropriate use of glandular products. He was particularly concerned that practitioners were pressured by exaggerated advertising or by desperate patients into trying out glandular derivatives against diseases for which they were never indicated.

> There prevails a widespread feeling that many practitioners are making use of endocrine products in therapy in an indiscriminate and haphazard way, taking no trouble to ask themselves in a given case why the administration of such products may be indicated, but administering glandular substances or derivatives, and especially 'mixed products,' in various abnormal states merely because advertising matter strongly commends their trial ... An extravagant use of these products must be hard to resist at a time when almost every layman has had his interest aroused in one way or another in the internal secretions, when even a considerable proportion of physicians hug the fallacy that because the myxoedematous child is backward mentally therefore most cases of mental deficiency can be cured if only the particular hormone that presumably has been lacking be administered, and when consultants are daily besieged by both laymen and physicians with requests to examine a great variety of patients who 'surely must have something wrong with their glands.'[36]

He acknowledged that this situation was not difficult to understand given the central place endocrine activities had come to occupy in normal and pathological physiology. Instead of this scattershot approach, he emphasized the principle of treating an endocrine deficiency by substitution with a transplant or the extract of a normal gland, which had resulted in some of the field's greatest therapeutic triumphs. In this context he referred to the insulin research, saying, 'The work of Toronto investigators on diabetes seems at this moment to be particularly promising.' This did not, however, mean that hormone treatments were necessarily limited to those which acted by replacement of a deficiency; for example, the treatment of asthma with adrenaline did not depend on a hypofunction of a gland.[37]

Clinician A.S. Blumgarten, MD, of Lenox Hill Hospital in New York, tried to argue for the other side, complaining, 'The recent appearance of a number of hypercritical articles on endocrinology tends to create a state of unwarranted skepticism toward this branch of medicine.' From the perspective of an interested practitioner, the debate between enthusiasts and conservatives was bewildering. He noted the many positive achievements in endocrine therapy, and added with cautious optimism, 'the recent work at the University of Toronto, where a substance, "insulin," which is capable of reducing hyperglycemia, has been prepared from the islands of Langerhans, seems to mark an important step in advance.'[38]

Through the summer of 1922, the Toronto researchers and the Lilly researchers struggled with production problems finding it difficult to reliably make insulin on a commercial scale.[39] By November physiologist W.B. Cannon was calling the work of the insulin team 'highly important' and spoke of it promising much light and new information on the physiological response of the pancreas.[40]

By 1923 tremendous publicity had been generated in Canada and the United States and hundreds of diabetics' lives had been saved. However, clinical testing had only begun in Britain in December 1922 and January 1923. Through the winter of 1922–3 fewer than fifty diabetics in eight hospitals in Britain received insulin.[41]

The bewildering debate between enthusiast and conservative that Blumgarten noted in America was also playing out in Britain. Historian Diana Long Hall argues that there was a crisis in British endocrinology in the 1920s, as personified by the views of two of the leading researchers in the field, Ernest Starling and Swale Vincent. In his Harveian Oration to the Royal College of Physicians in 1923, entitled 'The

Wisdom of the Body,' Starling took an optimistic view of the field, naming as noteworthy Banting and Best's discovery of insulin along with W.B. Cannon's work on adrenalin in emotional excitement and pain, Kendall's work on the chemistry of the thyroid, the isolation of thyroxine, and several pituitary hormones, and David Marine's work on goiter prevention. In contrast, Swale Vincent, Professor of Physiology at Middlesex Hospital, London, gave a major lecture to the Royal Society of Medicine on 9 January 1923, speaking of a 'crisis in the field of endocrinology' that threatened its existence as a respectable scientific medical specialty. He attacked physiological and dismissed the significance of insulin for lack of evidence.[42]

In contrast, U.S. endocrinologist Albert Rowe was unequivocal about the importance of insulin in therapeutics:

> The insulin treatment of diabetes mellitus made possible through the discovery of Banting and his associates, including Macleod, Best, Collip and others of the University of Toronto, occupies the centre of attention in the medical world today. Joslin writes in a recent article, 'the contribution of Banting and Best to the treatment of diabetes is greater than I ever expected to witness.' All diabetic specialists, including Allen, Joslin and Woodyatt have incorporated insulin into their treatments and can confirm the original conclusions of the Toronto group that with the use of insulin even the most severe diabetics can be restored to health and strength.[43]

The battle between enthusiasts and sceptics began to change in 1924. Julia Rechter argues that after 1924, when clinical reports on insulin were clearly demonstrating the efficacy of hormones in saving lives, endocrinologists could point to the incredible therapeutic power of endocrinology as cause for optimism about the potential of the field and proof that critics of glandular charlatans should not throw the baby out with the bathwater.[44]

In the 1924 presidential address to the Association for the Study of Internal Secretions, Walter Timme gleefully noted the impact of the insulin discovery on pessimists, reminding his audience of Cushing's remarks three years before:

> It was but a few years ago that a distinguished though discouraged gentleman told us that we were sailing uncharted seas, that we knew not whither we were bound, and that perforce we should stop until the depths were sounded and beacons erected – and by implication, the new

lands mapped ... His address left his hearers in a quandary and in depression. Was all this work, all their observations, all their conclusions, faulty? Was their world worthwhile? Ought they not stop and wait?

... Indeed, hardly was the ink of his address dry than the world was startled, and of course the medical part of the world cynically so, by the announcement from Toronto of Banting's great discovery of what has come to be called insulin, which I venture to say will prove to be one of the outstanding historical landmarks in medicine. The medical pessimists ran to cover, the therapeutic nihilists still think there must be some mistake. It is this spirit of – not conservatism, as by some it is called, for true conservatism, is not opposed to advance – but negativism, or nihilism, or even fetishism, that keeps medical progress tied to old masters, old thoughts and methods of thinking, with thongs as strong as superstition.[45]

Hans Lisser was able take the importance of insulin for granted: 'It is hardly necessary to comment on the value of insulin. Since its discovery and introduction, about two years ago, an amazingly rich literature has accumulated.'[46]

In 1925 J.B. Collip, one of the insulin discoverers, announced a new achievement: the preparation of an active extract of the parathyroid.[47] Hans Lisser and an associate carried out a successful trial using Collip's parthryoid extract in the treatment of a woman who had three parathyroid glands accidentally removed during goiter surgery.[48] In an editorial, Lisser placed Collip's achievement in the context of a field now unquestionably changed by the advent of insulin:

Organotherapy since several years has been bombarded with ridicule and censure. In the enthusiasm for applying this novel therapy endocrine extracts have been prescribed in innumerable conditions where the theoretical clinical indications for their usage have been of whimsical, flimsy texture. Rebuke for such hazy therapeutics has been warranted. More lamentable, however, was the failure to achieve improvement in endocrine deficiencies where fundamental indications for glandular therapy were positive and sound. It is but a short time since pancreatic therapy for diabetes mellitus was utterly futile. How different now with insulin. It is no simple matter to produce potent extracts. Hormones are delicate structures, easy to destroy in the process of manufacture and harmed sometimes by intestinal juices. It is therefore a matter of congratulation that Professor Collip of the University of Alberta, Canada (who it will be remembered contributed to the isolation of insulin), has added another potent extract to the field of organotherapy. Whether or no his extract contains a perfect parathyroid hormone or all the active principles, if there be more than one, is impossible to state at this time, but most emphatically *it does contain a something that does something.*[49]

Like insulin, this new parathyroid extract contained 'a something that does something,' that is, it had clearly defined physiological effects. Lisser decried the haphazard use of glandular products and especially what he called the 'pluriglandular three-ring circus,' that is, the use of popular commercial products containing a mix of extracts from several glands. This stemmed from the belief that the glands must interact with each other, and that many diseases might be the result of problems in many organs, but Lisser and others were concerned that the leap to using a mix of products without a clear understanding of the effects and correct dosage of each component was premature. He commented, 'Fortunately, the stampede into the "endocrine gold fields" (as merrily phrased by Abel) is beginning to wane, probably because much of the ore is low grade.'[50] Finally, he urged patience. 'It took thirty years of persistent endeavor by many scientists in many lands, from Minkowski in 1892 to Banting in 1922, before insulin was consummated. Meanwhile we must work with what we have. It is hoped, in the attempt to evaluate what we have to work with, that the writer has displayed neither ignorant credulity nor cynical intolerance. In endocrinology we have had too much of both.'[51]

## Institutional Development of Endocrinology

Because endocrinology is a field rather than a discipline, drawing upon and dominated by different disciplines in turn, it has been difficult for historians to clearly delineate its growth. Although insulin gave endocrinologists newfound confidence, if we look at some crude indicators, it is not readily apparent that the insulin discovery led to any sudden surge in actual research activity. For example, in looking at the numbers of papers delivered at the annual meetings of the Association for the Study of Internal Secretions from its institution in 1917 through the 1920s, there does not seem to be any marked increase in the few years after the insulin discovery. (Collip was the president of the society in 1924.) Well into 1927–8, Lisser recalled having to plead and prod colleagues in order to put together a short, reasonably respectable program.[52] The volume of published papers can perhaps be indicated by the growth of the association's official organ, *Endocrinology*, which began as a quarterly in 1917, became bimonthly in 1921, and only became a monthly in 1937. After 1938 the further growth of the field was demonstrated in the fact that the annual output had to be gathered in two volumes. The year 1941 marked the establishment of the *Journal of Clinical Endocrinology* and the splitting off of the clinical from the experimental papers. British endocrinologist Arthur Hughes charted the overall growth of laboratory endocrinology using statistics culled from *Biological Abstracts*. Unfortunately, his data start only in 1926, which makes his analysis less useful for our present purposes, but during the period after 1926, his chart supports the trends noted above, showing a definite expansion of the field only after 1940.[53]

## Suspect Motives

Perhaps an important part of the appeal of the insulin triumph lay not only in the fact that it was life-saving, often dramatically so, but that its patients were blameless innocents who had none of the suspect motives of the seekers of more sensational glandular treatments. Hans Lisser made it clear that endocrinologists must not brush aside the work on sex-gland transplants simply because of the overblown reports of these practices in the popular press. In fact, these therapies had had strikingly beneficial results such as increased size of genitalia, growth of hair, changes in weight, and alterations in skin and nails in men and boys suffering from hypogonadism. However, he warned, 'This judgment is not to be construed as applying to the same procedure when used in Ponce de Leon strivings for rejuvenation or longevity, the premature exploitation of which does not redound to the credit of some members of our profession.'[54] To Lisser and other leading endocrinologists, the field's credibility was tainted by those who treated glandular science as a fountain of youth, sexuality, and beauty.

Interestingly, Gertrude Atherton's personal motives were less simple and distasteful than perhaps critics might have assumed. Her professed goals and experience with the 'reactivation' treatment turn out to be more indicative of real women's concerns than those of her fictional counterpart, the Countess Zattiany. To Benjamin and Atherton's surprise, while the fairy tale of mystery and glamour had brought the rejuvenation work into the limelight, the majority of patients who came to take the treatment were professional and business women, nurses and schoolteachers, concerned that they were losing their ability to work, rather than society ladies seeking renewed beauty and romance. (Or at least they claimed this to be the case.) As a *New York Herald Tribune* article speculated, 'They have been in the majority, women whose hair is greying and who feel they are losing a grip on their work. It seems more essential for them to retain their vitality and strength than for married women of leisure.'[55]

Benjamin wanted to dissuade women from considering this a quick ticket to beauty and youth. He reported that he 'had to turn down a number of actresses who had an idea that his laboratory was a new sort of beauty parlour.'[56] In the case studies he reported, fitness for work was described among the principal results of his therapy. Women who were physically tired and emotionally depressed were said to be able to regain energy, enthusiasm, and mental alertness, and 'ten years of added usefulness.'

While sexual desire and potency were principal concerns for male regeneration patients, these concerns were not mentioned with respect to the female patients treated by Benjamin nor by Atherton herself. Even among male patients, Benjamin thought that references to sexual matters were more circumscribed in American medical circles than in European, because of a more puritanical mindset. He warned that, in America, 'business interests often replace or suppress love and sex interest, therefore the lack of data from patients with regard to increased libido and potency or even a direct denial of such must be accepted *cum grano salis*.'[57]

One of the characters in *The Black Oxen* voices a misgiving about the Countess Zattiany's transformation that was perhaps shared by Atherton herself: it seemed somehow distressingly unnatural that a woman could look young enough to attract the attentions of a young man, yet no longer be able to bear children, which, after all, should be the true function of youthful womanhood. More importantly, for Atherton, a mother of two grown children and a widow for over thirty years by this time, her writing career was the focus of her greatest passions. In an interview decades later, Benjamin revealed doubts about Atherton's interest in sex, even using the term 'frigid' and speculating that her writing took the place of procreation. He reported that she even joked about experiencing strange food cravings while preparing a novel and told Benjamin, 'I am the mother and you the father' of *The Black Oxen*, her most successful novel.[58] Together, the patient and physician seem to have chosen the imagery of pregnancy and birth to explain woman's passion for even these, her non-reproductive activities.

Emily Leider portrays Atherton as a woman of considerable vanity, who strove to reclaim her youthful looks long before the Steinach treatment. So sensitive was she about her age that she insisted on introducing her adult granddaughter as her niece rather than admitting that she was sufficiently old to be the young woman's grandmother. After the Steinach treatment, she continued to avail herself of other glandular therapies such as high-frequency stimulation of the pituitary and the surgical implantation of sheep ovary tissue. She carefully weeded out unflattering photographs of herself. Well into her seventies, she was portrayed in the press as regal in black silk, with 'a cloud of ... tulle about her milk-white shoulders,' ensconced amidst six young men.[59] However, sixty years later, when interviewed by Leider, Harry Benjamin was somewhat ironic about his patient's vanity, but restated his view that Atherton's principal concern, more than beauty or sexuality, was regaining her ability to work.[60]

Taking into account the proscriptions against women admitting physical vanity or sexual feelings, perhaps it is not entirely surprising that these patients chose to frame their motives in terms of utility rather than beauty and sexuality. Nevertheless, the motives of Atherton and her less-famous sisters in rejuvenation treatment suggest the complexity of the gender and class ideas associated with sex hormones. In endocrinology textbooks of the 1920s, normal womanhood was defined in terms of a correct balance of female hormones. This ideal of femininity was framed in terms of reproductive ability, heterosexual impulse, and traditional feminine appearance. A description of 'the normal woman' ended with her ability to produce offspring.[61] This limited vision of femininity contrasted with the multidimensional understanding of a woman's life that emerges from the patients themselves. The more complex motivations of the patients themselves, in particular, post-menopausal women, suggest an active engagement with physicians' notions about the functions of women and of women's hormones. These patients included a widow in charge of a large dressmaking establishment, a teacher suffering from overwork and mental depression, and a professional dancer of forty-eight who no longer had the full strength for her work. To the patients, hormone treatments may have held out the hopes for improved appearance and sexuality, but also, importantly, the ability to work and to support themselves financially. The ovaries were the source not only of traditional feminine characteristics but also of the ability to take on challenging roles in a man's world. Likewise, Atherton's heroine, the

Countess Zattiany, while momentarily tempted by the pleasures of youthful love, ultimately turns away from it and dedicates her miraculously renewed vitality to greater social and political ends. She forgoes the offer of marriage from her young lover and chooses to return to Europe, where she can make a contribution to politics.

Perhaps not surprisingly, the male physician and his male patients were in greater agreement on the meaning of rejuvenated manhood: renewed sexual potency, vigour, and the ability to once again be 'actively in charge of his office' and to climb mountains.[62] In an article describing the treatment of women patients, Benjamin was cautious to keep his clinical assessment clear of the patients' subjective accounts of their experiences. In addition to the patients' descriptions of their feelings, Benjamin included the more objective measurements of blood pressure, pulse, and weight. He warned that 'considering the mentality of patients undergoing a socalled rejuvenation treatment,' it was advisable to disregard whatever the patients said or wrote about their feelings, at least where there was no objective change to corroborate them.[63]

Although the field of endocrinology became well established, Hans Lisser bemoaned the fact that 'even as late as 1933, 11 years after the beneficent discovery of insulin, a world-famous investigator saw fit to express his derision for the clinical endocrinology' at a major medical meeting. Lisser quoted the researcher as saying, 'To be an endocrinologist among the practicing profession today means too often to be primarily concerned with making fat ladies thin,' which Lisser complained was 'a rather cheap and snide remark,' sighing, 'Anything for a laugh!'[64] The leading researchers and clinicians in endocrinology saw their field as vastly more than making fat ladies thin and old men virile. Hormones were the key to the body's fundamental processes, and as such held the promise for understanding growth, reproduction, and metabolism, perhaps even behaviour and psychology. These cautious commentators did not rule out the possibility that hormones could also be a great boon to the understanding and treatment of aging or weight gain, but they worried their field might be dragged into disrepute through overmuch attention being paid to these aspects at the expense of a more cautious, systematic approach to therapy. The price of popularity was in having too many overzealous practitioners and eager patients anxious to throw all varieties of glandular solutions at all sorts of problems. Insulin was clearly different. Insulin provided dramatic successes, but it was against a very specific disease. And it was no cure. Insulin therapy required painstaking attention to dosage and careful management of diabetic diets for the remainder of the patients' lives. There was no room for scattershot approaches here.

In a 1924 editorial entitled 'Patience in Organotherapy,' Hans Lisser urged attention to therapies that were less dramatic and immediate than stories of rejuvenation, but no less marvellous because of it. He called the 'veritable transformation' of myxoedema by thyroid extract 'probably the most wondrous, consistent and convincing example of successful gland therapy.' But was this change sudden? Certainly not. Just as one could see the slow, insidious development of the disease in the gradual changes to the features and body contours of the patient over many years, likewise, the symptoms did not disappear overnight once thyroid therapy was provided.

> Ordinarily in a course of a week or two increased warmth is noticed by the patient, then gradually increased strength, more alertness, less lethargy. The metabolic rate is gradually elevated. Hair begins to grow after a few weeks, the excess fat slowly disappears, and many other evidences of a return to thyroid normality appear from week to week. But the final consummation of a transformed individual, physically, mentally and emotionally, is not achieved for at least six months.'[65]

**The Long View**

The dramatic and colourful stories of the rejuvenators with their associations with sexuality, gender identity, and aging, have drawn considerable interest from historians. The 1920s is undoubtedly a fascinating era, full of dynamic changes, emerging trends, and striking contrasts. Yet, like Hans Lisser speaking about successful treatment of myxoedema by thyroid therapy, we must remember that wondrous changes are sometimes wrought not in a flash but by slow, almost imperceptible steps. Often, rejuvenation is written of as a historical episode that flares up then dies out, yet we must not forget that the personages involved often have many decades of life and vital work afterwards. The example of Michael Bliss's scholarship reminds us of the long, yet intimate, perspective gained through studying the individual life, a life that can span bewildering social and personal changes and encompass great ambiguities and conflicts.

Harry Benjamin lived to 101 years of age and in his later career engendered even more startling transformations as the pioneer of sex-change surgery for transsexuals in the 1950s. He is now regarded as the founding father of contemporary Western transsexualism.[66] Gertrude

Atherton lived for more than twenty-five years after her first reactivation treatment and remained a life-long correspondent with Benjamin. Starting in the 1940s, Benjamin practised in San Francisco during the summer months,[67] and Atherton's correspondence includes invitations to Benjamin and his wife to visit during their stays in California. Benjamin continued to be interested in the application of hormones to gerontology (he named the sub-specialty 'gerontotherapy'). Atherton often asked him for pills (Progynon) to help with her aches and complaints. In 1980, in an interview with Atherton's biographer, Emily Leider, Dr Benjamin was persuaded to reveal his perspective on rejuvenation, and he answered simply that he 'thought the single most important contributor to sustained, productive, and healthy life was heredity.'[68] The goal of creating a healthy, vital life continued to be something both Benjamin and Atherton valued, but decades later, instead of using the Steinach treatment, they were using vitamin shots and hormone tablets to attempt these ends. While historians might isolate this colourful strand of events, to the people who lived them these rejuvenation experiences were something they had to make sense of in their own lives and retell in their own personal narratives.

The aftermath of insulin was also one of less dramatic, long-term collaborative work. Nicolas Rasmussen notes that Eli Lilly and Company's 'spectacular success brought many other drug companies into closer collaboration with enterprising endocrinologists in an effort to repeat the insulin story with the hormones of other organs, and even spurred the establishment of whole new endocrine firms such as Organon in Holland.'[69] The development of an effective and consistent method of large-scale manufacture of insulin was a long, complex process involving the collaboration of teams of researchers from universities and pharmaceutical companies.[70] The creation of a standard insulin unit was the result of a transdisciplinary and transnational network, including academic scientists, the drug company Eli Lilly, and government regulatory bodies. The construction of insulin as a medication was, according to Christiane Sinding, 'a difficult and conflicted undertaking that triggered complex and heterogeneous processes of application/production of knowledge, along with administrative, legal and commercial procedures.'[71] For diabetics as well, the insulin discovery was most definitely not a simple event. Historian and physician Chris Feudtner speaks of the legacy of insulin as contradictory: the 'mythically-framed' accounts of the discovery of insulin as a modern medical miracle conceal the sober, mundane challenges faced by

diabetics living with what was now a chronic disease requiring dili-
gent management and still carrying the risk of devastating complications such as blindness, kidney failure, and amputation.[72]

## Conclusion

To the early leaders of endocrinology, sex hormones and rejuvenation
were just a tiny part of a range of issues that caught their interest and
concern. However, they were abundantly aware that the public associated their field with precisely these things. It is understandable that the
early 1920s feature numerous articles by prominent researchers asking
'Where are we as a field?' and railing against quackery and disreputable drug houses. Once the insulin triumph gave them a clear victory
against critics and pessimists – a life-saving drug of unquestionable
efficacy – they were able to move on from these incessant ruminations
and anxieties about the disreputable side of glands. It was not so much
that they were prudish and moralistic, but rather that they saw that the
real achievements of endocrinology were often not dramatic, newsworthy, or sexy. They knew that many of the most significant therapeutic achievements might not suggest resurrections from the dead but
were nonetheless changes that made real differences to the health and
well-being of their patients.

NOTES

1 Hans Lisser, 'Organotherapy, Present Achievements and Future Prospects,'
  *Endocrinology* 9 (1925): 1–20.
2 Hans Lisser, 'The First Forty Years (1917–1957),' *Endocrinology* 80 (January
  1967): 5–28, 7.
3 Ibid., 16.
4 Gertrude Atherton, *The Black Oxen* (New York, 1922).
5 Nicolas Rasmussen, 'Steroid in Arms: Science, Government, Industry, and
  the Hormones of the Adrenal Cortex in the United States, 1930–1950,'
  *Medical History* 46, 3 (July 2002): 299–324; J.E. Rechter, '"The Glands of
  Destiny": A History of Popular, Medical, and Scientific Views of the Sex
  Hormones in 1920s America,' PhD dissertation, University of California
  Berkley, 1997.
6 Michael Bliss, *The Discovery of Insulin* (Toronto: University of Toronto Press,
  1981), 11.

7 Brett A. Berliner, 'Mephistopheles and Monkeys: Rejuvenation, Race, and Sexuality in Popular Culture in Interwar France,' *Journal of the History of Sexuality* 13, 3 (July 2004): 306–25. Berliner argues that French popular culture used the literary metaphor of the Faustian myth to represent the rejuvenation movement, specifically Serge Voronoff's surgical treatment of older men by the transplantation of monkey testicles. Berliner suggests that the popular media celebrated but ultimately rejected rejuvenation therapy, insisting that people age gracefully. This conservative approach to the human life cycle is also mixed in the popular imagination with fears of miscegenation and racialized sexuality.

8 Diana Long Hall and Thomas F. Glick, 'Endocrinology: A Brief Introduction,' *Journal of the History of Biology* 9, 2 (Fall 1976): 229–33.

9 Victor Cornelius Medvei, *A History of Endocrinology* (Boston: MTP Press, 1982), 501–2.

10 Richard Welbourn, *The History of Endocrine Surgery* (New York: Praeger, 1990), 9–11.

11 Lisser, 'The First Forty Years,' 6.

12 Chandak Sengoopta, *The Most Secret Quintessence of Life: Sex, Glands, and Hormones, 1850–1950* (Chicago, London: University of Chicago Press, 2006), 4, 56–67, 75–94.

13 Chandak Sengoopta, 'Rejuvenation and the Prolongation of Life: Science or Quackery?' *Perspectives in Biology and Medicine* 37, 1 (1993): 55–66.

14 Chandak Sengoopta, '"Dr Steinach coming to make old young!": Sex Glands, Vasectomy and the Quest for Rejuvention in the Roaring Twenties,' *Endeavour* 27, 3 (September 2003): 122–6.

15 Rechter, '"The Glands of Destiny."' On the link with eugenics, see pp. 27–45. Julie Prebel, 'Engineering Womanhood: The Politics of Rejuvenation in Gertrude Atherton's *Black Oxen*,' *American Literature* 76, 2 (June 2004): 307–37.

16 'Mrs. Atherton Causes Amusement in Berlin – Newpapers Ridicule Her Suggestion for Rejuvenation of All Germany's "Supermen,"' *New York Times*, 6 April 1924, sect. 2, 7 (quoted in Sengoopta, '"Dr Steinach coming"').

17 'Women Here Made Younger, Like Heroine in "Black Oxen," By Rejuvenation Treatment,' *New York Herald Tribune*, 16 March 1924.

18 See Sengoopta, '"Dr Steinach coming."' In a 1932 review, Benjamin claimed to have either direct or indirect experience with almost 1000 cases, including 300 men upon whom he had operated himself, 100 more he had observed, and about 500 women he had treated or observed in the United States and abroad. Harry Benjamin, 'Steinach-Therapy against Old Age: A Review of Ten Years' Experience,' *American Medicine* 38 (December 1932): 467–72, 492.

19  Emily Wortis Leider, *California's Daughter: Gertrude Atherton and Her Times* (Stanford, CA: Stanford University Press, 1991), 292.

20  'Gertrude Atherton Claims Rejuvenation,' *New York Times*, 4 December 1935.

21  Gertrude Atherton, *Adventures of a Novelist* (New York: Liveright, 1932).

22  Rechter, '"The Glands of Destiny,"' 24.

23  Lisser, 'The First Forty Years,' 5–6.

24  Michael Bliss, *Harvey Cushing: A Life in Surgery* (Toronto: University of Toronto Press, 2005), 382–4. This critical attitude towards Harrower was already distinctly shown even within the association's official organ, *Endocrinology*. In 1920, Harrower's book *Practical Organotherapy: The Internal Secretions in General Practice*, was reviewed in *Endocrinology* by Murray Gordon as 'an ambitious book written by an optimistic endocrinologist' and dismissed as a commercial publication, 'readable and interesting,' 'but with no great success as to scientific accuracy.' Murray B. Gordon, review of *Practical Organotherapy*, by Henry R. Harrower, *Endocrinology* 4 (1920): 429. The following year, *Harrower's Monographs on the Internal Secretions. Hyperthyroidism: Medical Aspects* was criticized by Roy Hoskins as 'permeated with no little "pseudoscientific nonsense"' and 'apparently addressed to those unfortunately credulous clinicians who hope to get a command of present day endocrinology without the labour of serious study.' R.G. Hoskins, review of *Harrower's Monographs on the Internal Secretions. Hyperthyroidism: Medical Aspects* by Henry R. Harrower, *Endocrinology* 5 (1921): 613.

25  Lisser, 'The First Forty Years,' 9.

26  R.G. Hoskins, 'Editorial: What Is Endocrinology?' *Endocrinology* 5 (1921): 610–12.

27  Medvei, *History of Endocrinology*, 501–2.

28  Rechter, '"The Glands of Destiny,"' 21.

29  W.B. Cannon, 'Invitations to Research in Endocrinology,' *Endocrinology* 6 (1922): 745–59.

30  Medvei, *History of Endocrinology*, 454.

31  Ibid., 506.

32  Lisser, 'The First Forty Years,' 8.

33  Rasmussen, 'Steroids in Arms.'

34  Bliss, *Cushing*, 384.

35  Bliss, *Discovery of Insulin*, 164.

36  Lewellys F. Barker, 'The Principles Underlying Organotherapy and Hormonotherapy,' *Endocrinology* 6 (1922): 591–5.

37  Ibid.

38  A.S. Blumgarten, 'The Positive Achievements of Endocrinology,' *Endocrinology* 6 (1922): 811–32.

39  Bliss, *Discovery of Insulin*, 150–3.
40  Cannon, 'Invitations to Research in Endocrinology.'
41  Bliss, *Discovery of Insulin*, 166–7.
42  Diana Long Hall, 'The Critic and the Advocate,' *Journal of the History of Biology* 9, 2 (Fall 1976): 269–85.
43  Albert H. Rowe, 'The Insulin Control of Diabetes Mellitus and Its Complications,' *Endocrinology* 7 (1923): 670–80.
44  Rechter, '"The Glands of Destiny,"' 23.
45  Walter Timme, 'Relation between Clinical and Experimental Endocrinology,' *Endocrinology* 8 (1924): 719–26.
46  Hans Lisser, 'Organotherapy, Present Achievements and Future Prospects,' *Endocrinology* 9 (1925): 1–20.
47  Alison Li, 'J. B. Collip, A. M. Hanson and the Isolation of the Parathyroid Hormone, or Endocrines and Enterprise,' *Journal of the History of Medicine and Allied Sciences* 47, 2 (October 1992): 405–38.
48  H. Lisser and H.C. Shepardson, 'A Case of Tetania Parthyreopriva Treated with Collip's Parathyroid Extract,' *Endocrinology* 9 (1925): 383–94.
49  H.L. (Hans Lisser), Editorial, 'Parathyrin (Collip),' *Endocrinology* 9 (1925): 242–4.
50  Lisser, 'Organotherapy,' 16–17.
51  Ibid., 20.
52  Lisser, 'The First Forty Years,' 11–12. 1917 – 3 papers; 1918 – 4 papers; 1919 – 5 papers; 1920 – 9 papers; 1921 – 13 papers; 1922 – 10 papers; 1923 – 7 papers; 1924 – 10 papers; 1927 – 12 papers.
53  Hall and Glick, 'Endocrinology.'
54  Lisser, 'Organotherapy,' 11–12.
55  'Women Here Made Younger.'
56  Ibid.
57  Harry Benjamin, 'The Control of Old Age; with Special Reference to Gonadal Therapy,' *American Medicine* 22 (June 1927): 345.
58  Leider, *California's Daughter*, 294.
59  Ibid., 306.
60  Ibid., 294–307.
61  Robert Frank, *The Female Sex Hormone* (Springfield, IL: Charles C. Thomas, 1929), 198–205.
62  Harry Benjamin, 'The Steinach Method as Applied to Women: Preliminary Report,' *New York Medical Journal and Medical Record* 18 (1923): 750–3; also see Paul de Kruif, *The Male Hormone* (New York: Harcourt, Brace & Co., 1945).
63  Benjamin, 'The Steinach Method,' 753.
64  Lisser, 'The First Forty Years,' 6.

65 Hans Lisser, 'Patience in Organotherapy,' *Endocrinology* 8 (1924): 120–2.
66 Richard Ekins, 'Science, Politics and Clinical Intervention: Harry Benjamin, Transsexualism and the Problem of Heteronormativity,' *Sexualities* 8, 3 (2005): 306–28.
67 'Harry Benjamin (1885–1986),' Archive for Sexology, Humboldt-Universität zu Berlin, http://www2.hu-berline.de/sexology/GESUND/ARCHIV/COLLBEN1.HTM.
68 Leider, *California's Daughter*, 307.
69 Rasmussen, 'Steroid in Arms,' 302.
70 John Patrick Swann, 'Insulin: A Case Study in the Emergence of Collaborative Pharmacomedical Research,' *Pharmacy in History* 28, 1: 3–13, 65–74.
71 Christiane Sinding, 'Making the Unit of Insulin: Standards, Clinical Work, and Industry, 1920–1925,' *Bulletin of the History of Medicine* 76 (2002): 231–70.
72 Chris Feudtner, *Bittersweet: Diabetes, Insulin and the Transformation of Illness* (Chapel Hill, London: University of North Carolina Press, 2003), 10.

# 14 A History of Lobotomy in Ontario

GEOFFREY REAUME

The history of lobotomy in Ontario reflects the wider international context in which the practice developed and gradually declined after its first two decades. The enthusiastic reception that some leading Canadian medical figures, such as Kenneth G. McKenzie, gave this treatment matched that of their American counterparts. Doctors and some patients' families welcomed the promise of more active treatments for mental anguish here as elsewhere. However, the lack of either critical judgment on the part of many doctors or a standardized basis upon which the operation could be judged led to serious abuses of patients from which the reputation of lobotomy has never fully recovered – notwithstanding recent attempts at a comeback under the guise of a 'new psychosurgery.' Most important, the people upon whom this procedure was inflicted in Ontario still have not had their stories told as to how this notorious treatment affected them.

This essay will first examine the background of this topic by discussing how the perception and treatment of people with mental-health disabilities helped to lead to a radical, and devastating, new therapeutic approach. Then the main portion of this essay will deal with the practice of lobotomy in Ontario: why it spread, the reasons for its decline to a reduced scale, and its legacy in contemporary provincial mental-health policies. As will become evident, this paper will show how the hope for a 'cure' for people labelled as having a mental illness was overtaken by professional interests and management concerns within various institutions. In the long term, this short-sighted approach harmed rather than helped mentally disturbed people.

## The Historical Context and Background of Psychosurgery

Psychosurgery is an irreversible surgical procedure that permanently destroys healthy brain tissue in order to alter behaviour in a mentally disturbed individual. The basic theory behind this operation assumes the connection of certain areas of the brain with the termination of presumed mental disturbance.[1] There were different approaches to psychosurgery during its 'classical' period, from 1936 to 1954, including such well-known procedures as pre-frontal leucotomy, developed by the Portuguese doctor Egas Moniz, as well as standard and massive lobotomy operations advocated by Walter Freeman and James Watts. These procedures were performed on tens of thousands of people in mental institutions around the world.[2]

Generally speaking, the attending physician would insert one of a variety of specially designed devices through at least two strategically drilled burr holes on the side or top of a person's skull. Then he or she would cut away at various portions of the brain where it was thought that symptoms of mental anguish were located.[3] Of course, such an approach followed a strictly medical model and failed to consider the role of life circumstances, both past and present, in mental well-being. These lobotomizing physicians completely failed to consider the humanity of the people that they subjected to such horrifying ordeals. In order to understand how such a radical treatment developed and came to be accepted among so many eminent doctors, it is essential to understand the background of this period and the clinical attitudes towards the people being operated upon.

Psychosurgery developed and spread at a time when physically intervening in a person's body to supposedly 'relieve' him or her of mental disturbance was increasingly practised. These treatments included insulin-coma therapy, metrazol convulsion therapy, and electroconvulsive shock therapy.[4] Since mental illness was widely believed to be 'incurable,' psychiatrists and neurologists were eager to advance what they saw as a highly optimistic and activist approach. They hoped that this would increase the legitimacy of their work among the public and the medical community. They also wanted to demonstrate that psychiatrists – who were medically trained – had more to offer than psychoanalysts and psychologists – who were not medically trained.[5] In other words, they wanted to corner the market of treatment for mental problems and physical intervention was a good way to help push this agenda forward.

Another factor that helped to promote psychosurgery was the support it received from such prestigious figures such as Adolf Meyer, dean of American psychiatry, and Harvey Cushing, the leading American neurosurgeon.[6] Brain surgery was on the rise during this period and psychiatrists sought to adapt the model to their own purposes. Before the 1930s, many physicians showed great interest in the potential for brain surgery to alleviate mental disturbance. During the nineteenth and early twentieth centuries there had been reports of medical cases in which the alteration of behaviour occurred after the frontal lobes had been damaged. All these episodes were the unintentional results of accidents or of operations involving the removal of brain tumours.[7] Nonetheless, reports of such cases helped to encourage the view that surgical intervention in the brain might be one way of relieving mental anguish.

There had been two early attempts at psychosurgery in 1891 and 1910 in Switzerland and Russia, respectively. However, neither operation was considered successful by physicians.[8] As with so much of this history, finding out what the patients thought needs a great deal more research in files that are difficult to access and through first-person accounts, such as interviews of survivors or their relatives. Psychosurgery, or as it came to be called popularly in North America, lobotomy, really began after a 1935 meeting in London, England, of the International Neurological Congress, where the renowned American neurophysiologist John Fulton, along with the psychologist Carlyle Jacobsen, reported on the prevention of neurotic symptoms in two chimpanzees following the removal of their frontal lobes. Egas Moniz, a Portuguese neurologist, returned home and decided to try a modified version of this operation on people in mental institutions. On 12 November 1935 his colleague Almeida Lima did the first of about one hundred operations on hapless psychiatric patients.[9] Moniz reported on his first twenty patients in 1936 and claimed a 35 per cent 'cure' rate, with the best results being on individuals experiencing anxiety and depression, while people diagnosed with chronic schizophrenia were said to benefit the least. However, as Elliot Valenstein has shown, Moniz's postoperative follow-up reports failed to provide evidence for anything even approaching a 'cure' of the people subjected to this procedure. Nevertheless, medical colleagues quickly endorsed the 'impressive' results of these early reports.[10]

After Moniz published reports of his first operations, the practice spread. The main impetus for psychosurgery came from the United

States, where the neuropathologist and neuropsychiatrist Walter Freeman, aided by neurosurgeon James Watts, popularized their technique, although they eventually went their separate ways in 1948 over another, even more barbaric, procedure developed by Freeman.[11] Psychosurgery came to be practised from the late 1930s to the early 1950s on a large scale, partly because of Moniz and Freeman's ambitious, determined advocacy of an 'activist' physical treatment for mental illness. Their radical physical approach appealed to many ambitious doctors and some desperate families.[12] Furthermore, psychosurgery was seen as a cost-effective treatment that helped to reduce the number of institutionalized patients in underfunded and overcrowded mental institutions.[13]

Thus, a combination of factors helped to push psychosurgery over the edge of theoretical debate and into the eager hands of its aggressive medical promoters. Among these factors were wildly exaggerated optimism about the efficacy of surgical treatments for mental illness, prestigious supporters, strongly motivated advocates, and the desire to cut health-care costs on a population for whom few people had sympathy in the wider world. As will be seen, a particularly important factor was the desire for social control of the people subjected to this treatment, on and off the hospital ward.

## Psychosurgery in Ontario

A lack of historical research on psychosurgery in Canada makes it impossible to estimate the extent of the practice. It is clear, however, that Walter Freeman and Kenneth McKenzie were the central figures in spreading the use of lobotomies to and within Canada. According to Dr John Griffin, former general director of the Canadian Mental Health Association (1951–71), Freeman toured Canada and many other countries in the 1940s and 1950s to 'spread the gospel' of lobotomy, which he championed fanatically. Indeed, he is listed as having visited London, Ontario, as late as January 1951, four years after a lobotomy program had been initiated there.[14] While lobotomy was performed in provinces across Canada, here I focus on Ontario.

Kenneth G. McKenzie was the physician most responsible for initiating and carrying out lobotomies in Ontario.[15] McKenzie was well respected within the Canadian and American medical community, as he was Canada's first neurosurgeon in 1923, having studied under Dr Harvey Cushing in Boston. Among the numerous medical societies he belonged to was the Harvey Cushing Society, initially an informal

organization of neurosurgeons before it became the American Association of Neurological Surgeons, which aimed to transform neurology
into a 'dynamic' research-oriented profession.[16] McKenzie even served
as president of the Cushing Society.[17] Membership in this group and
introduction to members like Freeman's partner, James Watts, undoubtedly exposed McKenzie to proponents of psychosurgery. In the late
1930s, McKenzie was encouraged by Cushing and Fulton to consider
psychosurgery.

With all these influences and likely spurred on by his own interests,
McKenzie began his lobotomy operations. McKenzie and Dr Lorne D.
Proctor wrote about how psychosurgery was introduced to Ontario in
a 1946 article:

> Our interest in bilateral frontal lobe leucotomy was stimulated by Free-
> man and Watts and in 1939 we visited Washington and were kindly
> shown a number of their cases. In 1941 the research unit of the Toronto
> Psychiatric Hospital embarked upon the psychosurgical treatment of
> hopelessly mentally ill people. The first patient chosen was a mentally
> defective female, aged 58, suffering from an involutional agitated depres-
> sive state with paranoid features.[18]

Another source noted that Freeman visited Toronto in the early 1940s to
get things going. In any case, it is certain that the first psychosurgery procedure undertaken in Ontario (and perhaps in Canada) was on 23 July
1941.[19] Fourteen females and thirteen males were operated upon in
Toronto between 1941 and 1946. McKenzie and Proctor reported that
none of their first twenty-seven patients died from the operation – a telling admission, as if absence of post-operative death was in itself something about which to be self-congratulatory. The two doctors also
claimed that 85 per cent of the patients improved in their behaviour. Just
what this meant was explained in most detail in regard to the first person
lobotomized – the fifty-eight-year-old woman, noted above. She was
described as 'being ill for 2 years previous to the operation, having had a
remission of five years' duration from a prior mental illness.' She was
also reported to have been wishing to be dead due to little men pounding
on her brain; she cried and anxiously paced up and down the ward,
frightened about what was going to happen to her. This unnamed
woman had also lost her appetite and her weight had dropped to ninety-
two pounds by the time she was given a bilateral frontal lobotomy. Afterwards, what the doctors described as her 'delusions' went away, she did

not discuss feelings of anxiety unless it was raised by the person questioning her, she gained fifteen pounds in two months, and 'now was able to help in the care of convalescing patients in a boarding-out home, being limited only by her mental deficiency.' She died of breast cancer two and a half years after being lobotomized. Based on this 'remarkable improvement,' according to McKenzie and Proctor, they decided to proceed with further operations, choosing people with 'at least "pathological fear"' of some kind.[20] It is striking that the passing reference to this woman's 'mental defect' is so quickly referred to and then not elaborated upon or explained in any way. There is no social context of what was troubling her, only a catch-all medical-model label imposed by the attending physicians for whom such social context was irrelevant. The lack of any detailed comparison of pre- and post-operative cognitive abilities clearly indicates how doubtful these supposed 'success' stories are.

While it is not possible to determine how many other patients were lobotomized elsewhere in Ontario during this early period, another article specifically noted that 'many patients' had been operated upon in this manner by July 1943.[21] Though few operations seemed to have been done in the mid-1940s, by late 1947 and early 1948 psychosurgery was being carried out at Westminster Hospital for veterans in London as well as the Toronto General Hospital.[22] While available statistics are incomplete, it is possible to show that a disproportionate number of women were targeted for prefrontal lobotomies at the Toronto General Hospital between 1948 and 52. Of 147 people lobotomized at the TGH during this four-year period, and whose gender is known, 109, or 74 per cent, were women.[23] Since these patients were selected from other psychiatric facilities and sent to be operated upon by McKenzie, it is clear that more women than men psychiatric patients endured lobotomies during this period in Ontario.

Over the next few years, until the mid-1950s, psychosurgery reached the height of its popularity in Ontario. An important factor in stimulating the practice of psychosurgery was the belief in its value as a supposed 'therapeutic advance' by doctors claiming that they were trying to relieve patients of their mental torment. This view was shared by the popular press and the families of patients as well as doctors. No one seriously consulted the patients as to whether they thought the treatment appropriate or not.[24] No doubt there was public pressure on physicians to carry out these operations. But doctors were not robots being pushed about by public opinion. Indeed, at least one physician – Dr Stevenson of London – courted and received positive press coverage with outlandish claims of 'Amazing Results.'[25] Some other doctors expressed their opposition to the way things were going.

In a May 1949 meeting of physicians, Dr A.B. Stokes, professor of psychiatry at the University of Toronto and later director of the Toronto Psychiatric Hospital, expressed his dismay towards his colleagues – especially the ubiquitous Dr Stevenson of London – about meeting this growing demand for psychosurgery. Stokes insisted that

> this form of treatment has not been accepted as standard procedure and that very careful control was advisable in order to prevent things from getting out of hand, with the inevitable result that pressure would be brought to bear by relatives and, not infrequently, the Department would be forced to proceed with the operation even although [sic] medical evidence might be against such a course.[26]

This sort of opposition was likely due, in part, to the view of well-established figures like Stokes that physicians alone should decide who was to undergo the operation, in order to maintain their professional autonomy. In other words, it was a territorial dispute – the lay public in general, and the media in particular, should not be allowed to influence medical decision making. In spite of Stokes's arguments, the federal government agreed, in October 1949, to provide the necessary funds that allowed up to three more referrals per week for psychosurgery to the Toronto Psychiatric Hospital.[27] This was important as space was at a premium. McKenzie was based at the Toronto General Hospital, where he was head of the neurosurgical department (1933–52). As he was the recognized expert in Ontario for psychosurgery, patients were referred to him from outside Toronto, though he also did lobotomies in provincial hospitals. As soon as the patient was out of danger of dying from complications, such as a brain hemorrhage, he or she was sent to the Toronto Psychiatric Hospital for post-operative recovery.[28] The criteria for selection were rather elastic and included patients who were in the chronic category – over two years in a hospital – or who were considered uncooperative and aggressive.

Lobotomy was frequently used on those patients who were viewed as most difficult to control, from the staff's point of view, which thus clearly proves how social control within the ward was an important factor in the selection process. Dr Carscallen of London's Westminster Hospital illustrated this point in a 1948 report in which he noted: 'We find ourselves faced with a group which has stubbornly resisted psychotherapy, shock therapy, etc.' Accordingly, these chronic patients were 'targeted' for lobotomies.[29] The attitude encapsulated in this approach was hardly conducive to a therapeutic environment. Carscallen is clearly saying that it was the patients' own 'fault' for getting a lobotomy for daring to 'resist' other treatments. Such a 'lesson' could not have been lost on other patients and doubtless promoted submissiveness. Carscallen noted four cases where families adamantly and successfully refused the operation. But for people who had no advocates, there was no such luck. As Harvey Simmons has written, consent for psychosurgery in Ontario was flexibly used and abused.[30]

Regardless of the criteria employed at various mental institutions, it is clear that many of those who were lobotomized in Ontario were diagnosed as having schizophrenia: 76 per cent, according to three studies comprising 318 patients.[31] Ironically, it was this group of patients whom Moniz earlier stated had benefited the least from the psychosurgery that he had initiated in Portugal. What happened to people after they were lobotomized was crucial to determining its presumed success or failure. According to the minutes of a meeting of Ontario Hospital Superintendents, rehabilitation – a nebulous term in this context – was the responsibility of the parent hospital from which the patient had been referred, though another source claims this was done at the Toronto Psychiatric Hospital.[32] In any case, while patients' rehabilitation of any kind did not become standardized in Ontario, there was agreement that the first six months after a lobotomy was crucial for the patient in terms of what were described as professional support and maximum improvements. After this, according to the theory, encouragement from family and friends was essential for the person to readjust outside of hospital. How this theory was implemented is revealing. Hospitals, such as Westminster in London, developed their own programs, which were designed to take at least a year before the patient could be discharged. This included having the patient participate in sports and dances, wear their own clothes instead of hospital garb, visit the city, and undergo 're-education in personal and social habits and customs.'[33] The success ratio appeared to be based on how many patients were discharged and whether they could live and work in the community.

One long-term report by Dr Abraham Miller noted that, out of 116 patients, 67 per cent had improved enough to live in the community, although he acknowledged that there were less positive results in other studies. Furthermore, this same article reported that 91 per cent of lobotomized patients experienced personality 'defects' and another 12 per cent had developed epilepsy. While Miller disingenuously claimed that the origin of the personality changes was 'not clear,' in fact his description of the impairment of intellectual functions makes it quite obvious that lobotomy was the cause of these changes. His own words are worth quoting at length:

> A noteworthy clinical finding in this study of 116 patients was the frequency of significant personality defects. Only in nine patients was it not possible to recognize signs of personality defects. The defects were expressed in the patient's limited capacity for new learning, the restriction in the ability for positive planning, and a lack of flexibility in dealing with situations that required a shift in thinking or action. The consequence of this defect was a narrowing in the capacity to adapt to changing life situations. Thus even those patients who were functioning extremely well in terms of relationship with people, regular work and social activities, did so as long as conditions were stable and supportive relationships constant. It was the clinical impression that the reason for this restriction in personality function was an impairment in the capacity for abstract thinking. Whether this was primarily due to the patient's mental disorder or the result of prefrontal lobotomy is not clear.[34]

Evidence from other studies clearly shows that the above description of psychic impairment is a known outcome of lobotomies.[35] Miller's unwillingness to take clinical and, therefore, professional responsibility for this change in an individual's personality, and instead to try to attribute it to 'the patient's mental disorder' indicates the level of intellectual dishonesty that characterized some physicians who practised lobotomy.

The notion of 'success' was also applied to those patients who were unable to leave the institution. Those patients who, after the operation, were still uncooperative and thus continued to pose management problems for their overseers, were said to have been treated by the 'kindly attitude' of ward staff, according to Dr Carscallen at Westminster Hospital. This meant being 'rolled out of bed in the morning, pushed under the shower, and urged in the same manner for the rest of the day.'[36] The contrast between the doctor's words about staff being 'kindly' towards patients and the actions of staff while they 'rolled,' 'pushed,' and 'urged' patients during the post-operative period underlines the reality of how harsh treatment was for such individuals.

Patients who were no longer causing problems for the staff after the operation were judged improved – another clear example of the social-control function that lobotomy served.[37] Miller made this point when he noted that, out of the 33 per cent of post-lobotomy patients who remained in hospital, 'there were a number who showed some improvement, so that their adjustment in hospital was better. The significance of this improvement was particularly important in those patients who had presented severe problems in management because of destructive and impulsive behaviour.'[38]

Miller also noted that lobotomy did not always make a patient easier to handle. He wrote about one patient, whose sex is not mentioned, who 'had improved temporarily' after a prefrontal lobotomy. However, this person then became 'extremely disturbed and difficult to manage' and so another lobotomy was done to 'reduce assaultive behaviour'; but the second operation was of 'little value' – presumably referring to issues of staff management of this patient, who was at their mercy.[39] Lobotomy outcomes were increasingly being revealed as less 'impressive' than the first reports from Portugal in 1935 had indicated – or from Toronto a decade later. A plateau had been reached during the early 1950s in Ontario's lobotomy program.

The introduction of chlorpromazine, a powerful behaviour-altering drug, in Toronto in December 1953 was a major reason for the termination of the lobotomy program at the Toronto General Hospital the following year.[40] The fact that Dr McKenzie retired in 1952 may also have been a factor, though he continued to do psychosurgery elsewhere, notably at the Ontario Hospital, Whitby, from 1955–7. When he did these operations, McKenzie would have nothing to do with the patients on a personal level outside of the operating room.[41] In such cases, he relied on hospital staff to collect the research data, which he analysed and later published. This point accords with Simmons's view that the superintendent of each hospital made the decision on who was to be lobotomized.[42] It also leads to another disturbing feature of this history – the detached, cold way in which the *people* who were operated upon were looked upon by the physicians responsible for the lobotomy program. Patients, to them, were 'devitalized clinical objects' in the words of Joel Braslow.[43] This comes through clearly in a 1944 study by Dr L.S. Penrose, Ontario's director of psychiatric research, which described certain lobotomized patients as being 'extremely unpromising material' since he did not foresee the likelihood of their being permanently discharged.[44] Similarly, in a 1954 report, Dr Abraham Miller, who was heavily involved in the lobotomy program in Toronto, referred to the human beings who were operated upon as 'case material.'[45] The fact that this term was used in two different reports, ten years apart, from two leading psychiatrists in the field, indicates how common this attitude was among the doctors who ran this program. Describing people in mental institutions in this way, as disembodied matter, ultimately distances their humanity from the doctors responsible for the devastating consequences that surgical intervention could and did have on these individual patients. In the worst cases, the deaths of patients – and some patients did die as a direct result of having lobotomies done on them – are not discussed in these reports as causes for regret or reflection, because such people are, after all, clinical 'material.'[46]

Lobotomies were also performed at the Toronto Western Hospital and at Westminster Hospital in London, as well as at Ontario Hospital, Hamilton, from 1952–67, where Dr J.N. Senn was assisted at the outset by Dr McKenzie.[47] They were also done in the St Thomas, Kingston, and New Toronto (or Lakeshore) provincial psychiatric institutions.[48] Roger Caron, a former inmate at the prison in Penetanguishene, Ontario, for people judged 'criminally insane,' has written that he saw a number of fellow prison inmates in 1962 who had been lobotomized.[49] What impact did lobotomies have on people who underwent them in Ontario? In most cases we do not know, as their stories have yet to be unearthed. Mel Starkman, a psychiatric survivor who lives in Toronto, recalled the circumstances surrounding the 1956 lobotomy of his father, Theodore Starkman, at Whitby Psychiatric Hospital, where he was one of 183 people lobotomized by Drs McKenzie and Kaczanowski.[50] While he acknowledges that his memory for this period is 'hazy on details of what actually took place,' Mel Starkman nevertheless is able to recall the impact that his father's lobotomy had on him and his family when he was fifteen years old. The Starkman family lived at this time in North York, a suburb of Toronto. He described his father, Theodore, as 'a quiet, shy, unlearned working man who only wanted the best for his immediate family and had had a brain injury around 1940 which led to his sometimes upsetting behaviour and several incarcerations in the Toronto Psychiatric Hospital and the Queen Street asylum.'

At some time in 1956 he suffered another breakdown although I don't remember details of his behaviour or hospitalization. All I remember is that my mother got a call from someone and told me that we were going to go to Whitby hospital early in the morning to be with my father when he had the operation under Dr Mackenzie. I don't know if we or she had heard about the matter before that. We duly went and sat around a few hours without seeing my father ... We then left and I don't remember when I next saw my father but his iron black hair was shaved and to my possible queries he was mute as was my mother. In the ensuing years he became quieter than ever and never again had a 'psychotic' episode to my recollection. He had in the past not been in the habit of turning over his income to my mother and only occasionally giving her money for the household. I remember that he used to walk to the Hydro office on Carlton at Yonge to pay the bill. I don't think that he did this after his lobotomy ... He went back to work after the lobotomy but had to work in a non-union shop where he was paid piecework wages at a very low scale. He became less talkative after the operation despite my often asking him about his life and experiences. I was burning to know but he was uncommunicative with the exception of always saying that I should treat my mother well and that a father is a father whether good or bad ... When he wasn't working which was often he would look after the house, the grass and cutting the weeds and growth in the back yard ... All in all there was not a marked difference between the pre and post lobotomy phases of his life although one thing that stopped occurring was his earlier tendency to take umbrage at our sometimes renters of rooms in the house and forcing them to move.[51]

Theodore Starkman died of cancer in 1968, twelve years after the lobotomy operation.

Precisely how many other people underwent lobotomies in this province during this very dark period in psychiatric patients' history is not known for certain. It is also not known to what extent doctors protested the flagrant abuse of power that went on under their collective noses during this time. Jack Griffin claimed that his mentor, Dr Clarence Hincks, the founder of what would eventually become the Canadian Mental Health Association, was opposed to lobotomies.[52] Dr E.A. Clark, who was based in Woodstock, Ontario, and was secretary of the twice-yearly meetings of the Ontario Hospital superintendents, made his criticisms known in an appendix to the minutes of the 6 May 1949 conference. He criticized the majority of articles published on lobotomy as being 'devoid of any critical appraisal,' with no standardized 'table of values.' He went on to point out that it was 'meaningless' to base a satisfactory outcome of the operation on whether or not a patient was out of the hospital. Finally, he wrote, 'One wonders, because of the contradictory accounts, whether the period of confusion uniformly experienced post-operatively by the patients is confined strictly to them.'[53]

However, these criticisms appear to have had little effect, as psycho-surgery continued to be widely used in Ontario well into the following decade. The only institution that expressed reservations to lobotomy outside the medical profession during this period was the Catholic Church, which argued that because the procedure was irreversible and 'uncertain of success,' it was only justifiable in extreme cases – a position that allowed a certain leeway for interpretation.[54]

The introduction of the 'new generation' of drugs throughout North America came at a time of increasing scepticism about lobotomies within the medical profession. Consequently, the procedure began to decline in popularity.[55] By the time of his death at the age of seventy-one on 11 February 1964, Dr McKenzie had at long last realized the error of his ways – too late for the people he had lobotomized. In an article published after he died, McKenzie and Dr G. Kaczanowski of the Whitby mental institution reported on 183 operations done at this facility between 1955 and 1957: 'It is concluded that prefrontal leucotomy does not produce any rate of remission significantly beyond that to be expected without the operation.'[56]

The *Canadian Medical Association Journal*, in an editorial entitled 'Standard Lobotomy: The End of an Era,' eulogized McKenzie as a 'greatly loved Toronto neurosurgeon' who eventually decided to abandon psychosurgery, 'for which he was internationally known.'[57] Ironically, his obituary in local daily newspapers did not mention his central role in the history of psychosurgery in Ontario, and instead vaguely alluded to McKenzie being a 'pioneer of many techniques and developments in neurosurgery.'[58] Long-term studies, such as that carried out at Whitby, have clearly shown that lobotomies did not help the vast majority of patients who were subjected to this operation. Lobotomy irreversibly alters the human psyche, leading to negative and, not infrequently, devastating changes to an individual's personality. It was also known to cause serious medical complications for some people, leading to death in some cases; thus, lobotomies unquestionably did more harm than good to more than a few people who were operated upon.[59] Results such as this can hardly be construed as 'harmless' for the affected person's ability to think or comprehend when contrasted to their pre-lobotomized abilities.

Lobotomy was used to ease management difficulties for hospital staff, a point that has quite rightly aroused its most vociferous opponents. It was not until the negative portrayals of psychosurgery in the 1970s in films and the media that the treatment received widespread public condemnation, first in the United States and then in Canada. By this time, many in the medical profession had already abandoned and disowned the original forms of lobotomy.[60] While psychosurgery remains extremely unpopular among the wider public, it still has its supporters, though even they agree it should be used under very controlled and restricted circumstances. Advocates in the Canadian Psychiatric Association (CPA) have acknowledged the abuses of the past. They argue that improved methods are not aimed at the alteration of behaviour but rather at the relief of intense emotional anguish – an argument not at all far removed from the views of psychosurgery's earliest promoters.[61] It is in effect a way for psychiatrists to prevent their work from being more closely scrutinized by outsiders, even though the purpose of this scrutiny is to prevent past abuses from recurring.

In 1978 Ontario's *Mental Health Act* outlawed psychosurgery for involuntary or incompetent patients, even though the CPA argued that a review board should decide this matter on a case-by-case basis.[62] Conceivably, the 1982 *Canadian Charter of Rights and Freedoms* could also be used to ban psychosurgery as an attack on freedom of thought.[63] Given all these restrictions imposed upon psychosurgery and the negative view of it among the general population, it is unlikely that this crude and justifiably feared and despised procedure will be ever widely accepted. But that of course does not mean its use has disappeared altogether, for the history of lobotomy in Ontario is a chapter that continues under another, less obvious name.

By 1967, according to the estimates of Harvey Simmons, approximately one thousand lobotomies had been done in Ontario. It has not, however, disappeared entirely and has continued to be practised in the years since then, albeit on a much reduced scale, both in Ontario and elsewhere.[64] I attended a grand rounds at the then Clarke Institute of Psychiatry on 1 December 1989, where it was mentioned that an average of two psychosurgery operations a year were done in Toronto with a radio frequency needle.[65] More recently, psychosurgery – now commonly called cingulotomy and capsulotomy – has been on the rise again in North America, including Ontario, where it has been done on people diagnosed with obsessive-compulsive disorder, depression, and body-image disorders such as anorexia.[66] Accurate figures are not available, but there are nonetheless grounds for serious concern among psychiatric-survivor human rights advocates about the re-adoption of a practice that was so flagrantly open to abuse in the past – namely, the surgical alteration of personality. Given such developments, it is timely and instructive to reflect on the legacy of lobotomies during the 1940s and 1950s, when its use was most widespread in Ontario.

## Conclusion

Lobotomies flourished in Ontario during the late 1940s and early 1950s largely because of management concerns by hospital staff and the desire of physicians to show the relevance of their methods in treating psychiatric patients. As more doctors and some laypersons uncritically accepted the potential 'benefits' of psychosurgery, this operation spread without adequate critical studies or cautionary standards. Consequently, when its benefit to patients was eventually shown to be non-existent, lobotomies fell into decline among most medical practitioners and became synonymous with some of the worst excesses of twentieth-century psychiatry. Throughout these developments it is important to remember the central role that Dr Kenneth McKenzie played in the history of lobotomy in Ontario. Undoubtedly, the high regard in which he was held by his colleagues helps explain why many of them so blithely accepted this crude operation as having some legitimate purpose. However, by the time McKenzie disowned lobotomy, he reflected the majority opinion among medical authorities inside and outside of Canada on this issue. Indeed, what is surprising is that he took so long to disown this operation that he continued to inflict on patients after 1955, in the face of mounting professional opposition.

McKenzie, like many of the other physicians who practised lobotomy, was in the mainstream of his profession and was regarded not as an irresponsible maverick but as an expert in his field. At the top of his profession and free from the restraints of serious critical appraisal, McKenzie did as he pleased. While public pressure can be held partly accountable for the spread of lobotomies by the late 1940s, the doctors who actually practised it were the most responsible, from an ethical and legal point of view. They had the training, experience, and authority in their field to assess, better than anyone else, the irreversible risks and potentially damaging impact on patients that this operation entailed, without feeling pushed into it by relatives, the media, or the wider public. Since many doctors wanted to be seen to be actually 'doing something' about treating people who were mentally disturbed, their own critical judgment became impaired. Their patients paid a very high price indeed. Developments in more recent decades, into the

early twenty-first century, in which psychosurgery is once again rear-
ing its ugly head in Ontario and elsewhere, indicate the need to re-
learn historical lessons from the not too distant past. The fact that this
procedure is still being done, albeit on a more reduced scale than
before and with 'new' surgical techniques, is nevertheless a disturbing
indication that even with all that has happened, the irreversible
destruction of a person's brain tissue, with its devastating consequences, is still being advanced in some medical circles as an appropriate form of treatment for people experiencing mental anguish. The
story of the use and abuse of lobotomy in Ontario is thus not fully over,
as this history is still ongoing. What can be shown from the past, with
which this essay has been concerned, is that medical authorities and
the wider lay public need to be particularly critical of approaches that
present intervention in the brain as a legitimate treatment for mental
disturbance. Psychiatric patients have already travelled down that
road, and it is a dead end.

NOTES

An earlier version of this paper was prepared when I was an MA student in
Michael Bliss's seminar course 'The History of Medicine in Canada, 1800–
1989,' Winter 1989 term in the Department of History, University of Toronto. I
would like to thank Professor Bliss for his comments and encouragement on
this essay, which prompted me to study Canadian psychiatric and medical history with him for my PhD. I would also like to thank Robin Keirstead,
Archives of Ontario, for assistance in locating primary source material in the
AO. Much gratitude is expressed to Mel Starkman for sharing memories of his
father, Theodore, and his personal history of lobotomy. Thanks also to the editors and reviewers of this volume, particularly Elsbeth Heaman, for their helpful suggestions. All errors and interpretations are my responsibility.

  1 John Kleinig, *Ethical Issues in Psychosurgery* (London: George Allen and
    Unwin, 1985), 1; *Behaviour Alteration and the Criminal Law* (Ottawa: Law
    Reform Commission of Canada, Working Paper 43, 1985), 12.
  2 Besides Canada and the United States, psychosurgery was done in Europe,
    Asia, Australia, and Latin America. See Elliot S. Valenstein, 'Historical Per-
    spective,' in *The Psychosurgery Debate: Scientific, Legal and Ethical Perspectives*,
    ed. E.S. Valenstein (San Francisco: W.H. Freeman and Co., 1980), 25. For
    a discussion of the various surgical approaches to psychosurgery see

P. Flor-Henry, 'Psychiatric Surgery, 1935–1973: Evolution and Current Perspectives,' *Canadian Psychiatric Association Journal* 20, 2 (March 1975): 157–63.

3 Elliot S. Valenstein, *Great and Desperate Cures: The Rise and Decline of Psychosurgery and Other Radical Treatments for Mental Illness* (New York: Basic Books, 1986), 3; M. Girgis, 'The Biological Basis of Emotion,' in *Psychosurgery and Society,* ed. J.S. Smith and L.G. Kiloh (Oxford: Pergamon Press, 1977), 11–14.

4 Valenstein, *Great and Desperate Cures*, 45.

5 Ibid., 22, 41.

6 David Shutts, *Lobotomy: Resort to the Knife* (New York: Van Nostrand Reinhold Co., 1982), 70–1; Abraham Miller, 'Historical Review of Psychosurgery,' unpublished transcript of a talk presented to a 'Seminar on the History of Canadian Psychiatry,' Clarke Institute of Psychiatry, Toronto, 7 December 1977. I would like to thank Dr J.D. Griffin for bringing to my attention this transcript and accompanying audio-tape. A copy of it is available at the Centre for Addiction and Mental Health Archives, Toronto.

7 Ashley Robin and Duncan Macdonald, *Lessons of Leucotomy* (London: Henry Kimpton Publishers, 1975), 9–11; Valenstein, *Great and Desperate Cures*, 89–93.

8 Valenstein, *Great and Desperate Curses*, 43–4.

9 Ann Jane Tierney, 'Egas Moniz and the Origins of Psychosurgery: A Review Commemorating the 50th Anniversary of Moniz's Nobel Prize,' *Journal of the History of the Neurosciences* 9, 1 (2000): 22–36; P.K. Bridges and J.R. Bartlett, 'Psychosurgery: Yesterday and Today' (review article), *British Journal of Psychiatry* 131, 3 (September 1977): 249; Robert P. Feldman and James T. Goodrich, 'Psychosurgery: A Historical Overview,' *Neurosurgery* 48, 3 (March 2001): 649–52.

10 Valenstein, *Great and Desperate Cures*, 107–13.

11 Larry O. Gostin, 'Pre-Frontal Lobotomy,' *Journal of Medical Ethics* 6, 3 (September 1980): 149; Shutts, *Lobotomy*, 147–8, 159.

12 While some families undoubtedly did want to help their relatives, there were others who did not care and used lobotomy in a punitive, vicious manner. See, for example, the cruelty of Joseph Kennedy in relation to his daughter Rosemary: Gerald O'Brien, 'Rosemary Kennedy: The Importance of a Historical Footnote,' *Journal of Family History* 29, 3 (July 2004): 227–8. See also the following Internet link for a heart-rending first-person account by a man who was twelve years old at the time he was lobotomized by Dr Freeman with the collusion of his parents: 'My Lobotomy: Howard Dully's Journey,' 23 min., National Public Radio, 16 November 2005, http://www.npr.org/

templates/story/story.php?storyId=5014080. Thanks to Agatha Barc for informing me about this radio documentary and providing the link.

13 Valenstein, *Great and Desperate Cures*, 154.

14 Ibid., 323n.

15 Harvey Simmons, 'Psychosurgery and the Abuse of Psychiatric Authority in Ontario,' *Journal of Health Politics, Policy and Law* 12, 3 (Fall 1987): 540. See a revised version of this article in Harvey Simmons, *Unbalanced: Mental Health Policy in Ontario, 1930–1989* (Toronto: Wall and Thompson, 1990), 209–24.

16 Jack D. Pressman, 'Sufficient Promise: John F. Fulton and the Origins of Psychosurgery,' *Bulletin of the History of Medicine* 62, 1 (Spring 1988): 19. For a revised version of this article see Jack D. Pressman, *Last Resort: Psychosurgery and the Limits of Medicine* (Cambridge: Cambridge University Press, 1998), 47–101.

17 For bibliographic information on McKenzie, see his obituary in *Toronto Daily Star*, 11 February 1964 (evening edition), 23; and *Globe and Mail*, 12 February 1964, 33. For reference to McKenzie being past president of the Harvey Cushing Society, see Howard A. Brown, 'The Harvey Cushing Society: Past, Present and Future,' *Journal of Neurosurgery* 15, 6 (November 1958): 600. For Cushing's view of McKenzie while a student, see Michael Bliss, *Harvey Cushing: A Life in Surgery* (Toronto: University of Toronto Press, 2005), 387–8. See also Thomas P. Morley, *Kenneth G. McKenzie and the Founding of Neurosurgery in Canada* (Markham, ON: Fitzhenry and Whiteside, 2004).

18 Kenneth G. McKenzie and Lorne D. Proctor, 'Bilateral Frontal Lobe Leucotomy in the Treatment of Mental Disease,' *Canadian Medical Association Journal* 55, 5 (November 1946): 435. Dr Mary Jackson recalled that Dr C.B. Farrar was also involved with McKenzie in bringing psychosurgery to Ontario: Miller, 'Review of Psychosurgery,' 8.

19 Miller, 'Review of Psychosurgery,' 8–9; K.G. McKenzie, 'Results of Bilateral Frontal Leucotomies, July 23, 1941 – July 31, 1944,'*American Journal of Psychiatry* 100 (September 1944): 281.

20 McKenzie and Proctor, 'Bilateral Frontal Lobe Leucotomy,' 435, 438 – see table II, 4th 'case' listed on p. 438 for reference to the death of the woman who was the first person lobotomized in Ontario.

21 McKenzie and Proctor, 'Bilateral Frontal Lobe Leucotomy,' 437, 440; Lloyd H. Ziegler, 'Bilateral Prefrontal Lobotomy: A Survey,' *American Journal of Psychiatry* 100 (September 1943), 178–9.

22 Archives of Ontario (AO), RG 10, file 40, item 12A, H.B. Carscallen, 'Preliminary Report on Prefrontal Lobotomy at Westminster Hospital' (paper given at a meeting of the Ontario Neuropsychiatric Association at Ontario Hospital, Whitby, 7 May 1948), 17; Simmons, 'Psychosurgery,' 540.

23  A. Miller, 'Analysis of Case Material before Lobotomy' in *Lobotomy: A Clini-cal Study*, ed. A. Miller (Toronto: Ontario Department of Health, 1954), 4; Simmons, 'Psychosurgery,' 540. Simmons is criticized by Joel Braslow for not providing evidence of the 'relative frequencies of men and women' under care in the TGH, thus supposedly not proving his point that more women than men were lobotomized during this period. Joel Braslow, *Mental Ills and Bodily Cures: Psychiatric Treatment in the First Half of the Twentieth Century* (Berkeley: University of California Press, 1997), 153. This criticism is irrelevant, as lobotomy patients were brought to the TGH from psychiatric facilities to be operated upon there, and thus the overall rates of males and females at the TGH would not tell us anything, as this was not the originating hospital from which they came. It is clear from the statistical evidence that those doctors engaged in this decision-making process of selecting patients from psychiatric hospitals for lobotomies at the TGH during these years were choosing more women than men, and so Simmons's point is proved, (though his related speculation about female predominance being due to manic-depressive diagnosis is not proved as this evidence is not available).

24  The optimistic, though at times cautious, attitude towards the early psycho-surgery operations in Ontario is obvious from some of the early reports: L.S. Penrose, 'Results of Special Therapies in the Ontario Hospitals, Coma, Convulsion and Leucotomy up to November 1944' (Ontario: Ontario Department of Health, 1944), 9–13; AO, RG 10, file 2, item 27, Minutes, Ontario Neuro-Psychiatric Association Meeting, Toronto, 15 January 1943 (reprinted in pamphlet 'Recollections from the First Fifty Years,' Ontario Psychiatric Association, 1970, no page numbers, though reference is under 'Therapeutic Advances'); Simmons, 'Psychosurgery,' 541–2; Valenstein, *Great and Desperate Cures*, 174–7.

25  Cited in Roger Baskett, 'The Life of the Toronto Psychiatric Hospital,' in *TPH: History and Memories of the Toronto Psychiatric Hospital, 1925–66*, ed. E. Shorter (Toronto: Wall & Emerson, 1996), 133.

26  AO, RG 10, Series 20-A-1, box 1, file 2, Ministry of Health, Psychiatric Hospitals Branch, Minutes of Superintendents Conference, 1930–1957, 6 May 1949, 8.

27  Ibid., 14 October 1949, 4.

28  Miller, 'Review of Psychosurgery,' 9, 15.

29  Simmons, 'Psychosurgery,' 542–3; AO, Carscallen, 'Lobotomy at Westminster,' 12–13.

30  Carscallen, 'Lobotomy at Westminster,' 13–14; Simmons, 'Psychosurgery,' 544.

31 The data from three Ontario studies show that out of 318 patients, 242 had
a diagnosis of schizophrenia, while the remaining people had diagnoses ranging from manic depressive to neurotic. K.G. McKenzie and G. Kaczanowski,
'Prefrontal Leucotomy: A Five Year Controlled Study,' *Canadian Medical Association Journal* 91, 23 (5 December 1964): 1195; A. Miller, 'The Lobotomy Patient
– A Decade Later: A Follow-up Study of a Research Project Started in 1948,'
*Canadian Medical Association Journal* 96 (15 April 1967): 1098; McKenzie, 'Bilateral Frontal Leucotomies,' 281.
32 AO, RG 10, Series 20-A-1, box 1, file 2, Ministry of Health, Minutes of
Superintendents Conference, 14 October 1949, 4; Miller, 'Review of Psychosurgery,' 15–16.
33 A. Miller, 'Some Aspects of Lobotomy Response in Post-Operative Period,' in
*Lobotomy: A Clinical Study*, 37; AO, Carscallen, 'Lobotomy at Westminster,' 15–16.
34 Miller, 'The Lobotomy Patient,' 1101–3.
35 Braslow, *Mental Ills and Bodily Cures*, 144–6; Valenstein, *Great and Desperate
Cures*, 250–3.
36 AO, Carscallen, 'Lobotomy at Westminster,' 17.
37 Raj Anand, 'Involuntary Civil Commitment in Ontario: The Need to Curtail
the Abuses of Psychiatry,' *Canadian Bar Review* 57 (1979): 268.
38 Miller, 'The Lobotomy Patient,' 1101.
39 Ibid., 1100.
40 AO, RG 10, Series 20-A-1, box 1, file 5, Ministry of Health, Minutes of
Superintendents Conference, 23 April 1954, 1; Miller, 'Review of Psychosurgery,' 11. For a discussion of the discovery of the 'new generation' of 'anti-
psychotic' drugs, see David Healy, *The Anti-Depressant Era* (Cambridge,
MA: Harvard University Press, 1997), 42–77; and Robert Whitaker, *Mad in
America: Bad Science, Bad Medicine, and the Enduring Mistreatment of the Mentally Ill* (Cambridge, MA: Perseus Publishing, 2001), 141–59.
41 Interview with Dr J.D. Griffin, 30 March 1989.
42 Simmons, 'Psychosurgery,' 539, 542–3.
43 Braslow, *Mental Ills and Bodily Cures*, 145.
44 Penrose, 'Results of Special Therapies,' 9.
45 Miller, 'Analysis of Case Material before Lobotomy,' 4. This degrading reference to 'material' comes up a number of times in *Lobotomy: A Clinical
Study*, ed. Miller: see, for example, subsections in the two-page 'List of
Contents' and p. 54, where Miller again refers to 'studying the case material
subjected to lobotomy.'
46 Penrose makes reference to 'one case which died probably as a result of
the operation [leucotomy]'; 'Results of Special Therapies.' See also note 59
below, which refers to a 2% mortality rate recorded by Dr Miller.

47  AO, RG 10, Series 20-A-1, box 1, file 4, Ministry of Health, Minutes of Superintendents Conference, 1 February 1952, 10; ibid., 17 April 1953, 8; Miller, 'Review of Psychosurgery,' 1.

48  Baskett, 'Toronto Psychiatric Hospital,' 133.

49  Roger Caron, 'Psychotreatment,' in *Shrink Resistant: The Struggle against Psychiatry in Canada*, ed. Bonnie Burstow and Don Weitz (Vancouver: New Star Books, 1988), 137.

50  For reference to the Whitby lobotomies, see McKenzie and Kaczanowski, 'Prefrontal Leucotomy,' 1195.

51  Mel Starkman, Toronto, personal written communication to the author, 15 February 2006. For first-person accounts about lobotomy from the United States, see http://www.psychosurgery.org.

52  Griffin Interview.

53  AO, RG 10, Series 20-A-1, box 1, file 2, Ministry of Health, Minutes of Superintendents Conference, 6 May 1949, appendix B, 'Prefrontal Lobotomy: A Brief Review of Selected Literature' by Dr E.A. Clark, 1, 5.

54  'Ethical and Religious Directives for Roman Catholic Hospitals' (no author), *The Canadian Hospital*, May 1949: 31; Walter Freeman and James W. Watts, *Psychosurgery in the Treatment of Mental Disorders and Intractable Pain*, 2nd ed. (Springfield, IL: Charles C. Thomas, 1942, 1950), 379–80.

55  Valenstein, *Great and Desperate Cures*, 254–8, 278.

56  McKenzie and Kaczanowski, 'Prefrontal Leucotomy,' 1193.

57  'Standard Lobotomy: The End of an Era' (editorial), *Canadian Medical Association Journal* 91, 23 (5 December 1964): 1229.

58  *Toronto Daily Star*, 11 February 1964, 23; *Globe and Mail*, 12 February 1964, 33. McKenzie wrote about one of these so-called achievements – his lobotomy technique – and includes photographs of brains from patients who died after the operation: K.G. McKenzie, 'Neurosurgical Technique,' in *Lobotomy: A Clinical Study*, 8–12.

59  Besides the figures already mentioned in this paper from his later study, Dr Miller recorded a 2% mortality rate and 3.3% rate of severe postoperative hemorrhage. A small number of other patients were also recorded as having complications, such as one person who had a fatal brain abscess, seven people who had severe post-operative dementia as well as incontinence of bowel and bladder in a small number of other people. A. Miller, 'Surgical Complications with Lobotomy,' in *Lobotomy: A Clinical Study*, 53.

60  Simmons, 'Psychosurgery,' 545–6, 549.

61  J.D. Earp, 'Psychosurgery: The Position of the Canadian Psychiatric Association,' *Canadian Journal of Psychiatry* 24, 4 (June 1979): 353–7, 361.

62  David N. Weisstub, ed., *Law and Psychiatry in the Canadian Context* (New York: Pergamon Press, Inc., 1980), 815.

63  Harvey Savage and Carla McKague, *Mental Health Law in Canada* (Toronto: Butterworths, 1987), 126.

64  Dr Miller reported that more than 400 people were lobotomized outside of Toronto between 1952 and 1967: Miller, 'Review of Psychosurgery,' 11; Simmons, 'Psychosurgery,' 540–5; Simmons, *Unbalanced*, 210.

65  It is worth noting that one doctor sitting in the audience at this 1989 symposium wondered aloud after the presentation whether a forty-year-old man who had had this operation done on him was chronically depressed because he was homosexual, even though nothing was said about the man's sexual orientation in the presentation or tape clip of him that was shown to the audience. Nevertheless, the doctor in the audience 'deduced' this interpretation from the man's supposed femininity and involvement in the local arts scene. Another doctor in attendance denounced this view as a harkening back to the times when homosexuality was pathologized as a 'mental illness,' and further stated that people who accept themselves as homosexuals are better off than people who don't accept their sexual orientation. Author's personal notes on 'Psychosurgery: Its History and Present Practice in Toronto,' presented by Dr John Fairwell, 1 December 1989, Clarke Institute of Psychiatry, Toronto. Thanks to Dr John Griffin for telling me in advance about this presentation.

66  Danielle Egan, 'Magical Mystery Cure,' *This Magazine*, January–February 2005; see: http://www.thismagazine.ca/issues/2005/01/magicalmystery.php. Thanks to Lana Frado for this source. See also G.A. Mashour, E.E. Walker, and R.L. Martuza, 'Psychosurgery: Past, Present and Future,' *Brain Research Reviews* 48, 3 (2005): 409–19. Thanks to Erick Fabris for this reference. For criticisms of the 'new psychosurgery' see Dr Peter Breggin's comments at http://www.breggin.com/lobotomy.htm. Thanks to Don Weitz for this reference. It should be noted that 'cingulotomy' is not a new clinical term for lobotomy – this is one of seven different surgical lobotomy procedures that Dr Miller identified in 1967 as having been used on patients since 1948 in Ontario, where it was called 'cingulectomy'; Miller, 'The Lobotomy Patient,' 1096. Breggin also points out in his above citation that both surgical lobotomy procedures now in vogue – cingulotomy and capsulotomy – were first introduced in 1948 and 1949.

# 15 Limitations Exposed: Willem J. Kolff and His Contentious Pursuit of a Mechanical Heart

SHELLEY MCKELLAR

From the 1950s to the 1990s, Dutch physician Willem J. Kolff (b. 1911), inventor of the artificial kidney,[1] led an ambitious artificial-organ research program in the United States. Kolff advocated organ replacement by mechanical means – or the replacement of diseased human organs with artificial devices – at a time when most medical researchers dismissed such ideas as impractical. Yet Kolff believed that it was both feasible and desirable to pursue the development of artificial organs.[2] His success with the artificial kidney machine motivated Kolff to begin work on an artificial heart, which dominated his research program for forty years. A driven, stubborn, and resourceful man, Kolff worked tirelessly to promote and garner support for his artificial-heart research. At the Cleveland Clinic and later the University of Utah, Kolff led a team that finally succeeded in developing a device – the Jarvik artificial heart – that moved from laboratory testing to human implantation. In December 1982 Barney Clark, a sixty-one-year-old dentist from Seattle, Washington, became the celebrated first patient to undergo the experimental procedure, living 112 days with this artificial heart.[3] Thereafter medical practitioners, scientists, and bioethicists debated whether this clinical case could be labelled a 'success,' with many arguing that there were indeed limits to the mechanical replacement of diseased body parts.

This article examines Kolff's contentious pursuit of a mechanical heart, exploring the obstacles, gains, and attitudes that emerged in this researcher's lab, the larger themes reflected in the development and use of artificial hearts, and the changing characterization of disease and the body within American medicine and society in the second half of the twentieth century. During Kolff's career, the utilization of machines and devices to fight disease became a dominant aspect of American medicine and the conceptualization of the body as an entity of replaceable parts was adopted by medicine and society. Technological shifts in medicine contributed to reconfiguring the body as a site for intervention, yet this should not be misunderstood as a form of technological determinism. For example, the engaging work of historians Stanley Reiser, John Pickstone, and Stuart Blume, among others, explores the shape of medical technology and its meanings within the larger socio-economic and political contexts where medicine is found.[4] Sociologists have embraced the body as a site for both medical intervention and invention, exploring such themes as identity, normality, surveillance, and objectivity.[5] These themes emerge in Kolff's artificial-heart research, with its debatable outcomes, conflicts, and uncertainty, highlighting the contested and negotiated process of medical-device research and development.[6] Kolff's pursuit of an artificial heart was contentious. Debate, disagreement, and challenge emerged from within his own research team as well as from the medical community, government regulators, bioethicists, and journalists. In the end, however imperfect the device, an additional limitation to Kolff's artificial heart research lay in the growing discrepancy between Kolff's narrow technological optimism and increased misgivings by others surrounding such 'experimental' technologies.

## Kolff's First Artificial Hearts: The Cleveland Clinic (1950–67)

At the early meetings of the American Society for Artificial Internal Organs (ASAIO), a scientific forum attended by 'disciplined scientists and free-spirited, gadgeteer-geniuses,' members discussed the future development of the artificial kidney and the heart-lung machine, the two artificial organs of primary interest in the 1950s.[7] ASAIO president Peter Salisbury challenged members to think beyond the short-term use of the artificial kidney or heart-lung machine.[8] What about treating chronic renal failure? How about a pumping device to assist failing human hearts? Could a mechanical heart machine be developed for use beyond the operating table? At the time, the heart-lung machine demonstrated the feasibility of mechanical circulatory support; that is, replicating a patient's heart and lung function by pumping and re-oxygenating blood outside the body. The machine, however, caused blood trauma in the form of blood-cell damage and bleeding, and therefore was limited to short-term use for surgical procedures. Could a machine be developed to overcome these problems, possibly for long-term use? In Cleveland Kolff had been working on experimental blood oxygenator devices, transferring his knowledge and experience with blood flow (through his work with artificial kidneys) to this project. Not surprisingly, Kolff took up Salisbury's 1957 challenge by heading back to his lab at the Cleveland Clinic to design a total artificial heart.

Kolff's aim was to develop an artificial heart to replace the human heart inside the chest. He envisioned the natural heart as a double pump; the right side (right ventricle) pumped the body's unoxygenated venous blood to the lungs for aeration and the left side (left ventricle) pumped the reoxygenated blood back into the general circulatory system of the body. Kolff set out to build a mechanical double pump small enough to fit inside the body.[9] Working with medical researcher Tetsuzo Akutsu at the Cleveland Clinic, Kolff experimented with plastic replacements of aortic and mitral valves in the hearts of dogs. Similar research had been conducted by Selwyn McCabe at the National Institutes of Health, with whom the Cleveland group consulted. After twenty-seven experiments implanting plastic valves in the hearts of dogs, Kolff and Akutsu moved in an ambitious direction: they built an entire plastic heart, composed of two polyvinyl chloride pumps, which contained the necessary plastic valves. It was a simple pneumatically driven device, built from a plastic cast impression of the heart of a 20 kg dog. The heart was connected to an air compressor by plastic tubes. This air-driven heart was tested first in mock circulation on the bench (to ensure mechanical function), then implanted into a dead dog (to study surgical procedure and fit), and finally placed into a living dog in December 1957. The device worked; the dog moved, breathed, and exhibited reflexes for ninety minutes.[10]

Kolff and Akutsu reported to the professional community the first successful implant of an artificial heart in an animal in the Western world.[11] This case demonstrated the feasibility of mechanically replacing the heart, yet it also revealed device and procedural limitations.[12] The most obvious technological limitation was that the device was pneumatically driven, necessitating connection to an outside air compressor to power it. Equally problematic was the surgical procedure, which needed refinement. Heart removal was difficult and painstaking, and implanting the device required the tedious and time-consuming surgical connection of five blood vessels to the mechanical heart. This was due to the design of this early device, which was modelled on the natural heart and the complexity of blood vessels surrounding this organ.

Researchers questioned the suitability of the human heart as the ideal form for a mechanical heart model. During the next several years, the Cleveland group developed different artificial heart devices that varied in form and method of operation. These medical researchers and bioengineers were looking for the best biocompatible materials and reliable components, the best source of energy, the best driving mechanism, and the best regulating controls. In the end, all the early artificial heart devices were abandoned owing to technical complexity, poor durability, biomaterial problems, and their large size. Two examples of the flawed but interesting designs that emerged in this period were the 'solenoid artificial heart' and the 'pendulum artificial heart.'

The solenoid-driven artificial heart involved a magnet-driven pump. This heart was a six-sided flat box, about 2 inches high and 4 inches across, and only 3½ pounds in weight. Five coordinated electromagnets, arranged in a rosette, were activated by electric current, that entered through two wires, creating mechanical energy. The electromagnets (or solenoids) pushed disks inward, compressing hydraulic fluid that squeezed two collapsible plastic ventricles, situated on either side of the rosette, thereby simulating diastole (filling stroke) and systole (emptying stroke) of the heart.[13] The pendulum artificial heart was an electromotor-driven pump based on a pendulum principle. It contained a motor, suspended by pivots, which swung back and forth within a rigid housing. This compressed each ventricle alternately. The pendulum heart was implanted in a dog, maintaining circulation for over five hours, with Kolff reporting that the animal breathed spontaneously and retained reflexes.[14] Both the solenoid and the pendulum hearts were electrically driven, but battery power was limited to only a few hours before the devices needed to be recharged through an electric converter plugged into a wall socket. As Kolff acknowledged, the solenoid-driven heart was inefficient and produced heat at a level intolerable to the body, while the pendulum heart was too bulky and heavy within the body and the energy derived from the driving power was limited.[15]

Engineers from the National Aeronautics and Space Administration (NASA) convinced Cleveland researchers to return to pneumatically driven devices. Air power was plentiful, simpler, and resulted in less heat production in comparison to electrically driven hearts. Pulsating air pressure, generated outside the body, could be easily channelled through small flexible tubings to any device in the chest. At first Kolff 'recoiled' at the thought of returning to air-driven hearts. He stated,

'That idea would commit us to a system in which the power supply would have to be outside the body. I had visions of the possessor of an artificial heart walking around with something like a garden hose sticking out of his chest!'[16] Kolff eventually agreed that efforts should be concentrated on building a reliable heart-pump mechanism and only later an improved energy source developed. Soon thereafter, Akutsu and Kolff came up with a 'sac-type artificial heart,' a flexible plastic ventricle fitted into a slightly larger rigid housing.[17] Air pressure directed into the space between the ventricle and housing resulted in the compression and release of the sac-type ventricle, moving the blood in and out of the device. After bench testing and animal implants, Kolff reported the sac-type heart as reliable, small, light, and easy to fit into the chest cavity. Dogs survived up to twenty hours with this device. However, technical difficulties became apparent. Most important, Kolff documented the common occurrence of thrombosis and emboli as a result of blood clotting on the plastic components of the device. In dogs who survived more than twelve hours, emboli dislodged causing infarction, stroke, and other neurological conditions.[18] The Cleveland group enlisted the help of chemists to help them find a plastic not conducive to the formation of thrombi. Research also continued into alternative designs, new biomaterials, and power sources.[19]

Kolff was not alone in the development of an artificial heart during the late 1950s and early 1960s. In 1957 Bert Kusserow of Yale University implanted a small blood pump into the abdomen of a dog, which took over the function of the right side of its heart; the pump did the work of delivering deoxygenated blood from the body to the lungs for oxygenation, bypassing the right side of the heart. In 1959 Kusserow reported a similar replacement pump for the left side of the heart.[20] Both his pumps, however, destroyed red blood cells (hemolysis), so his lab worked to revise the pump design as well as to investigate new power sources, surgical implant procedures, and anticoagulant therapy to control blood clotting. Frank W. Hastings, William H. Potter and John W. Holter developed a mechanical heart device driven by a reciprocating fluid column at Miners Memorial Hospital in Harlan, Kentucky. It was a two-chambered diaphragm pump that was only implanted in one dog, with unsuccessful results.[21] At the University of Cordoba in Argentina, Domingo Liotta and his research team began implanting artificial hearts in dogs in 1959, experimenting with various types of pumps and materials. He recorded dogs surviving up to thirteen hours, although none regained consciousness.[22] Liotta remarked that 'from a mechanical point of view, the ventricular function of the heart-pump is not difficult to replace; the problem is to preserve the functional integrity of the rest of the circulatory system.'[23] There were a handful of other research teams also experimenting with mechanical circulatory support systems, including Michael DeBakey's at the Baylor College of Medicine in Houston, Texas, who were developing bypass pumps situated inside and outside the body.[24] Regardless of device specifications, these researchers recognized that building an artificial heart was a complex undertaking; there were mechanical malfunctions, problems with device tolerance within the human body, the delicate surgical procedure and fitting of the device, thrombosis and blood-clotting difficulties with these devices, and more. It required substantial research expertise and resources.

During the 1960s, Kolff's artificial-heart research continued, but it was far from clinical application, which was the interest of Cleveland Clinic administrators. (Artificial-kidney research had developed into a successful clinical program involving remunerative patient treatments and improved procedures for transplantation and home dialysis.) Nonetheless, Kolff pushed Cleveland Clinic administrators to give him more staff and more space.[25] His request was denied. Kolff accused the Cleveland Clinic of trying to limit his research at a time when artificial-heart research promised to expand substantially as a result of the newly established U.S. Artificial Heart Program, a targeted research initiative supported by the U.S. government through the National Institutes of Health (NIH).[26] Funding for artificial-heart research was expanding at the very time Kolff felt that institutional support for his research was diminishing. Feeling frustrated and constrained at the Cleveland Clinic, Kolff began to look elsewhere. Within a short time, he received an attractive offer from the University of Utah in Salt Lake City, which he eagerly accepted.[27]

### Grander Research Aims: The University of Utah (1967–97)

In 1967 Willem Kolff left the Cleveland Clinic and shifted his research program to the University of Utah, where he was promised the opportunity to build an outstanding interdisciplinary institute devoted to artificial-organs research and development. When Kolff moved to Salt Lake City, so did many of his researchers, who were convinced of Kolff's ability to build a grander, successful research program. The University of Utah administrators responded enthusiastically to Kolff's proposed outline for the new Institute for Biomedical Engineering and Division of Artificial Organs, facilitating his plans to bring together medical research with the science and engineering disciplines.[28] The university provided space, staff, and some equipment for the institute, while Kolff secured research funding through government grants, contracts, and private donations, among other sources.

Under Kolff's direction, the Institute for Biomedical Engineering and Division of Artificial Organs developed rapidly, supporting a broad artificial-organ research program. There were research projects on artificial kidneys, artificial limbs, artificial ears, and artificial eyes as well as artificial hearts and circulatory assist devices. Kolff recruited and welcomed any researcher who had creative and feasible ideas. Within a few short years, staff numbered over one hundred and included internists, surgeons, engineers, chemists, physicists, machinists, medical students, veterinarians, and others. Kolff convened regular morning conferences in which members of this diverse group gave brief reports of their work, generating discussion and new approaches to solve immediate problems. Known as a domineering taskmaster, Kolff nonetheless encouraged young investigators to pursue their own ideas within the confines of the Utah research program's objectives and available funding. During the late 1960s and 1970s, Kolff successfully secured funding from NIH grants, contracts, and other sources for his artificial-organ research projects. With adequate staff and funding, Kolff managed a productive research program that introduced numerous device innovations, such as the Wearable Artificial Kidney.

Made available to dialysis patients in 1979, the Wearable Artificial Kidney promised to grant these individuals greater mobility to travel, take a vacation, or treat themselves at home. Kolff took great pride in this device and the institute's 'Dialysis in Wonderland' program, a recreation-therapy program for dialysis patients with Wearable Artificial Kidneys at Lake Powell, Canyonlands, National Parks, and other local areas.[29] Kolff boasted, 'These were people who once felt that they were dependent on dialysis for the rest of their lives – that is, treatment with an artificial kidney, three times per week for four hours and being constrained to be dialyzed either in a hospital, a limited care facility or at home. Now, these people suddenly are able to go in a raft down the rapids of the Colorado River and are dialyzed on shore. They see a whole new world and begin to realize that life still has a lot to offer.'[30] It was this aim of restoring patients to an enjoyable lifestyle, returning them to activities in the community, that motivated Kolff in his artificial-organ research.

In Utah, Kolff's primary research project remained the development of an implantable total artificial heart. During the 1970s, numerous mechanical-heart designs emerged out of Kolff's lab, such as the Kralios artificial heart (1970), the Lyman artificial heart (1972–3), the Donovan artificial heart (1973), and the Unger artificial heart (1974), named after the designers on the team working on the devices at the time.[31] These hearts were short-lived owing to design and biomaterials problems, but they demonstrated Kolff's open approach to experiment in different directions. If a design worked, it was pursued; if it did not work, it was abandoned. Some projects Kolff abandoned reluctantly, as in the case of the nuclear-powered artificial heart (1971–6).[32] Referred to as the AEC (Atomic Energy Commission) artificial heart and later ERDA (Energy Research and Development Administration) artificial heart after the government agency supporting this device, the nuclear-powered artificial heart achieved limited animal success before funding was halted. The device was large, complicated, and expensive, and raised significant social anxiety regarding the risk associated with implanting plutonium in patients.[33] In the end, Kolff's lab returned to air-driven hearts, a simple power source that had been used since 1957 with his first successful animal implant. Thus, the most promising artificial hearts to emerge out of Kolff's labs were two pneumatically driven devices: the Kwan-Gett artificial heart (1967–71) and the Jarvik artificial heart (1972–90).

Clifford Kwan-Gett was an Australian engineer and physician who had joined Kolff's lab as a research fellow at the Cleveland Clinic in 1966. The following year he relocated as part of Kolff's research team to the University of Utah, where he contributed to the design, construction, and testing of artificial hearts. In the lab Kwan-Gett performed surgical implants of artificial hearts in animals, supervised engineers in the research program, designed a heart monitoring system that could regulate cardiac output, and invented a diaphragm-type mechanical heart, the Kwan-Gett total artificial heart.[34] He laid the groundwork for the artificial-heart system that would be used in the first permanent implant case in a human.

The Kwan-Gett heart was large and round, measuring 7 cm (later 8 cm) in inner diameter, and functioned adequately with air power. It had two ventricles, each hemispherical in shape, which connected at the base to form a spherical heart device. The outer casing or housing of the pump was made of Dacron-reinforced Silastic. There were inflow and outflow connections with valves that were continuous with

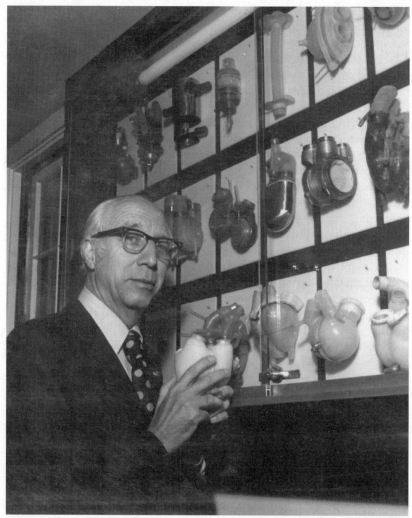

Dr Willem J. Kolff proudly displays the numerous artificial heart models developed in his laboratory during his 40-year career. Many prototypes (such as the nuclear-powered artificial heart) did not move beyond bench testing, several models (such as the pendulum artificial heart) were tested in animals, but only one artificial heart (the Jarvik-7 artificial heart) was ever implanted in humans. (Photo courtesy of Special Collections, J. Willard Marriott Library, University of Utah)

the housing, positioned so as to permit the surgeon to stitch these connections to the patient's remaining heart tissue and surrounding vessels. Within each ventricle, a diaphragm made of a thin layer of Dacron-reinforced Silastic expanded and collapsed by means of compressed air delivered through a metal tube at the base of the device. The driving system used applied pulses of compressed air to each ventricle through two six-foot drive lines. Compressed air passed between the diaphragm and base, expanding the diaphragm towards the housing and moving blood through the outflow valve. The diaphragm collapsed when air in the heart and connecting lines was vented to the atmosphere, thus allowing blood to enter into the device through the inflow valve.[35]

Kwan-Gett's innovation was the use of a diaphragm as the pumping element to move the blood through the device. This marked a significant development in the Utah artificial-heart program. In the early 1970s, the Kwan-Gett heart tested well in mock circulation systems, did not demonstrate problems with mechanical breakage, and did not damage the blood (hemolysis). In animal implant cases, the Kwan-Gett successfully functioned for one week in 1971, improving to two weeks in 1972, setting new survival records in the field. Problems, however, did emerge with this device. First, the device caused excessive clotting of the blood; small clots formed when the blood came in contact with any substance foreign to the body, and these clots then circulated throughout the body with sometimes fatal results. To address this, Kwan-Gett transformed the smooth silicone rubber material of the inside of the heart into a non-smooth surface by attaching tiny fibers of Dacron to anchor these small clots. The clots would form a smooth layer of fibrin (a protein that helps to form a web-like mesh that traps platelets and red blood cells and holds a clot together), hopefully preventing clot dislodgement into the blood stream where it could cause serious problems. More significantly, the problem of 'right-heart failure syndrome' (attributed to an imperfect fit obstructing venous return of blood into the heart) occurred in calves living more than ten days with the Kwan-Gett heart. To overcome this problem, Kolff challenged another researcher, Robert Jarvik, to improve the design.[36] (A common practice of Kolff's was to pit one researcher against another to either test or improve another's device; Kolff's version of 'healthy' competition to stimulate new directions led to animosity among some researchers. Kwan-Gett later challenged Jarvik's alleged sole credit for the Jarvik total artificial heart during the 1980s clinical implants of this device.)[37]

## Success at Last? The Jarvik Artificial Heart

Robert Jarvik joined the Utah lab as an assistant design engineer in 1971, and as directed by Kolff, he modified the Kwan-Gett artificial heart in several significant ways. Like the Kwan-Gett artificial heart, Jarvik's heart consisted of two ventricles with diaphragms that were powered by compressed air. Inflow and outflow valves and connectors ensured the unidirectional flow of blood into the pump and back to the body. One notable difference was the elliptical shape of the Jarvik artificial heart, which did not compromise the lung space, leaving plenty of room for the venous structures above the heart (avoiding right-heart failure syndrome). More importantly, rather than use Silastic, Jarvik experimented with various other blood surface materials in different models, eventually settling on the polyurethane Biomer, to create surfaces on the inside housing that prevented blood thrombosis or clotting. For the diaphragm, Jarvik again used Biomer in three, and later four, thin layer sheets that improved the flexibility and durability of this component. Lastly, Jarvik designed a quick-connect system in which the inflow and outflow cuffs joined coated rigid polycarbonate segments. Dacron vascular prosthetic grafts then connected the artificial heart to the patient's vessels.[38]

In 1972 Donald Olsen, a veterinarian who had earlier consulted for Kolff, joined the Utah artificial-heart research team full-time to direct animal care and device implants. The animal barn and experimental surgery cases required improved management since animals continued to die of infections, convulsion, hemorrhaging and other causes that could have been avoided. Olsen imposed proper animal-care protocols to be followed before, during, and after all animal operations. Calf sitters were hired to keep animals clean and fed. Often pre-med or science students at the university, calf sitters were trained to administer drugs, take blood pressure readings and blood samples, and be prepared for any emergency that might occur during their shift.[39] Animal survival rates dramatically improved thereafter. In 1974 animal implants with the Jarvik-3 artificial heart set new animal survival records: one calf named Bruce lived eighteen days and another, called Crocker, survived twenty-four days.[40] In 1975 calves Tony and Burk survived thirty-six and ninety-four days respectively with their Jarvik-3 hearts.[41] The lab soon discovered that their calves were outgrowing the device; calves grew from approximately two hundred pounds at surgery to more than three hundred pounds five to six months later. So

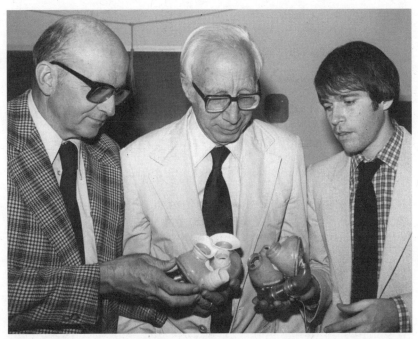

Drs Donald Olsen, Willem Kolff, and Robert Jarvik examine the Jarvik-7 artificial heart, the first FDA-approved total artificial heart for permanent implant (or destination therapy) in humans. In 1982–3, the first Jarvik-7 artificial heart recipient, Barney Clark, survived 112 days with this device implanted in his chest. After his death, the medical community, bioethicists, and others debated the technological and sociological 'success' of the Jarvik-7 artificial heart. (Photo courtesy of Special Collections, J. Willard Marriott Library, University of Utah)

Jarvik designed the larger Jarvik-5 artificial heart, which pumped more blood with each stroke to meet the growth of calves. This model allowed Abebe, the calf, to survive six months.[42] Still, at autopsy, recurring problems presented, including mechanical failures, infection, hemorrhaging, thromboemboli, and pannus (uncontrolled growth of connective tissue at suture points, which spread across the inflow openings of the device). Jarvik observed a wearing of the diaphragm in the device, so he added another thin layer to this component. He then designed another smaller model – the Jarvik-7 total artificial heart – for improved anatomical fit in a human. The Jarvik-7 heart, implanted in both calves and sheep, kept Phred (calf) alive for 169 days and Ted E.

Bear (sheep) alive for 297 days.[43] By the early 1980s, the Utah artificial-heart research team had implanted more than 350 animals with total artificial-hearts. Was the timing right to move from animal to human implant cases?

As argued by medical sociologists Renee Fox and Judith Swazey, 'the decision that "the time is right" to move a new device, procedure, or drug from laboratory and animal testing to human testing is seldom an unambiguous, certain one, either at the time it is made or in retrospect.'[44] Kolff's goal had always been to develop a device for human implant. During the late 1970s and early 1980s, the Utah artificial-heart research team appeared close to implanting their device in a human, but key individuals – Kolff, Jarvik, DeVries, and Olsen – sent mixed signals to each other and to the public about their readiness to proceed. For example, Kolff, Jarvik, and several other lab members formed Kolff Medical Associates, an independent proprietary company, in 1976 to market the artificial heart device.[45] Within a matter of a few years, Jarvik successfully raised needed venture capital, reorganized its management structure, and reduced Kolff's control of the company.[46] Kolff later remarked, 'If I were a lot younger, I would have resisted it.'[47] Simultaneous to Jarvik's actions, Kolff promoted the artificial heart by writing to most cardiac surgery centres, asking them to consider using the device in their hospitals. Kolff wrote, 'The implantation of an artificial heart in man is very close,' and indicated he would provide a Jarvik heart and training for implantation in animals, and later humans.[48] Perhaps Kolff felt pressured to move to clinical cases to ensure continued funding and support of his artificial heart research in Utah. Government funding and support was shifting from research on total artificial hearts to research on ventricular assist devices, which were nearing clinical trials at this time.[49]

Public expectations of a forthcoming total-artificial-heart clinical case were fuelled by newspaper reports. In July 1980 headlines announced 'Utah Doctors to Try Mechanical Heart' and 'Surgeons Are Ready for Mechanical Heart Transplant.'[50] One month previously, William DeVries, a cardiac surgeon who had been part of the Utah artificial-heart research team since he was a medical student, submitted an application to the University of Utah Institutional Review Board (IRB) to explore the possibility of implanting an artificial heart in a patient. As per government funding guidelines and university research procedures, all research involving the use of human subjects required review and clearance by, first, the research institution and, then, the

U.S. Food and Drug Administration (FDA). Once the artificial-heart IRB application became public knowledge, Kolff, DeVries, and other team members received a barrage of inquiries, most significantly questions from NIH's funding agency, which had been supporting much of Utah's research. To the director of NIH's Artificial Heart Program, Kolff wrote: 'The unintentionally started publicity is mostly incorrect, and regrettable. We are indeed talking with the Committee for Human Experimentation [University of Utah Institutional Review Board]. We want the Committee for Human Experimentation to take their time and advise us. We are not ready.'[51] Publicly, Kolff and DeVries admitted they were not ready at that moment, but both envisioned their human implant case to occur soon. Their successful animal implants motivated them to begin navigating the regulatory process to avoid delays later.

In July 1981, at the Texas Heart Institute in Houston, Denton Cooley successfully implanted an Akutsu total artificial heart, developed in his lab by Tet Akutsu, as a bridge to transplantation into a patient.[52] *Life* magazine ran the cover story 'The Artificial Heart Is Here,' publishing photos of Cooley's historic operation as well as photos of DeVries's surgical team 'standing ready for their implant of a Jarvik-7 heart' in Utah.[53] This media coverage was similar to the heroic reporting of the early heart transplantation operations in 1967 and 1968.[54] The first successful heart transplantation took place in December 1967 in South Africa, by Christiaan Barnard, who transplanted a young women's heart into fifty-nine-year-old Louis Washkansky. Washkansky died eighteen days later from pneumonia.[55] Within months, American surgeons began performing heart transplant operations; Denton Cooley, at Houston's St Luke's Episcopal Hospital, accomplished the first successful heart transplant operation in the United States in early 1968.[56] However, few patients survived these early transplant operations due to organ rejection, and a moratorium on the procedure was declared in the early 1970s, lasting throughout the decade. The history of artificial hearts is intertwined with the history of heart transplantation, as both procedures demonstrated the feasibility of replacing the diseased heart in a patient. Furthermore, the challenge of heart-transplant researchers to overcome organ rejection and immunity issues fuelled mechanical replacement as a viable alternative. By the early 1980s, improved anti-rejection drugs (notably cyclosporine) encouraged surgeons to perform heart transplantation operations once again with significantly improved results. Surgeons, such as Cooley, performing heart transplantation operations became more open to using artificial hearts as temporary (or bridge-to-transplant) devices to keep dying heart patients alive until a donor heart could be secured.[57] This created a potential new role for the mechanical heart, in addition to Kolff's intended purpose of the artificial heart as a permanent replacement device.

At a board of directors' meeting of Kolff Medical Associates, Kolff argued that Cooley's implant could help the Utah group gain federal and public approval to move ahead to clinical cases.[58] The team would not attempt to repeat Cooley's bridge-to-transplant operation, but remained committed to implanting the Jarvik artificial heart as a permanent device in a cardiac patient ineligible for a heart transplant. Nonetheless, both Jarvik and Olsen voiced their caution. Despite his business actions with Kolff Medical Associates, Jarvik stated that 'neither the Jarvik-7 nor any of the several other total artificial hearts being developed is yet ready to permanently replace a human heart, even on a trial basis, but the pace of improvement in the technology suggests that the day may not be long in coming.'[59] Olsen, who was most familiar with animal successes and failures, wrote to a colleague: 'I can now say that we are closer to being ready to implant the artificial-heart in man, but unfortunately we are not yet confident enough to do so.'[60] The tension within the artificial heart team surrounded the issue of acceptable risks in clinical research. To Kolff, the animal results suggested an acceptable level of risk for patients who would die in any case owing to heart disease, whereas Jarvik and Olsen were not as accepting of this risk, expecting similar problems, such as clot formation, resulting in animals to present in humans as well. Although not explicitly drawn along engineer-against-clinician lines, those working most closely with the device in the laboratory expressed their reservations more so than either Kolff or DeVries, who saw the device as possibly helping a dying patient. This tension within the team was further increased when Kolff and DeVries decided to apply for institutional and FDA approval of the artificial heart for clinical use.

## The First Clinical Case: Barney Clark

Kolff and the artificial-heart research team began the labourious process of securing institutional and FDA approval for a clinical implant in 1980. Cardiac surgeon William DeVries applied to the University of Utah IRB for permission to implant the Jarvik-7 device in a human suffering from terminal heart disease as a permanent therapy. The proposal was lengthy and included historical background information on the goal of artificial hearts, the testing results of the Jarvik-7 heart, patient selection criteria, surgical procedures, post-operative care measures, and an informed-consent form. The IRB committee found no fault with the technical aspects of the device, but did have a number of problems with the patient selection criteria and the informed-consent form. There was extensive debate around the definition of what was meant by 'virtually facing death,' which was used as the final patient criterion for proceeding with the implant. How certain would the attending physician be that the patient was indeed facing imminent death? Also, the IRB committee raised questions regarding patient lifestyle and operation costs which they felt were not clearly presented in the consent form. What if a not-so-fully informed patient awakened post-operatively to a drastically altered lifestyle with extremely limited mobility, not to mention enormous medical bills? The IRB committee was emphatic that the patient would have to realize what life would be like after the implant of a Jarvik-7 total artificial heart.[61] A stricter protocol needed to be worked out, most significantly a limiting of the potential patient population eligible for this experimental procedure. DeVries complied and altered the application accordingly. After six months of meetings and amendments, the university IRB approved the application, granting permission for a clinical implant in early 1981.

Next, DeVries submitted an Investigation Device Exemption (IDE) application to the U.S. Food and Drug Administration as a first step on the long road to final FDA clearance for marketing and widespread clinical use of the artificial heart. Federal regulatory control of medical devices was first enacted with the U.S. *Food, Drug, and Cosmetic Act* of 1938 in an effort to protect the public against the misbranding of medical devices. Later, the Medical Device Amendments of 1976 required pre-market review of all new devices to ensure their safety and efficacy.[62] The FDA issued investigational-device exemption status to experimental devices approved for use in a limited clinical study in order to collect this safety and effectiveness data, which was required before the FDA approved devices for general practice.[63] The FDA did not approve DeVries's first IDE application, responding with a long list of specific deficiencies, for example, that the informed consent did not accurately present all possible complications and that the scientific protocols of assessing the adequacy of cardiac output needed to be tightened in order to produce sound data.[64] A six-man IRB subcommittee at the university, chaired by Dr F. Ross Woolley, was struck to work with DeVries towards amending the FDA proposal for re-submission. After notable changes and re-submission, the FDA approved the amended application in September 1981.[65]

At this point, the Utah team now had permission to implant a Jarvik-7 total artificial heart in a human. However, both the IRB and FDA approved only a narrow, select patient population for this procedure. That is, only a surgical patient whose heart had stopped while on the operating table and could not be restarted would be eligible for a Jarvik-7 heart implant. Over the next six months, several possible recipients for a Jarvik-7 consented to the implant should their surgery result in failure to restart their hearts. None of these cases provided these circumstances; all recovered successfully from their cardiac operations without the need of an artificial heart. As a result, DeVries was anxious to expand the patient category to include not only patients who died on the operating table but also non-surgical patients dying of severe heart disease with no other options. At this time, a well-publicized case with a patient who was demanding a Jarvik-7 implant assisted DeVries by providing the impetus for an expanded protocol.[66]

In March 1982 Dale Lott begged the University of Utah's IRB committee and the FDA to allow him to become the first recipient of the Jarvik-7 total artificial heart.[67] A Florida fireman, thirty-seven-year-old Lott was dying from cardiomyopathy, a progressive degeneration of the heart muscle that cannot be repaired surgically. Both the IRB and FDA re-stated the criteria for an artificial heart implant as applying only to those patients whose heart stopped on the operating table. Lott threatened to sue the university for denying him this treatment, urging the IRB and FDA to expand the patient category to those, like him, who suffered cardiomyopathy. University officials accused Lott of attempting to circumvent clinical research protocol by using the news media and intimating legal proceedings to access treatment, and furthermore indicated he was not qualified as a candidate even under the expanded criteria.[68] Nonetheless, the media favoured Lott's position that a bureaucratic obstruction prevented him from receiving a potential life-saving treatment.[69] While Lott never did sue the university, this case as well as DeVries's earlier inclination to expand the patient category did result in IRB deliberations and an agreement to include a new category of patient for the Jarvik-7 artificial heart. Patients suffering from cardiomyopathy were added as well as surgical patients. The University of Utah submitted a revised protocol for implanting an artificial heart in a human, which included this new group of heart patients, to the FDA. In June 1982 the FDA approved this expanded protocol.[70] By this time Dale Lott had withdrawn his request for the Jarvik-7 artificial heart; his condition had deteriorated and multiple complications made him ineligible even under the expanded category of patients.[71]

Dale Lott was not the only heart patient to request a Jarvik-7 implant.[72] Many individuals in poor health as a result of heart disease requested more information on the device. Family members contacted DeVries, Kolff, and other members of the Utah artificial-heart team directly, asking if their loved ones could be considered candidates.[73] One woman wrote, 'My husband would like very much for you to try the plastic heart on him ... We both understand the chances he would be taking and we are still willing to try anything.'[74] Many of these desperate people were responding to favourable media coverage of the device. As *Life* magazine reported, 'The Artificial Heart Is Here.'[75] *People* magazine announced, 'Utah Surgeon William DeVries Seeks a Patient Who Could Live with a Man-Made Heart.'[76] Although the device captured the imagination of many families and individuals, most patients did not meet the strict criteria for being considered a candidate for this experimental operation.[77]

The patient ultimately selected as the first implant recipient was sixty-one-year-old Barney Clark, a retired dentist from the Seattle area. The evaluation committee, which was chaired by DeVries and included two cardiologists, a psychiatrist, a social worker, and a nurse, approved Clark as a candidate for a Jarvik-7 implant. Several years earlier, Clark had been diagnosed with cardiomyopathy-myocarditis by his local cardiologist, who treated Clark's illness with drug therapy. Over time, Clark's condition worsened and his doctor sent him to Latter Day Saints Hospital in Salt Lake City to undergo treatment with the experimental drug Amrinone in October 1981. Clark, however, could not tolerate the drug. He was also not a candidate for heart transplantation owing to his age. With no other options to pursue, Clark's doctor suggested the possibility of a total artificial-heart implant procedure in late 1982.[78] Barney Clark and his wife Una Loy met with DeVries, Kolff, and other members of the Utah artificial-heart research team to discuss the artificial heart implant. According to Una Loy Clark, they 'spared us nothing in explaining the highly experimental nature of the implantation.'[79] When seeing the calves and sheep with artificial hearts, Kolff remembered Barney Clark telling him, 'These animals cannot speak, but I believe they feel a lot better than I feel at this time.'[80] After discussing the experimental procedure with his family, Clark agreed to the operation.

On 29 November 1982, Clark was admitted to the University of Utah Medical Center, where he signed an eleven-page consent form twice, twenty-four hours apart. The consent form outlined the procedure as experimental, with no guarantee of a successful outcome, and listed many potential complications including device malfunction, infection, and machine-dependency with limited mobility.[81] According to Una Loy Clark, her husband 'was astutely aware of his critical physical condition and the highly experimental nature of the implantation and DID NOT expect any great personal miracle; he knew FULL WELL that by volunteering, he would be submitting to a totally unpredictable future ... There were absolutely no promises made to him.'[82] Yet Clark was a very ill man within weeks, if not days, of dying. He was diagnosed as being in class IV heart failure, with a heart working at one-sixth capacity of a healthy heart. It is not unreasonable to assume that many, probably including Clark himself, expected the operation to go one of two ways, either as (1) a failure – he would not survive the implant surgery or tolerate the device beyond a few hours; or, conversely, (2) a success – the implant would work, delivering a moderately improved quality of life compared to the patient's grave circumstances beforehand. No one, including the medical team, anticipated the extent of complications that resulted.

On 1 December 1982 Clark was rushed into surgery in advance of the 3 December scheduled operation because of his heart's deterioration. In a nine-hour operation, DeVries removed Clark's diseased heart and implanted a Jarvik-7 artificial heart. Clark survived the surgery, opening his eyes and moving his arms and legs only three hours after the operation. On the second day after the operation, now extubated (removal of breathing tube), Clark communicated with his family and the medical team. Then a series of complications ensued. On day 3 after the operation, DeVries was forced to re-operate on Clark to repair ruptured air sacs in his lungs. On day 6 Clark started experiencing seizures. On day 13 he went into left-heart failure resulting from a broken valve in the artificial heart, necessitating that DeVries replace the left ventricle of the device in yet another surgery. Clark was listed as being in 'extremely critical condition.' Then, near the end of December, Clark appeared to be recovering – standing for the first time, taking his first few steps, even eating soft food by mouth.[83] The hospital released photos of Clark with his physical therapist; Clark was standing on his own and exercising on a stationary bicycle. The Utah artificial-heart team began to receive congratulations from inside and outside the medical community. Feeling uncomfortable with these accolades but still optimistic about Clark's recovery, Kolff wrote: 'I will remain very concerned as long as we have not restored Dr Clark to an enjoyable existence. We still have a reasonable chance to accomplish this ... [and] we fervently hope that we will succeed in getting him well.'[84]

Complications returned to plague Barney Clark. In mid-January 1983 he underwent surgery to control recurring nosebleeds due to his aggressive anticoagulant therapy to prevent blood clotting in the artificial heart. In February 1983 Clark suffered from various kidney and respiratory problems, which were never satisfactorily overcome, and he battled pneumonia, diarrhea, shortness of breath, bloody stool, and fever, among other conditions.[85] Una Loy Clark told friends and family that 'Barney keeps valiantly trying and we pray we may soon reach the point when things will turn in our favor but the days are hard.'[86] By March Una Loy wrote, 'The days pass and we are still trying to climb a big hill. This last bout with pneumonia was discouraging.'[87] Clark was back on the respirator, making communication with friends and family difficult. As Una Loy Clark acknowledged, 'He can't talk and it is difficult ... when all you can do is nod your head and grin.'[88] On 23 March 1983 Clark died as a result of severe pseudomembranous colitis and sepsis, which led to circulatory and organ failure.[89] Dr Barney Clark had lived 112 days with the Jarvik-7 artificial heart.

The Jarvik-7 artificial heart was removed at autopsy and studied for signs of device malfunction, deterioration, or blood clotting. None were reported, an outcome that supported the technological feasibility of mechanically replacing the heart. For the Utah artificial heart team, the Barney Clark case was deemed a scientific success – the Jarvik-7 heart had worked, as it gave this patient and his family 112 extra days of life. Yet success measured as an improvement of patient quality of life had clearly not been achieved.[90]

In 1984–5 in Louisville, Kentucky, DeVries implanted a Jarvik-7 artificial heart in three more patients – William Schroeder (survived 620 days), Murray Haydon (survived 488 days), and Jack Burcham (survived 10 days) – before the FDA withdrew permission for further permanent implant clinical cases.[91] In addition to these implants, the Jarvik-7 artificial heart was also FDA-approved and used widely in conjunction with heart transplantation from 1985 to 1990 as a bridge-to-transplant device for deteriorating patients on the heart transplant list.[92] Then in 1990 the FDA recalled the device and withdrew its earlier IDE approval, citing record-keeping and quality-control problems by Symbion, Inc. (formerly Kolff Medical Associates), now a publicly owned company.[93] The commercialization of the Jarvik-7 necessitated that Kolff and his team move the artificial heart from being a lab device to a commercial product, and for Kolff this foray into the medical-device industry was a costly and volatile process. Kolff was no businessman, and slowly lost control of this device to Kolff Medical, later Symbion Inc. Symbion held the exclusive rights from the University of Utah to distribute this mechanical heart, and when this company lost FDA approval, so ended the clinical use of the Jarvik-7 total artificial heart in the United States.[94] Kolff was ill prepared for a very different medical marketplace than that encountered during his artificial-kidney years and.was unable to navigate the business environment of medical devices in the 1980s.

**Limitations Exposed**

Kolff never faltered in his optimism for the artificial heart. He repeatedly asserted that artificial hearts would someday prove more effective than their natural counterparts, and that future marathon winners would be disqualified for bearing such a device.[95] For Kolff, the feasibility of mechanically replacing the human heart was demonstrated in his animal experiments of the 1960s and 1970s, and later confirmed with the clinical cases of the 1980s. Without equivocation, Kolff asserted that the Barney Clark case was a success for medical science. 'What we learned from Barney Clark was that when he was not sick from any of the many complications he had, his brain worked perfectly well, he retained his joy from life and all his mental capacity, that he still loved his family, and that he still wanted to serve mankind. So all the properties that really make life worth living were preserved for 112 days ... When Barney Clark came to the gates of heaven, St Peter looked down on him and said, "Barney Clark, you're 112 days late."'[96]

Critics – including bioethicists, journalists, and many medical professionals – labelled these early clinical cases as borderline human experimentation and questioned the consent procedure, the therapeutic value of the device, and the patient's real quality of life.[97] In 1988 a *New York Times* editorial dubbed the artificial heart the 'Dracula of Medical Technology' and applauded the NIH decision to halt total-artificial-heart funding, arguing that the total artificial heart had long sucked money out of heart research for little gain. 'At long last, the institute has found the resolve to drive a stake through its voracious creation.'[98] In other editorials, researchers and policy-makers argued that medical research funding was better spent on disease etiology study or preventative programs than on applied technology pursuits. Most urged redirection of research money to prevention programs rather than high technology or heroic cures, arguing that the health-care system could not afford the artificial heart, perfected or otherwise.[99] Yet within weeks, NIH funding for the total artificial heart was reinstated under political pressure from U.S. Senators Orrin Hatch (Utah) and Edward Kennedy (Massachusetts), who threatened to withhold federal funds for other NIH research unless current multi-year artificial-heart contracts were honoured.[100] Not coincidentally, research laboratories in Utah and Massachusetts received the majority of NIH artificial-heart funding at this time. Issues of cost, access, and the limited number of heart-disease patients who might benefit from this technology (estimates ranged from 10,000 to 50,000 U.S. heart patients each year) continued to be debated among bioethicists and medical professionals. At the cost of $60,000 for the device and surgery, as well as the hospital stay (Barney Clark's bill was over $200,000), and with insurance companies declining payment owing to the experimental nature of the procedure, who would be able to afford this treatment?[101]

In the beginning, the media delivered the artificial-heart story as a medical breakthrough with heroes and saved lives. Yet the miracle that was sought remained elusive. The critical views of bioethicists and others in the media appeared to convey public anxieties regarding this device, particularly regarding the issue of quality of life. Reports of Clark's suffering and difficulties with the artificial heart challenged the message that medicine could rebuild diseased bodies. As one reporter wrote, 'The marriage of machinery with flesh and blood is finding the road rough going. With every implant of an artificial heart, physicians are uncovering new obstacles – strokes, hemorrhages, kidney failure, and respiratory distress, among others.'[102] Poor results in these early clinical cases disturbed the public and threatened research programs.

The criticism against the total artificial heart upset Una Loy Clark and infuriated Kolff. After Barney Clark's death, Mrs Clark toured the country as a spokesperson for the American Heart Association, supporting greater heart-disease research and defending the artificial heart. To critics she replied, 'It is easy for those of us standing here with healthy hearts to criticize and to say what we would or would not do –

it is quite another thing to be facing death because our own heart is giving out and have to make a decision about whether to die or to have an artificial heart and prolong our lives and have a chance of survival. My husband wanted to live – he also wanted to help others to live – he took that chance.'[103] Kolff was frustrated that others did not recognize the 'trial-and-error' of clinical investigation. He stated, 'It is unfair to assume that the first patient treated with an artificial heart inside the chest would be an all-out success' and reminded others that 'Of the first 16 patients treated with artificial kidneys, 15 died and only number 17 owed her life to the treatment.'[104] According to Kolff, 'No matter how many successful animal experiments you have, you can still lose your first patient when you attempt something new clinically. You must have some leeway for some failures when you are beginning something new and worthwhile.'[105] What Kolff failed to realize was that his 'leeway' translated into 'sacrificial patients,' which was not acceptable in late-twentieth-century clinical cases in America. His comparison to the first artificial-kidney patients was not apt owing to the changes that had occurred in research conduct and reporting, clinical- trial protocols, acceptable patient risks, and evolving patient rights since the 1940s.[106]

After a half-century in the field of artificial organs, Kolff closed his lab at the University of Utah in 1997 and donated the lab's numerous artificial heart models to the Smithsonian Institution.[107] Citing personal family reasons, Kolff moved across the country to Newtown Square, Pennsylvania.[108] Today, in 2006, he remains convinced that the total artificial heart will finally be developed and accepted as the best permanent therapy for patients dying of heart disease. He concedes that artificial hearts and ventricular assist pumps may be used mainly as temporary devices (as bridges to heart-transplantation devices), but reminds people that 'we will never have enough donor hearts for transplantation.'[109] As a result, the permanent use of the artificial heart must return.[110] In his own words: 'Inevitably this will come; it has to come; but it requires a different way of thinking by the medical profession. I have heard from all those medical advisors involved with putting in artificial kidneys, hearts, heart-lung machines ... [adding] "I would rather be dead!" You never hear that from a patient!'[111] Kolff firmly believes that people would always choose to live rather than die, and that medical research is close to offering a viable mechanical device as a permanent treatment for heart-failure patients. Patients, such as Barney Clark, are actors in the development of heroic therapies whose courage is often not rewarded in any personal recovery. Their decision to participate is influenced, knowingly or unknowingly, by the technological imperative in medicine, the role of the media and 'medical miracle' reporting, their fear of death, and the technological optimism of medical researchers like Kolff.

Kolff's forty-year pursuit of a mechanical heart was contentious. Within his own research team, there were clashes over device design, manufacturing processes, clinical use, and marketing. The medical community debated the use of total artificial hearts as permanent or temporary replacement devices, with the majority advocating its use only as a bridge-to-transplantation device. Kolff's team struggled to meet both institutional-review-board and FDA regulatory standards to gain limited clinical approval for the Jarvik heart. Bioethicists and the media voiced their concerns regarding continued government funding for artificial heart research, a device that seemed more monstrous than miraculous. Issues of access, cost, and quality of life needed to be addressed if this device was to be introduced into clinical use. Kolff's perseverance in his artificial-heart research demonstrated minimal change and poor adaptability to shifting research practices, clinical-use guidelines, and society's limited tolerance of 'experimental' devices, thus contributing to the less-than-satisfying outcomes of the Jarvik-7 clinical cases of the 1980s. Kolff did not succeed in delivering a mechanical heart as a viable treatment to patients in heart failure. Examination of his artificial-heart research program exposes clear limitations surrounding the device itself as well as the growing discrepancy between Kolff's narrow technological optimism and increased misgivings by others surrounding such 'experimental' technologies.

My use of this biographical framework – that is, attempting to understand the motivations of this individual, his contribution to the larger artificial-heart research field, and the broader medical issues or themes therein – will come as no surprise to Michael Bliss, who continues to act as mentor to me through his most recent publications, *William Osler: A Life in Medicine* (1999) and *Harvey Cushing: A Life in Surgery* (2005). Whereas Osler and Cushing are towering historical figures within medicine, Kolff will most likely be remembered only by a handful of current artificial-organ researchers who, armed with new biotechnology and bioengineering advances, respectfully acknowledge Kolff as an early but antiquated 'tinkerer' in their field. Whereas they may be pursuing new mechanical circulatory support devices with similar fervour and commitment in the fight against heart disease, their research practices demand a level of rigour, interdisciplinarity, and regulation that, if required of Kolff during the immediate post-war decades, almost certainly would have thwarted his research program sooner.

NOTES

1  Kolff developed the first clinically successful artificial kidney machine, crediting researchers Abel, Rowntree, and Turner for describing the mechanics of dialysis, and coining the term 'artificial kidney,' in 1913. These early artificial kidney machines failed owing to a lack of reliable anticoagulants and of good dialysing members and to the insufficient capacity of dialysing equipment. See Willem J. Kolff, 'Artificial Organs beyond the First 40 Years,' *Life Support Systems* 2 (1984): 1; Willem J. Kolff, 'First Clinical Experience with the Artificial Kidney,' *Annals of Internal Medicine* 62, 3 (March 1965): 608; J.J. Abel, L.G. Rowntree, and B.B. Turner, 'On the Removal of Diffusible Substances from the Circulating Blood of Living Animals by Dialysis,' *Journal of Pharmacology and Experimental Therapy* 5 (1913–14): 275.
2  Marie-Claude Wrenjn, 'The Heart Has Its Reasons,' *Utah Holiday*, July 1982, 32.
3  For more on the media frenzy surrounding the Barney Clark case, see Barron H. Lerner, *When Illness Goes Public: Celebrity Patients and How We Look at Medicine* (Baltimore: Johns Hopkins University Press, 2006), chap. 9, 'Hero or Victim? Barney Clark and the Technological Imperative,' 180–200.
4  S.J. Reiser, *Medicine and the Reign of Technology* (Cambridge: Cambridge University Press, 1978); J. Pickstone, *Ways of Knowing: A New Science, Technology and Medicine* (Manchester: Manchester University Press, 2000); S. Blume, *Insight and Industry: On the Dynamics of Technological Changes in Medicine* (Cambridge: MIT Press, 1992) and 'Land of Hope and Glory: Exploring Cochlear Implantation in the Netherlands,' *Science, Technology and Human Values* 25 (2000): 139–66.
5  Most well known is Michel Foucault's emphasis on the body as a site of social contest and power, which has attracted both proponents and critics. See M. Foucault, *The Birth of the Clinic* (London: Tavistock, 1976); B. Turner, *The Body and Society*, 2nd ed. (London: Sage, 1996); M. Lock, A. Young, and A. Cambrosio, eds, *Living and Working with New Medical Technologies* (Cambridge: Cambridge University Press, 2000); and N. Brown and A. Webster, *New Medical Technologies and Society: Reordering Life* (Cambridge: Polity Press, 2004). Feminist writer Donna Haraway explores body–identity relationships in *Simians, Cyborgs and Women: The Re-invention of Nature* (New York: Routledge, 1991).
6  As taken from Bruno Latour and his work, including *Laboratory Life* (Princeton: Princeton University Press, 1979) and *Science in Action* (Milton Keynes:

Open University Press, 1987). See also 'On Recalling ANT,' in J. Law and J. Hassard, eds, *Actor Network Theory and After* (Oxford: Blackwell, 1999), 15–25.

7 F.A. Gotch, 'The Evolution of the Society,' *Transactions of the American Society for Artificial Internal Organs* 25 (1979): 534–8.

8 Taken from S. McKellar and M. Kurusz, 'Reflections and Visions: 50 Years of Presidential Addresses,' *ASAIO Journal* 50, 6 (November/December 2004): 629–34.

9 Willem J. Kolff, 'An Artificial Kidney inside the Body,' *Scientific American* 213, 5 (November 1965): 41.

10 T. Akutsu and W.J. Kolff, 'Permanent Substitutes for Valves and Hearts,' *Transactions of the American Society for Artificial Internal Organs* 4 (1958): 230; Josephine Robertson, 'Substitute Heart of Plastic Pushed by Clinic Team,' *Cleveland Plain Dealer*, 15 April 1958; 'The Artificial Heart: Progress toward Its Implantation in Man,' *JAMA* 185, 13 (28 September 1963): 24.

11 Years later, Kolff and Akutsu learned that a Soviet scientist, Vladimir Demikhov, had performed a similar experiment in 1937. See George M. Pantalos, 'A Selective History of Mechanical Circulatory Support,' in *Mechanical Circulatory Support*, ed. T. Lewis and T.R. Graham (London: Edward Arnold, 1995), 6; H.B. Shumacker, Jr, 'A Surgeon to Remember: Notes about Vladimir Demikhov,' *Annals of Thoracic Surgery* 58 (1994): 1196.

12 P.M. Portner, 'Permanent Mechanical Circulatory Assistance,' in *Heart and Lung Transplantation*, 2nd ed., ed. W.A. Baumgartner et al. (Philadelphia: W.B. Saunders Co., 2002), 533. Portner also takes issue with the term 'total artificial heart,' stating that a more accurate description would be a 'biventricular replacement device.'

13 W.J. Kolff, T. Akutsu, B. Dreyer, and S.H. Norton, 'Artificial Heart in the Chest and Use of Polyurethane of Making Hearts, Valves and Aortas,' *Transactions of the American Society for Artificial Internal Organs* 5 (1959): 298.

14 C.S. Houston, T. Akutsu, and W.J. Kolff, 'Pendulum Type of Artificial Heart within the Chest,' *American Heart Journal* 60 (1960): 723.

15 Cleveland Clinic Foundation Archives, folder 3-PR20 Artificial Organs, news release, 15 April 1958; University of Utah, MS 654, Willem J. Kolff Collection, 'Early Types of Artificial Hearts,' n.d.; 'The Artificial Heart: Progress toward Its Implantation in Man,' *JAMA* 185, 13 (28 September 1963): 25–6; W.J. Kolff, 'The Artificial Heart: Research, Development or Invention?' *Diseases of the Chest* 56 (1969): 314–29.

16 Willem J. Kolff, 'An Artificial Heart inside the Body,' *Scientific American* 213, 5 (November 1965): 45.

17 T. Akutsu, V. Mirkovitch, S.R. Topaz, and W.J. Kolff, 'Silastic Sac-type of Artificial Heart and Its Use in Calves,' *Transactions of the American Society for Artificial Internal Organs* 9 (1963): 281.
18 'The Artificial Heart: Progress toward Its Implantation in Man,' *JAMA* 185, 13 (28 September 1963): 25–6.
19 W. Seidel, T. Akutsu, V. Mirkovitch, F.D. Brown, and W.J. Kolff, 'Air-driven Artificial Hearts inside the Chest,' *Transactions of the American Society for Artificial Internal Organs* 7 (1961): 378; K.W. Hiller, W. Seidel, and W.J. Kolff, 'A Servo-Mechanism to Drive an Artificial Heart inside the Chest,' *Transaction of the American Society for Artificial Internal Organs* 8 (1962): 125; K.W. Hiller, W. Seidel, and W.J. Kolff, 'Electro-Mechanical Control for an Intrathoracic Artificial Heart,' *American Journal of Medical Electronics* 2 (1963): 212; S.H. Norton, T. Akutsu, and W.J. Kolff, 'Artificial Heart with Antivacuum Bellows,' *Transactions of the American Society for Artificial Internal Organs* 8 (1962): 131; E.K. Panayotopoulous, S.H. Norton, T.Akutsu, and W.J. Kolff, 'A Special Reciprocating Pump to Drive an Artificial Heart inside the Chest,' *Journal of Thoracic and Cardiovascular Surgery* 48 (1964): 844; Y. Nose and W.J. Kolff, 'The Intracorporeal Mechanical Heart,' *Vascular Disorders* 3 (1966): 25.
20 B.K. Kusserow, 'The Use of a Magnetic Field to Remotely Power an Implantable Blood Pump. Preliminary Report,' *Transactions of the American Society for Artificial Internal Organs* 6 (April 1960): 292–8.
21 F.W. Hastings, W.H. Potter, and J.W. Holter, 'A Progress Report on the Development of a Synthetic Intracorporeal Blood Pump,' *Transactions of the American Society for Artificial Internal Organs* 8 (1962): 116–17.
22 D. Liotta et al., 'Artificial Heart in the Chest: Preliminary Report,' *Transactions of the American Society for Artificial Internal Organs* 7 (1961): 318–22.
23 'The Artificial Heart: Progress toward Its Implantation in Man,' *JAMA* 185, 13 (28 September 1963): 27.
24 C.W. Hall, D. Liotta, W.S. Henly, E.S. Crawford, and M.E. DeBakey, 'Development of Artificial Intrathoracic Circulatory Pumps,' *American Journal of Surgery* 108, 5 (November 1964): 685–92.
25 University of Utah, MS 654, W.J. Kolff Collection, box 380, folder 5, Correspondence Fay A. LeFevre to W.J. Kolff, 17 October 1961; box 380 folder 2, Correspondence W.J. Kolff to Research Projects Committee, Cleveland Clinic, 12 January 1965; box 381, folder 1, W.J. Kolff, Proposal: Institute of Artificial Organs for the Cleveland Clinic Foundation, 5 May 1965.
26 The NIH established the Artificial Heart Program in 1964, which served as a catalyst for mechanical circulatory support research and funding in the

United States. The program objective was to develop a 'family' of cardiac devices for emergency, temporary assist, permanent assist and replacement devices. NIH awarded investigator research grants as well as development contracts to encourage industry expertise.

27 University of Utah, MS 654, Willem J. Kolff Collection, box 381, folder 12, Correspondence W.J. Kolff to F.A. LeFebre, Chairman, Board of Governors, Cleveland Clinic Foundation, 23 March 1967; Correspondence Leonard L. Loveshin, Board of Governors, Cleveland Clinic Foundation, to W.J. Kolff, 13 April 1967.

28 University of Utah Archives, Faculty Files: Willem Kolff, Correspondence J.C. Fletcher to W.J. Kolff, 11 April 1967; Correspondence W.J. Kolff to B.G. Dick, 11 February 1974.

29 University of Utah Archives, Accession 475, box 22, folder 12, Institute for Biomedical Engineering: Some of Its Projects; Some of Its People, University of Utah, 1981. See also Trudy McMurrin, 'Artificial Organs Research at the University of Utah Medical Center,' in *Medicine in the Beehive State 1940–1990*, ed. Henry P. Plenk (Salt Lake City: University of Utah Press, 1992), 453–9.

30 'Artificial Organ Pioneer Says Star Wars Siphoning Funds,' *FAHS Review*, July/August 1986: 23.

31 Interestingly, there is no Kolff artificial heart since Kolff generously named these devices after the lead investigator in his lab working on the design at the time. This system later raised jealousy among some researchers when publicity surrounding the Jarvik heart spotlighted designer Robert Jarvik. Kolff countered this emphasis on Jarvik by stating that the work of more than 247 researchers had contributed to this device. University of Utah, MS 654, Willem J. Kolff Collection, box 2, folder 4, W.J. Kolff, 'Mankind and Life with Artificial Organs,' unpublished (n.d.).

32 University of Utah, MS 654, Willem J. Kolff Collection, box 169, folder 8, Correspondence Allan T. Howe (House of Rep., Utah) to W. Kolff, 2 May 1975.

33 L. Smith, K. Backman, G. Sandquiest, W.J. Kolff, K. Schatten, and T. Kessler, 'Development of the Implantation of a Total Nuclear-Powered Artificial Heart System,' *Transactions of the American Society for Artificial Internal Organs* 20 (1974): 732–5; L. Smith, G. Sandquist, D.B. Olsen, G. Arnett, S. Gentry, and W.J. Kolff, 'Power Requirements of the AEC Artificial Heart,' *Transactions of the American Society for Artificial Internal Organs* 21 (1975), 540–4. For opposing views on the development of a nuclear-powered artificial heart, see *The Totally Implantable Artificial Heart: Economic, Ethical, Legal, Medical, Psychiatric and Social Implications*, A Report by the Artificial Heart Assessment Panel, National Heart and Lung Institute (DHEW Publication no. [NIH] 74-191),

June 1973; Albert R. Jonsen, 'The Artificial Heart's Threat to Others,' *Hastings Center Report*, February 1986: 9–11; and Harold P. Green, 'An NIH Panel's Early Warnings,' *Hastings Center Report*, October 1984, 13–15.

34  University of Utah, MS 654, Willem J. Kolff Collection, box 149, folder 2, Departmental Report; Robert Jarvik, 'The Total Artificial Heart,' *Scientific American*, January 1981, 79.

35  D.J. Lyman, C. Kwan-Gett, H.H. Zwart, A. Bland, N. Eastwood, J. Kawai, and W.J. Kolff, 'The Development and Implantation of a Polyurethane Hemispherical Artificial Heart,' *Transactions of the American Society for Artificial Internal Organs* 17 (1971): 456–63; C. Kwan-Gett, D.K. Backman, F.M. Donovan Jr, N. Eastwood, J.L. Foote, J. Kawai, T.R. Kessler, A.C. Kralios, J.L. Peters, K.R. Van Kampen, H.K. Wong, H.H. Zwart, and W.J. Kolff, 'Artificial Heart with Hemispherical Ventricles II and Disseminated Intravascular Coagulation,' *Transactions of the American Society for Artificial Internal Organs* 17 (1971): 474–81; C.S. Kwan-Gett, K.R. Van Kampen, J. Kawai, N. Eastwood, and W.J. Kolff, 'Results of Total Artificial Heart Implantation in Calves,' *Journal of Thoracic Cardiovascular Surgery* 62, 6 (December 1971): 880–9.

36  University of Utah, MS 654, Willem J. Kolff Collection, box 149, folder 2, Departmental Report.

37  Personal interviews by author.

38  Robert Jarvik, 'The Total Artificial Heart,' *Scientific American*, January 1981, 79; R. Jarvik, J. Volder, D. Olsen, S. Moulopoulos, and W.J. Kolff, 'Venous Return of an Artificial Heart Designed to Prevent Right Heart Syndrome,' *Annals of Biomedical Engineering* 2, 4 (December 1974): 335–42; R.K. Jarvik, D.B. Olsen, J.H. Lawson, H. Fukumasu, T.R. Kessler, and W.J. Kolff, 'Recent Advances with the Total Artificial Heart,' *New England Journal of Medicine* 298, 7 (February 1978): 404–5.

39  University of Utah, MS 654, Willem J. Kolff Collection, box 221, folder 7, Manual for Calf Sitters.

40  H. Oster, D.B. Olsen, R. Jarvik, T.H. Stanley, J.G. Volder, and W.J. Kolff, 'Survival for 18 Days with a Jarvik-type Artificial Heart,' *Surgery* 77, 1 (January 1975): 113–17.

41  University of Utah, MS 654, Willem J. Kolff Collection, box 174, folder 1, table I: Historical (Animal) Records of Total Artificial Heart Research at the University of Utah.

42  University of Utah, MS 654, Willem J. Kolff Collection, box 226, folder 1, table: Longest Surviving Animals with a Total Artificial Heart (Over 100 days) at the University of Utah.

43  Ibid.

44 Renee C. Fox and Judith P. Swazey, *Spare Parts: Organ Replacement in American Society* (Oxford: Oxford University Press, 1992), 104.

45 For the changing entrepreneurial culture of university research, see Sheldon Krimsky, *Science in the Private Interest: Has the Lure of Profits Corrupted Biomedical Research?* (New York: Rowman and Littlefield Publishers, Inc., 2003).

46 In 1983 Jarvik severed ties with Kolff and allegedly squeezed him out of control of the company. Kolff returned to the university, while Jarvik left the university to become the company's president and chief financial officer. Jarvik promoted the Jarvik-7 total artificial heart as a temporary device for transplant patients deteriorating on waiting lists. In 1983 Kolff Medical went public, but struggled to make a profit. In 1984 Kolff Medical was renamed Symbion, Inc. (derived from symbiosis and bionic). In 1987 Jarvik was fired by the Symbion board of directors. He moved to New York to establish his own medical-device company, Jarvik Heart Inc., promoting his left ventricular assist device, the Jarvik 2000. See Fox and Swazey, *Spare Parts*, 103–4; 'The Inc. 100 Portfolio: King of Hearts – Has Jarvik Found a Heart of Gold?' *Inc.*, May 1986, 51; Mike King, 'Jarvik Fired as Chairman of Mechanical Heart Firm,' *Courier Journal*, 28 April 1987.

47 University of Utah, MS 654, Willem J. Kolff Collection, box 309, folder 11, Kolff's Four Companies, October 1984.

48 University of Utah, MS 654, Willem J. Kolff Collection, box 294, folder 1, Artificial Heart Program in Other Centers – Purchase Equipment through Kolff Associates document; Correspondence Jacques G. Losman to W.J. Kolff, 28 December 1980; Correspondence W.J. Kolff to Robert L. Replogle, 3 September 1980; Correspondence W.J. Kolff to Denton Cooley, 19 January 1982.

49 P.M. Portner, 'Permanent Mechanical Circulatory Assistance,' in W.A. Baumgartner et al., *Heart and Lung Transplantation*, 2nd ed. (Philadelphia: W.B. Saunders Co., 2002), 536–40.

50 A sample of news clippings include: 'Mechanical Heart Test,' *Sentinel* [Hanford, CA], 23 July 1980; 'Utah Doctors to Try Mechanical Heart,' *Dallas Times Herald*, 23 July 1980; 'Temporary Heart Implant Is Sought,' *Rocky Mountain News* [Denver], 23 July 1980; 'Artificial Heart Ready for Test,' *Fresno Bee* [Fresno, CA], 23 July 1980; 'Surgeons Are Ready for Mechanical Heart Transplant,' *Tribune* [Cheyenne, WY], 23 July 1980; 'Mechanical Heart Transplant Surgery Due,' *Democrat* [Sherman, TX], 23 July 1980.

51 University of Utah, MS 654, Willem J. Kolff Collection, box 292, folder 1, Correspondence W.J. Kolff to John Watson, NHLBI, 23 July 1980.

52 Willebrordus Meuffels, age 36, lived 39 hours with an Akutsu artificial heart before he was transplanted with a human heart, which his body

rejected within days. This was the world's second artificial-heart implant case. The first implant case, performed also by Dr Denton Cooley and also as a bridge to transplantation, occurred in 1969; Haskell Karp, age 47, received 64 hours of mechanical circulatory support from a Liotta artificial heart. Although the implant operation was technically successful, the patient died 32 hours after his human-heart transplant operation. University of Utah, MS 654, Willem J. Kolff Collection, box 322, folder 6, Correspondence Denton A. Cooley to W.J. Kolff, 10 August 1981.

53 'The Artificial Heart Is Here,' *Life Magazine*, September 1981, photo of DeVries's surgical team on p. 35.

54 'Gift of a Human Heart' [cover story], *Life Magazine*, 15 December 1967; however, reporting turned more critical with the poor results of transplantation by the early 1970s, as seen in 'The Tragic Record of Heart Transplants' [cover story], *Life Magazine*, 17 September 1971.

55 See Barnard's autobiography, Christiaan Barnard and Curtis Bill Pepper, *One Life* (New York: Macmillan Press, 1969).

56 Daniel J. DiBardino, 'The History and Development of Cardiac Transplantation,' *Texas Heart Institute Journal* 26, 3 (1999): 198–205.

57 Denton A. Cooley, 'Transplantation versus Prosthetic Replacement of the Heart,' *Biomaterials, Medical Devices, Artificial Organs* 3, 4 (1975): 481–8.

58 Dr Denton Cooley responded to Kolff's congratulations with words of encouragement – 'I only hope that the FDA will lift their restrictions on your project so we can learn how much practical knowledge we can gain now without waiting for years or until subsequent generations have the experience. I wish you and your team success when you get the green light.' University of Utah, MS 654, Willem J. Kolff Collection, box 322, folder 6, Correspondence Denton A. Cooley to W.J. Kolff, 10 August 1981; box 534, folder 5, Minutes of Kolff Associates Board of Directors' meeting, 27 July 1981.

59 Robert Jarvik, 'The Total Artificial Heart,' *Scientific American*, January 1981: 74; cited in Fox and Swazey, *Spare Parts*, 105.

60 University of Utah, MS 654, Willem J. Kolff Collection, box 354, folder 1, Correspondence Don Olsen to Larry Smith, 11 May 1979.

61 Ibid., box 350, folder 7, E.J. Eichwald et al., 'Case Study: Insertion of the Total Artificial Heart' (ca. March 1981).

62 Peter Barton Hutt, 'A History of Government Regulation of Adulteration and Misbranding of Medical Devices,' *Food, Drug, Cosmetic Law Journal* 44 (1989): 99–117. See also Philip J. Hilts, *Protecting America's Health: The FDA, Business, and One Hundred Years of Regulation* (Chapel Hill: University of North Carolina Press, 2003).

63 Data collected from IDE-approved clinical cases is used to support a Premarket Approval (PMA) application or a Premarket Notification [510(k)] submission to FDA, necessary for widespread distribution.

64 University of Utah, MS 654, Willem J. Kolff Collection, box 350, folder 10, Correspondence Victor Zafra (FDA) to Lee M. Smith (Kolff Associates), 29 March 1981.

65 Ibid., box 534, folder 5, Correspondence Victor Zafra (FDA) to Lee M. Smith (Kolff Associates), 10 September 1981.

66 University of Utah Archives, Accession 92–62, box 20450, Correspondence John Dwan to Willem J. Kolff, 25 June 1982; Correspondence Willem J. Kolff to Dale Lott, 21 June 1982; 'Dale Lott Cheering for Man Who Got Heart He Wanted,' Salt Lake Tribune, 5 December 1982.

67 'Dying Man Begs U. for Heart,' Salt Lake Tribune, 16 March 1982.

68 University of Utah Archives, Accession 475, Vice President for Health Sciences Records 1945–1960, Correspondence Chase N. Peterson, VP Health Sciences, to IRB Members, 18 March 1982.

69 'Floridian Waits as Lawyer Fights U. on Jarvik Rules,' Salt Lake Tribune, 21 March 1982; 'U. Surgeon Visits Doctors of Dying Floridian,' Salt Lake Tribune, 23 March 1982; 'CBS' Slurs against Medical Center Lacked Osgood's Rhyme, Reason,' Salt Lake Tribune, n.d.

70 University of Utah, MS 654, Willem J. Kolff Collection, box 350, folder 7, Artificial Heart Fact Sheet, 3 September 1982.

71 'Lott Abandons Quest for Artificial Heart,' Salt Lake Tribune, 28 May 1982. For an ethical discussion of this case, see 'A Volunteer for Utah's First Artificial Heart,' Hastings Center Report 12, 2 (April 1982): 2.

72 University of Utah Archives, Accession 475, Vice President for Health Sciences Records 1945–1990, Correspondence Chase N. Peterson, VP Health Sciences, to IRB Members, 18 March 1982.

73 University of Utah, MS 654, Willem J. Kolff Collection, box 292, folder 1, Correspondence W.J. Kolff to Chase N. Peterson, VP, 3 April 1981; box 354, folder 1, Correspondence Gerry Casey (Manchester, Eng.) to W.J. Kolff, 1 May 1984; Correspondence Mrs Milan Ganser (North Dakota) to W.J. Kolff, 23 August 1982; Correspondence J.M. Flake (Provo, UT) to W.J. Kolff, 3 February 1981; Correspondence Patricia Bullwinkel (Freeport, NY) to W.J. Kolff, 21 October 1980.

74 University of Utah, MS 654, Willem J. Kolff Collection, box 354, folder 1, Correspondence Mrs John I. McKillip (Lima, OH) to W.J. Kolff, 7 October 1975.

75 'The Artificial Heart Is Here,' Life, September 1981, cover page.

76 Frank W. Martin, 'Utah Surgeon William DeVries Seeks a Patient Who Could Live with a Man-Made Heart,' People 18 (19 July 1982): 30–1.

77 In one case, a New York City cardiac patient was evaluated as a fit medical candidate for a Jarvik-7 implant, but was ultimately rejected owing to the lack of a strong, supportive family, deemed crucial to the experiment's success. See Lawrence K. Altman, 'Heart Team Drawing Lessons from Dr Clark's Experience,' *New York Times*, 17 April 1983, 1.

78 University of Utah, MS 670, Barney Clark Collection, box 1, folder 30, Correspondence Una Loy Clark to Robert H. Ruby, M.D., 12 March 1987.

79 Ibid.

80 University of Utah, MS 654, Willem J. Kolff Collection, box 2, folder 4, Willem J. Kolff, 'Mankind and Life with Artificial Organs,' unpublished, p. 5.

81 Margery W. Shaw, ed., *After Barney Clark: Reflections on the Utah Artificial Heart Program* (Austin: University of Texas Press, 1984), 195–201.

82 University of Utah, MS 670, Barney Clark Collection, box 1, folder 30, Correspondence Una Loy Clark to Robert H. Ruby, M.D., 12 March 1987.

83 University of Utah, MS 670, Barney Clark Collection, box 1, folder 29, Chronology of Barney Clark's Transplant Saga, n.d.; box 7, folder 4, List of Dates and Times of All Operations Performed on Dr Clark, n.d.; box 7, folder 8, Artificial Heart Press Releases – Postoperation News Conference, n.d. See also William C. DeVries et al., 'Clinical Use of the Total Artificial Heart,' *New England Journal of Medicine* 310, 5 (2 February 1984): 273–8.

84 University of Utah, MS 654, Willem J. Kolff Collection, box 351, folder 3, Progress Report on Dr Barney Clark, 17 January 1983.

85 University of Utah, MS 670, Barney Clark Collection, box 1, folder 29, Chronology of Barney Clark's Transplant Saga. See also DeViries et al., 'Clinical Use of the Total Artificial Heart.'

86 University of Utah, MS 670, Barney Clark Collection, box 2, folder 1, Correspondence Una Loy Clark to Birdie and Erie Baurman, 17 January 1983.

87 Ibid., box 1, folder 30, Correspondence Una Loy Clark to Birdie and Erie Baurman, 9 March 1983.

88 Ibid.

89 William C. DeVries et al., 'Clinical Use of the Total Artificial Heart,' *New England Journal of Medicine* 310, 5 (2 February 1984): 273–8; William C. DeVries, 'The Permanent Artificial Heart: Four Case Reports,' *Journal of American Medical Association* 259, 6 (12 February 1988): 849–59; William C. DeVries and Lyle D. Joyce, 'The Artificial Heart,' *Clinical Symposia – CIBA* 35, 6 (1983).

90 DeVries et al., 'Clinical Use of the Total Artificial Heart,' 278. See also M.W. Shaw, ed., *After Barney Clark: Reflections on the Utah Artificial Heart Program* (Austin: University of Texas Press, 1984).

91 In 1984 William DeVries left Utah to continue his clinical cases at Humana Hospital in Louisville, Kentucky, where he was promised financial and bureaucratic support (which he felt was not forthcoming in Salt Lake City). DeVries, 'The Permanent Artificial Heart,' 849–59.

92 Don Olson, 'Bridge-to-Transplant Experience with the Jarvik-7 and the Jarvik-7–70 Total Artificial Heart,' *Artificial Organs* 11, 1 (1987): 63–8. See also Kristen E. Johnson et al., 'Use of Total Artificial Hearts: Summary of World Experience, 1969–1991,' *ASAIO Journal* 38 (1992): M486–92, which states that 230 total artificial hearts (of which there were 11 different models) had been implanted in patients in this 22-year period. The Jarvik heart had been implanted the most – 5 permanent implants (destination therapy) and 181 temporary implants (bridge-to-transplantation).

93 'FDA Recalls Jarvik Heart, Scolds Firm,' *Salt Lake Tribune*, 12 January 1990; University of Utah, MS 654, Willem J. Kolff Collection, box 551, folder 3, News Release from Symbion, 14 March 1990.

94 In late 1990 CardioWest Technologies Inc. purchased the technology and assets of Symbion, Inc. They further developed the Jarvik-7 total artificial heart or Symbion heart into the CardioWest C-70 total artificial heart. Within a few years SynCardia Systems Inc. purchased the CardioWest heart technology, and in 2004 this company received FDA market approval for the CardioWest™ temporary Total Artificial Heart (TAH-t) System as a bridge-to-transplantation device.

95 University of Utah, MS 654, Willem J. Kolff Collection, box 2, folder 4, Willem J. Kolff, 'Mankind and Life with Artificial Organs,' unpublished, n.d.; box 1, folder 11, Excerpt from Willem Kolff biography in *Innovators and Discoverers: Changing Our World*, written by Carole Douglis.

96 Ibid., box 1, folder 17, News clipping, Brian E. Albrecht, '"Scavenger" Is Creator of Medical Miracles,' *Plain Dealer*, 5 June 1983, 1C, 2C.

97 George J. Annas, 'Consent to the Artificial Heart: The Lion and the Crocodiles,' *Hastings Center Report*, April 1983, 20–2; Thomas A. Preston, 'Who Benefits from the Artificial Heart?' *Hastings Center Report*, February 1985, 5–7; George J. Annas, 'No Cheers for Temporary Artificial Hearts,' *Hastings Center Report*, October 1985, 27–8. See also Shaw, ed., *After Barney Clark*; and B.J. Bernstein, 'The Misguided Quest for the Artificial Heart,' *Technology Review*, November/December 1984, 13–63.

98 'The Dracula of Medical Technology,' *New York Times*, 16 May 1988, A16.

99 A sample of these editorials includes Daniel Callahan, 'The Artificial Heart: Bleeding Us Dry,' *New York Times*, 17 September 1988; Philip M. Boffey, 'Battling with Congress over Priorities on Heart,' *New York Times*,

8 July 1988; David T. Nash, 'Let's Invest in the Prevention of Heart Disease,' *New York Times*, 16 June 1988.

100 Philip M. Boffey, 'Federal Agency, in Shift, to Back Artificial Heart,' *New York Times*, 3 July 1988, 1, 12; 'Senators Doctors Kennedy and Hatch,' *New York Times*, 15 July 1988, A30.

101 See Gideon Gil, 'The Artificial Heart Juggernaut,' *Hastings Center Report*, March/April 1989: 24–31; and Fox and Swazey, *Spare Parts*.

102 'Artificial Hearts: An Uneasy Marriage of Machinery and Flesh,' *Medical World News*, 27 May 1985, 40–6, 49, 53, 55, 57.

103 University of Utah, MS 654, Willem J. Kolff Collection, box 353, folder 7, Correspondence Una Loy Clark to W. Kolff, 12 March 1984.

104 Ibid., box 2, folder 4, Kolff, 'Mankind and Life with Artificial Organs.'

105 Allen B. Weisse, *Heart to Heart: The Twentieth Century Battle against Cardiac Disease – An Oral History* (New Brunswick, NJ: Rutgers University Press, 2002), 251.

106 See Harry M. Marks, *The Progress of Experiment: Science and Therapeutic Reform in the United States, 1900–1990* (Cambridge: Cambridge University Press, 1997).

107 The Kolff Collection includes more than 250 objects, 5 boxes, and 2 binders of supporting material and complements the museum's existing artificial organ collection. See Willem J. Kolff Collection, American Museum of Natural History, Smithsonian Institution, Washington, DC.

108 Weisse, *Heart to Heart*, 269.

109 University of Utah, MS 654, Willem J. Kolff Collection, box 2, folder 4, Kolff, 'Mankind and Life with Artificial Organs'; see also Willem J. Kolff interview, *Dialysis and Transplantation* 16, 6 (June 1987): 306–9.

110 The AbioCor™ implantable replacement heart, the first completely self-contained total artificial heart, is currently in an FDA-approved 15-patient clinical study. In 2001 59-year-old Robert Tools became the first recipient of the AbioCor total artificial heart, manufactured by AbioMed Inc, and survived 151 days. Seventy-year-old Tom Christerson survived almost 17 months (September 2001 to February 2003) with his AbioCor total artificial heart, returning home to live for the last 10 months of his life. To date, 14 patients have received the implant; all have died.

111 Weisse, *Heart to Heart*, 268.

# 16 History, Memory, and Twentieth-Century Medical Life Writing: Unpacking a Cape Breton Country Doctor's Black Bag

SASHA MULLALLY

The white lab coat and the stethoscope are the most widely recognized symbols of contemporary medicine, but there is an equally powerful iconography built around the country doctor carrying a simple black bag. Embodying populist ideals of rugged self-reliance, community service, and personal sacrifice, the country doctor's folksy, homespun exterior belies an acute medical acumen and a calm, professional competence. Though this figure is easily recognizable in popular culture, historians still know relatively little about the rural medical practices with which this icon is associated.

The history of rural medicine is nonetheless a field of growing interest. Since the mid-1990s a new rural medical historiography has sought primarily to describe and define rural practice as distinct from medical practices in 'the city.' From Jan Coombs's demographic profile of nineteenth-century rural doctors in Wisconsin, for instance, emerges one of the first twentieth-century overviews of general practitioners at the state level. Coombs's project was culled from several years of research into the history of public health, and it was among the first studies that consciously explored the differences between urban and rural medical demographies.[1] Others choose to examine microcosms of rural medicine. In Jacalyn Duffin's intensive exploration of James Miles Langstaff's case books, we see an individual's specific responses to therapeutic change, patient and community demands, and the changing political environment of small-town life. Duffin's work is notable in that it points to the degree to which the small-town politics and the idiosyncratic medical habits developed over a lifetime of practice informed the therapeutic approach of her subject, Langstaff.[2] Even more recent works have focused on sources that reveal the interior life of physicians in order to understand their practices and political contexts. Judith Walzer Leavitt's study of turn-of-the century rural physicians' diary entries explores the personal preoccupations of doctors on their rural rounds. Her descriptions and analysis of these entries challenge our notions of late-nineteenth-century gendered spheres of labour by showing how rural physicians focused on domestic concerns when tending to patients and making arrangements for their care.[3] In a similar vein, the most recent contributors to this historiography explore the idea of 'authority' in rural practice and the interrelationship between informal traditional medicine and the formalized professional care offered by allopathic physicians. Sandra Barney's book on the social transformation of Appalachian health care is one example of such a work that examines the process by which a group of 'authorized' healers took over and institutionalized health-care services from a disparate group of lay practitioners.[4] By describing the scientific and therapeutic, business and economic, as well as psychological and emotional parameters of typical general practices, these works are reshaping our assumptions about the profession of medicine and its allopathic character. This paper contributes to this literature with a focus on an important historical source for the new rural historiography: life writing.

The enormous popularity of life writing, in particular medical autobiography and biography, make it important to the history of medicine. This popularity extends to rural medical practices. By the 1940s, rural physicians were increasingly taking up pen and paper to write about their life experiences in autobiographies or cooperate in the construction of biographical projects. As a result, rural medical life writing comprises a substantial corpus of literature. Approximately 130 titles have been published in the English language over the past century.[5] This makes rural medical life writing one of the richest sources of information about non-urban practices available to the historian. Nonetheless, like the country-doctor archetype, this body of writings has thus far either not interested or escaped the notice of most professional historians.[6]

Just because something is popular does not mean it is easily accessible. Perhaps historians have avoided discussing country-doctor tales because medical life writing as a whole is a very large literary genre, replete with overlapping themes that defy easy categorization. Some scholars have dipped into this well of memoirs to reveal the aspects of social and political medical history. S.E.D. Shortt used the opinions, observations, and claims in the autobiographies of general practitioners to present a demographic profile of this group of doctors. He plumbed their educational experiences, detailed the political activities in which they involved themselves, and offered an analysis of therapeutic change and continuity in their practices. Overall, Shortt uses physician memoirs to narrate the 'rise, fall, and rebirth of general practice' in early-twentieth-century Canadian medicine.[7]

Shortt's approach does fall victim to a categorization problem, however, in that he depicts 'general practice' as one undifferentiated sort of medical life.[8] He is not alone in subsuming the rural voice in medical life writing. In his work on the social history of the medical autobiography, anthropologist Donald Pollock attempts to outline the various 'subgenres' in medical life writing. Like Shortt, Pollock does not appreciate the extent and number of rural medical narratives, and allocates only a few lines to a discussion of these autobiographies. Instead, he focuses on 'the training tale,' exemplified by such works as *Under the Ether Dome*. Pollack assumed that most medical autobiography, including that produced by rural doctors, is motivated by the same 'cultural project' as the training tale, in that depictions of rural practices wish to critique medical bureaucratization. Pollack speculates that rural physicians engage in life writing to express a nostalgic desire to return to a 'traditional doctor–patient relationship.'[9] This, I will argue, is also a problematic interpretation. Like Shortt, Pollock conflates the experiences and messages in rural medical life writing with those expressed by other twentieth-century doctors. Nostalgia for a more straightforward or 'simple' doctor–patient relationship may be a part of their message. Yet there appear to be specific cultural projects for rural medicine and health care embedded in country-doctor life narratives that require discussion.[10]

The methodological problems of uncovering the cultural projects behind life-writing are well appreciated in the historical field. Especially since the 'linguistic turn' of the 1980s, most historians have been hesitant to make historical claims from biographical and autobiographical texts. Influenced by the new cultural history, many scholars focus instead on what such texts can tell us about the contemporary preoccupations of the writer.[11] This approach has considerably deepened our understanding of life writing as a human endeavour. By virtue of the work of many literary theorists, we may now carefully contextualize autobiography as a social activity. Historians now understand the many ways that life writing in general, and autobiography and biography in particular, are historically contingent on both the literary milieu of the individual author, as well as the political understandings about the importance of 'the self' and 'the individual' at any given point in our cultural past.

Building from this rich scholarly debate, the historian may now take and apply the work of cultural critics to a more sophisticated understanding of social history with life writing as a central focus. Social historians now find themselves able to not only use life writing to understand contemporary preoccupations of the writer, but to take these insights and apply them in an analysis and evaluation of the textual elements – the discrete memories, interpretations, and claims – made about an individual experience and an individual life. In other, more specific, words, uncovering the cultural projects that motivated country-doctor life writing is a very useful historical undertaking if the historian first attempts to analyse and understand them on their own terms. The preoccupations of the physicians and their publishers being revealed, these very biases can act as a guide to understanding important political messages built into the personal narratives. Clearly, an autobiography or biography is more than just a tale about the self/the individual, inasmuch as it is also a story about the various institutions that relate to the self or the individual. Especially when these forms are packaged as 'memoirs,' they represent a 'life and times' rendering of personal experience, usually through the eyes of someone whose social position gave them what Pollock calls an 'experience near' perspective. It seems clear that rural doctors wrote their memoirs primarily to highlight the conditions and problems unique to rural medicine – the degree to which they identify with and use the phrase 'country doctor' in their titles is the first indication of this. While I agree with Shortt that such works reveal much about changes in the emerging specialty of family medicine, and concur with Pollock's observations about how medical life writing is often ambivalent about medical 'progress,' I also believe that the rural aspect needs to be brought to the fore in order to represent these works with greater authenticity.

The genre of rural medical life writing has a history of its own. Country-doctor tales date back to the late nineteenth century.[12] But for North Americans, the first autobiography to reach a mass audience was Arthur Hertzler's *Horse and Buggy Doctor*, published in 1938 by New York's Harper and Brothers.[13] A title that is still widely available in print after a 1970 release by the University of Nebraska Press, Hertzler's book popularizes the work of 'forgotten' rural physicians labouring in obscurity throughout small-town America. *Horse and Buggy Doctor* gives a real-life edge to the romantic iconography of the country doctor emergent, as we shall see, in the same period. And it is significant in that it tells the story of early-twentieth-century social and scientific transformations of medicine from the perspective of a rank-and-file Kansas practitioner. Before him, this epochal transition was handled almost exclusively in the medical biographies and writings of elite physicians. His populist stance and critiques of medical standardization notwithstanding, Hertzler was himself not a typical country doctor. A professor of surgery at the medical school associated with the University of Kansas, Hertzler was an established scientific writer by the time this autobiography went to print. He had already written over eighteen books on surgical topics before *Horse and Buggy Doctor*, including a series on surgical pathology.[14] Neither did his publishing career end with this memoir of his country doctoring days. Hertzler would publish four more books in his later career, ranging from a treatise on sexual ethics to a textbook on the proper uses of anesthesia.[15] Aside from his autobiography, most of these would be self-published. Yet many rural physicians followed in Hertzler's footsteps in the production of an autobiography.

Another well-known example of the successful country-doctor tale is a Canadian story – the 1939 biography of Allan Roy Dafoe, the physician credited with 'delivering' the Dionne quintuplets, entitled *The Little Doc*. Dafoe's relationship with the quintuplets is central to his biography, but the narrative also details his life and career as an obscure country doctor in northern Ontario during the first decades of the twentieth century.[16] In this case, the divide between real life and Hollywood fiction becomes blurred, as the book is largely a response to the popularity of a 1936 film based on the story of Dafoe and the five famous little girls.[17] But as with *Horse and Buggy Doctor*, this autobiography also set a precedent for published success. Table 16.1 shows just how many subsequent rural physicians and their biographers were inspired to write and publish retrospectives of their careers

The table allows one to make three important observations about this body of literature. The most obvious of these is the increasing popularity of rural medical life writing, or at least the increasingly common practice among rural physicians of committing their memoirs to paper as the twentieth century unfolds. Before the 1930s, there were only a handful of books by and about rural physicians in print. The genre produced more and more titles during the 1950s, 1960s and 1970s, culminating in an exponential rise in rural medical life writing by the end of the century. By the 1990s the reading market saw three new titles published per year. Over this period there has been a consis-

Table 16.1
Rural medical life writing – by period of setting and decade of publication

| Decade of publication | Period of setting | | | | | |
| --- | --- | --- | --- | --- | --- | --- |
| | 19th century | | Early- to mid-20th-century | | Mid- to late-20th-century | |
| | A | B | A | B | A | B |
| 19th century | 2 | | | | | |
| 1900s | 0 | | | | | |
| 1910s | 1 | | | | | |
| 1920s | 2 | 1 | 1 | | | |
| 1930s | 2 | | 5 | 1 | | |
| 1940s | | 1 | 4 | 2 | | |
| 1950s | 1 | 1 | 3 | 7 | | |
| 1960s | | 1 | 9 | 3 | | 1 |
| 1970s | 2 | 2 | 10 | 4 | | |
| 1980s | | 1 | 4 | 5 | 15 | 1 |
| 1990s | | 2 | 5 | 6 | 20 | 3 |
| Total publications | 9 titles 14.8% of genre | | 69 titles 53.9% of genre | | 40 titles 32.3% of genre | |

A = autobiography; B = biography

tent and growing number of rural doctors engaged and invested in the production of their life stories. The second trend refers to authorship. The ratio of autobiographies to biographies consistently favours the autobiography. Although rural doctors have gained increasing attention from writers, journalists, and others interested in penning their life stories, country doctors have as a group consistently expressed an equal and greater interest in writing about themselves.

The third trend brought to light in this table is the decided generational focus represented in the genre. Despite the fact that the 1980s and 1990s witnessed the greatest output of country-doctor memoirs and biographies, and that most of these physicians were writing about their own lives in the mid to late twentieth century, it is actually the generation before them that garners the greatest attention. The table shows a strong and consistent representation of rural physicians who practised between 1900 and 1950. When one charts the publication of country-doctor tales into three broad categories – the nineteenth century, the early to mid-twentieth century and the mid- to late twentieth century – there is a clear dominance of early- to mid-twentieth-century medical lives. In fact, the majority of works published by and about country doctors are written by and about Hertzler's and Dafoe's contemporaries, whose practices roughly spanned the interwar period through to the 1950s – the 'last' generation of physicians to practise largely peripatetic medicine.

Apart from the generational focus, do these works have anything thematically in common? Certainly, when one examines rural medical life writing on its own terms, and reads through the memoirs, it is quickly apparent that country-doctor tales employ certain narrative strategies that are absent from other forms of medical life writing. Most prominent of these is 'the heroic travel tale,' an organizational device utilized exclusively by the rural memoirs. Although Judith Waltzer Leavitt's work on nineteenth-century rural Wisconsin points to a preoccupation with the domestic sphere in diary writings of physicians, in their public narratives the focus is definitely on travel.[18] By highlighting heroic travel, it appears that rural physicians are attempting to underscore the special conditions and obstacles they faced as 'country doctors.' The travel tale thus serves a moral function, in that it highlights a rural physician's dedication to practice and to the well-being of his community. Travel tales also foreground the difficulty of the doctors' work and are evidence of the demand and need for their services. It becomes the defining characteristic of the genre, particularly among North American physicians.

Why do physicians rely so heavily on these stories to organize their narratives? What does this focus on the travel tale represent? Why don't they and their biographers, as one might have expected, explore the deep doctor–patient relationships cultivated over years practising rural and small-town medicine? To answer these questions, this chapter will move from a macro-view of rural medical life writing to one that explores the microcosm. By outlining the process involved in bringing a physician's memoir to press, it will discuss and interpret apparent tensions between how physicians conceived of themselves and their work and how they and their work were ultimately packaged in book form. This tells us more than the fact that editors will edit – indeed, narrative fault lines reveal upheavals in the arena of early- to mid-twentieth-century medical politics.

## The Making of a Life Story

A quintessential example of rural medical life writing was produced in
Nova Scotia. C. Lamont MacMillan published *Memoirs of a Cape Breton
Doctor* through McGraw-Hill Ryerson of Toronto in 1975. In many
ways, *Memoirs* represents an ideal case study through which we can
metaphorically unpack the black bag. A 1927 graduate of Dalhousie
University, MacMillan established a private practice in Baddeck, Nova
Scotia, which became his base of operations for a practice that would
grow to cover hundreds of square miles throughout Victoria County.
Unsurprisingly, the travel tale figures prominently in his narrative. He
had only tenuous access to hospital services before the end of the Second World War, and lived at a time of significant technological
changes in medical practice. His career spanned almost forty years,
lasting until a heart condition forced his retirement in the 1960s.
Although MacMillan's practice extended well into the middle decades
of the twentieth century, most of his medical stories and anecdotes in
*Memoirs* are taken from his first, formative years in practice. This focus
on early years highlighted the arduous travel demanded of general
medicine that still revolved around the peripatetic rhythms of rural
house calls. It would seem that the inter-war years, when roads were
poor and travelling difficult, made a greater impression on MacMillan,
and on his identity as a country doctor. These elements, particularly
the narrative focus on the inter-war period, are representative of the
rural life-writing genre, and MacMillan was certainly an excellent representative of the 'last' generation of medical peripatetics.

The publisher foregrounds the country-doctor iconography in the
packaging of MacMillan's *Memoirs*. The first edition featured a water-
colour sketch on the cover, a scene where a young physician abandons
an automobile mired in mud on a country road. Grasping a black bag,
he continues his journey on foot. On opening the book, the reader is
greeted first by a map of Cape Breton, outlining the extensive geographical parameters of MacMillan's Baddeck-based practice. In a
glowing foreword, Canadian senator Henry Hicks (a Nova Scotian
himself) holds MacMillan up as an exemplar of national civic virtue.
The senator calls 'Dr. Monty' a 'real humanitarian' who spent his life
caring for 'small and rugged communities' in his medical sphere. He
extols the country doctor's virtues, brought out in the face of 'difficulties imposed by the terrain, the seasons, the weather, and the scattered
population.' Hicks also praises MacMillan for embodying a sturdy

sense of duty and adherence to communitarian values, bolstered by good humour and a positive outlook. The untiring task of practising medicine in such a context, in Hicks's opinion, 'makes it easy for one to understand why the country doctor of a generation ago was held in such high regard, and, indeed, why he was a citizen of such great importance to the people he served.' The senator closes his preface by remarking that MacMillan's story is important social history, the kind that Canadians 'ought to have of their country and its people.'[19]

This typical country-doctor tale promises a close encounter with a bedrock citizen of Canadian society. Doctors like MacMillan, portrayed in such flattering terms by individuals like Hicks, are depicted as key players in the ongoing twentieth-century process of nation building, and as such must necessarily embody political values and messages. In addition, as the senator comments at the end of his preface, 'there is something extremely charming about the delight he took in his first car ... or the pride he took in his mare, Gypsy Queen.'[20] These bedrock values are therefore fundamentally populist as well as communitarian. Even though he is an admirable physician of some standing in his community, MacMillan as a country doctor is at the same time 'delightful' in the obvious esteem he has for his horse. In this way, the senator paints MacMillan as an approachable hero. The model presented by his life offers a 'common man' version of great doctor tales, without challenging any of the great doctor's works or the broader profession of which he is a part.

These observations offer some insight into the appeal of MacMillan's *Memoirs*, at least from the perspective of those who designed the title pages and packaged the message, but they offer little insight into how or why he wrote his life story. As the saying goes, one cannot judge a book by its cover, and the methods used by his publishers and promoters reveal little about the physician's own intentions for this work. What message did MacMillan hope to send by committing his memoirs to paper? Is this even possible to ascertain?

**The Preface Makes Perfect**

For C. Lamont MacMillan, the autobiographical project was indelibly marked by the interaction with his editors and publishers at McGraw-Hill Ryerson. As it turns out, *Memoirs of a Cape Breton Doctor* is an altered version of MacMillan's original manuscript, which he had called 'Hang the Lantern on the Gate.' MacMillan's first title refers to a local practice where Cape Bretoners, upon receiving word that the doctor was travelling through their community, would signal to the physician that his services were needed by leaving a lantern lit at the end of their driveway or at the front gate. The original, unabridged manuscript is housed in the Nova Scotia Archives and Records Management Office in Halifax. It is a fascinating document containing many candid asides, frank discussions of community life, and the doctor's own medical foibles. Comparing the original and the published version allows for two very different readings of *Memoirs* as an autobiographical representation of the rural physician and his work.

It also sheds light on the autobiographical project. The original introduction describes how MacMillan, tape recorder in tow, spent the first six years of his retirement visiting communities of Victoria County, reliving stories of his early years in practice. He recreated his medical rounds, inviting former patients, friends, and travelling companions to tell their side of the story of his medical practice. The resulting assemblage of anecdotes in 'Hang the Lantern on the Gate' is an annotated collection of seemingly random cases roughly organized into a chronology covering the 1920s and 1930s, with some reminiscences from later decades thrown in. One is left with the strong impression that reliving his former peripatetic route, this time with a tape recorder in his hand instead of a black bag, and oral history instead of medicine on his mind, was a pilgrimage of sorts for the doctor. MacMillan set out on his oral-history project in order to make sense of a period in his career that was particularly arduous – remembered as a blur. And it is clear from the outset that he wants to answer a larger historical question: why were his early experiences so difficult?

Considering the lack of hard-surface roads and hospital facilities in Victoria County during the inter-war years, the answer might appear obvious to some: his experiences were difficult because he was the only physician in an extremely isolated location with challenging weather and terrain. But MacMillan reveals a decent understanding of the medical history in his region. Combining his oral-history project with archival sources, he illustrates the progressive history of medicine on the island. In the opening pages of his book, he gives evidence of early doctors' professional qualifications, details medical and surgical 'firsts' on Cape Breton, and describes the civic positions held by physicians.[21] This discussion, accomplished over a scant dozen pages in the published *Memoirs*, diverges significantly from the historical conclusions made in the eighty-eight-page preface in the manuscript. It is

clear from reading the original that he believes he practised at a particularly challenging juncture in the history of medicine. MacMillan,
for instance, is quick to point out in the original that medicine
appears to have been a part-time practice for his forebears. 'From stories I heard when I first came here, many times a doctor was called
only as a last resort,' he tersely observes in the manuscript.[22] One
physician who practised in the late nineteenth century, a Dr S.G.A.
McKeen, 'was regarded by the public as a demi-god to be avoided'
unless desperately ill.[23] And no physician felt it behooved him to
attend to obstetrical cases in nineteenth-century Cape Breton.

In his manuscript, but *only* in his manuscript, MacMillan recognizes
that midwives attended all the birthing in Victoria County. His praise
of their efforts is passing, and accompanied in the original by
humourous caricatures of their various personality types gleaned
from a nineteenth-century physician colleague.[24] He nonetheless
acknowledges their contribution to the health needs of women and
children in the colonial pre-Confederation era. This acknowledgment
is tempered by some descriptions of perineal tears he found while
examining older women in communities where he worked. These, he
states, were the unfortunate result of women's accepting attitudes
toward traditional methods of birthing. But MacMillan does not
blame the 'untrained' midwives for these lapses as much as he points
to a lack of professional interest among physicians in surgical post-
partum care. The contrast to his own practice is quite clear – he is concerned and does operate where his forebears feared to treat.

Despite these observations of inferior skill among lay medical practitioners, MacMillan finds reason to praise the intentions of his historical
confreres in the profession by highlighting the heroic image of the
intrepid travelling doctor. Travel is the ultimate marker of a physician's
dedication for MacMillan, and he expends a great deal of writerly
energy in the original document extolling his predecessors' bravery and
dedication through the details of travel exploits from the century before.
MacMillan draws parallels from these tales to his own life and work.
After detailing the adventures of previous Cape Breton doctors, he
writes, 'From my own experience on trips during winters such as we
used to have before good roads were built, I know no amount of money
could ever pay a man for this service.'[25] These depictions of previous
physicians from his district are also leading up to a comparison of medical generations, and in entertaining the reader with tales of heroic travel,
he is setting a benchmark against which he compares himself.

In his published *Memoirs* MacMillan seldom complains about the difficulties encountered travelling around the region, writing, 'despite the weather and road conditions, my years in Victoria County were happy ones. I feel my "Memoirs of a Cape Breton Doctor" is part of our heritage and should be preserved.'[26] But in the manuscript version he constantly refers back to the increased demands for obstetrical and other medical work made of him. In fact, MacMillan concludes in his manuscript's preface that rural physicians of his own generation worked harder than any of these pioneers.[27] In the published *Memoirs* there is no mention of why the doctor's immediate predecessor, Dr J. Angus MacIvor, left the Baddeck area in 1923. But the manuscript quotes relatives still living in Baddeck who explained that 'the pace of the practice was getting too hard for him.'[28] MacIvor's decision to leave was based on an increasing demand for his services, a 'pace' that he could no longer accommodate. Yet MacMillan would establish a practice in this territory just five years later. Uninterested in colouring himself as a national icon, MacMillan instead claims that his medical generation suffered from a unique juxtaposition of social and medical developments that laid an especially difficult communitarian burden upon early-twentieth-century rural medical practices:

> The work of the pioneer doctors in the wintertime was exactly the same as I did years later. I was no better off than they were that number of years before. We know that there were five doctors in Baddeck at the turn of the century; but I handled the practice alone for over 30 years when many more people used doctors. Our work was pretty much the same although I think I was on the go all the time.[29]

Although his *Memoirs* rely upon heroic travel tales, actual laments about being 'on the go all the time' are largely edited out.[30] But we know from a comparison of the manuscript to the published version that MacMillan considered himself to be part of a watershed medical generation, equally rewarded and harried by the burden of duty. This appears to be the main message he wanted to convey in his autobiography, and how he conceptualized his life and practice in the context of Cape Breton's medical history.

This is not the only message lost in the editorial process. It is also interesting to see which anecdotes are selected from the seven-hundred-page manuscript to adequately portray MacMillan's life as a 'part of our heritage that should be preserved.' From an examination of both copies, we find that most of MacMillan's most protracted and difficult travel tales do make the final cut for the published version. Many significant details, however, ended up on the cutting-room floor. In the manuscript MacMillan is forthright about many medical mistakes; in the long typewritten texts of the manuscript version there are many incidents of poor judgment, bad luck, and plain tomfoolery. Many of these never made it past the editorial desks of McGraw-Hill Ryerson. When the missing details are examined as an edited whole, it appears that the selection of anecdotes for publication was based primarily on maintaining an unassailable image of medical competence and confidence, in regards to the physician himself, the contexts in which he practised, and how he was viewed by his community and colleagues.

### Anecdotal Evidence in MacMillan's *Memoirs*

The anecdotes collected in 'Hang the Lantern on the Gate' are clinical case reconstructions from a physician's memory, sometimes enhanced with the corroboration or extra information supplied by the patient, a family member, or another physician or health-care provider who was on the scene at the time. Many cases highlighted in the published *Memoirs* revolve around childbirth, with the physician rushing to assist women in labour. In most cases, the difficult details of MacMillan's obstetrical cases recorded in the manuscript come through to the printing press. What is edited out are the anxieties of the physician himself. In his manuscript MacMillan bluntly writes that his first case of *placentia previa*, encountered when he was a young doctor, 'scared the hell out of me.'[31] The waiting, first for full dilation, and then for the arrival of assistance from a more experienced physician from North Sydney, only heightens the physician's anxiety as he is faced with the limits of his training and expertise. By contrast, in his *Memoirs* he merely recognizes the need for assistance and sends for a specialist from North Sydney. Then he calms the mother and waits.[32]

Other practical limitations to the country practice are also missing from the published version. In another case, MacMillan delivered a premature set of twins with the assistance of a nurse-midwife named Mrs Baker. His *Memoirs* recounts the episode as a milestone, the first internal manipulation of the baby's position he performed himself. This 'internal version' was written up in *Memoirs* as a 'good experience' of learning to perform a procedure that he would be called upon to accomplish on many occasions in the future. In *Memoirs* we learn that the doctor hired an airplane from the Cape Breton Flying Club to get him up to remote Ingonish in time to perform the delivery. In this published account of the story, a charming aside by Mrs Baker about how she kept the preemies warm in milk boxes, and called them 'Borden' and 'Carnation' after the milk brands, completes the anecdote.[33] It is only in the manuscript that one learns that the babies died.

In the manuscript there is no implication that this is the fault of the doctor; the twins were delivered live. Mrs Baker, the nurse-midwife, explains in the unedited copy that owing to the cold weather, the poor health of the mother, and 'home conditions not the best' the premature infants only survived a few weeks.[34] Like the slight reworking of MacMillan's first case of *placentia previa*, the omission of such details does not compromise the veracity of the published version in a strict sense. But leaving out the fear and self-doubt of the physician is a significant alteration of the meaning the clinical encounter had for him. Similarly, the omission of the negative outcomes of rural care leaves the reader to assume that none of the doctor's labours, particularly his heroic travel, are in vain. In fact, even the most skilled country doctor, adept at turning fetal positions *in utero* and managing complications during the birth of premature twins, cannot substitute for hospital facilities. Neither can the good will and care of dedicated nurses offset the combined effects of cold and poverty. Throughout the published *Memoirs*, poverty in Cape Breton is elided by the drama of medical intervention, and the reader is distracted by the heroic travel. This distraction is certainly evident in the story of 'Borden' and 'Carnation.'

'Another story that perhaps should be swept under the rug' according to MacMillan's more candid manuscript describes the time he left medication for an elderly woman with pneumonia out in Plaster Mines. 'I picked out a bottle of black medicine, syrup of white pine.' But the labels had detached from his bottles, and the woman was actually fed Lysol, two teaspoons every four hours for several days. On another occasion, some people in an isolated part of the island swabbed a sick man's throat with a concoction the doctor had left as cough medicine, but which was actually labelled iodine. The family spoke only Gaelic and could not read the label. The doctor returned after several days to find the patient 'yellow as goldenrod.' In *Memoirs*, the presence of Gaelic-speakers is mentioned only to provide local flavour to descriptions of MacMillan's Cape Breton practice; the language barrier is not an obstacle at the bedside. These stories are also meant to be amusing, but one wonders if he would have related the tales at all if

the patients had fallen ill or been poisoned by the mistaken medication. At the close of each anecdote, MacMillan accepts responsibility,
remonstrating himself for not being more careful, but also notes how a
later generation of patients would probably not have hesitated to sue
him for negligence.[35]

The obstacles and difficulties MacMillan encountered as part of his
isolated rural practice are ultimately organized in such a way that the
doctor's ingenuity is highlighted. *Memoirs of a Cape Breton Doctor* offers
several instances where the doctor's capacity for innovation overcame
the difficulties of practising with few medical supplies and no trained
personnel. A case in point is the time MacMillan used a speedometer
cable to dislodge a piece of meat stuck in a patient's gullet.[36] This episode had already become a well-known story when, in 1952, *Maclean's
Magazine* printed the details in their 'Canadianecdote' section. But the
physician's manuscript bears evidence to his own unease with these
episodes requiring medical 'innovation.' In 'Hang the Lantern on the
Gate,' MacMillan recounts the time he treated a young woman with a
severe facial laceration. She and her male companion had been looking
for him and caught up with the doctor on the return leg of a house call.
MacMillan was out of suturing medium for a facial case, and so went
around to the back end of his horse and pulled some hairs out of its tail
to use as a substitute. Meeting the woman years later in Halifax, he
congratulated himself on leaving only a very slight scar. An abbrevi-
ated version of this case made it into the published autobiography,[37]
but in the original the physician admits to a good deal of worry over
the case. Highlighting the difficulty in keeping supplies in a rural practice, he takes great care in the manuscript to detail how he boiled the
tail hairs for forty-five minutes, and then he took his time. Although he
'made quite a good job of the suturing,' he nonetheless admitted, 'It
was a bit of a worry for me for a long while that this particular material
I used for suturing might not have been boiled long enough.'[38] The vis-
cera of an automobile may be incorporated into surgical procedures
written up in *Maclean's* and MacMillan's *Memoirs*, but it is clear from
MacMillan's manuscript that not all improvisational episodes felt satisfactory to the physician at the time.

The stories of MacMillan's on-the-spot medical innovation cannot be
read as counter-technology narratives. As Donald Pollock has noted,
this kind of tale is a celebration of scientific progress by 'a kind of
inversion.' Writing about rural practices where the lack of surgical
equipment and trained personnel force the physician to innovate with

a limited medical armamentarium and in less than ideal surroundings 'celebrates technological advances through their absence, and the creativity of physicians who must do without.'[39] I would also add that these accounts convey a secondary message of equal importance. Over time, it is argued, physicians like MacMillan 'hone' this medical creativity. Ingenuity becomes, with the passage of the years and with experience, a skill unto itself. Thus, the message conveyed by such cases is relatively clear: MacMillan and country doctors like him become a special breed of physician. After years of practice, it is inevitable that such physicians become innovative enough to make do and provide adequate and safe care to patients. One wonders, after reading MacMillan's manuscript, if he would have agreed.

If the tales of innovation are selectively chosen to highlight the skill of ingenuity, the travel tales are similarly selected to highlight the physician's dedication. In this way, the demands of rural medicine also 'bring out' human virtues – as Senator Hicks's preface promises. Certainly, MacMillan's *Memoirs* are typical country-doctor tales in that they, too, revolve around the doctor's travel, particularly in winter. But the real strain on the doctor is largely absent. In the book's last chapter the reader learns that a heart condition forces him to retire. Nights like the one when he stopped at a house en route to a call, desperate to get warm and weeping bitterly from the cold, have all been edited out.[40] The workload cannot be seen as dangerous to the general public if it is heroic in a literary sense. This is likely why extreme fatigue in the *Memoirs* is often couched in humourous terms – patients he transports to the hospital jabbing him in the ribs to keep him awake and on the road; driving down treacherous Smokey Mountain so tired he could only keep one eye open – instead of dwelling on the physician's own anxieties about his inability to manage exhaustion. On a thirty-six-hour call in the early years of his practice, MacMillan blacked out from exhaustion on the way home. Both *Memoir* and manuscript recall that the doctor kept driving, although 'I didn't know who I was. I didn't seem to know anything. All I did realize was that each car I passed seemed to be getting a little closer to me all the time.'[41] In *Memoirs* the doctor musters up the will to get the car out of harm's way and parked. In the manuscript getting off the road was more a matter of luck. He wrote, 'I don't know how long it was before it dawned on me that I really should stop the car.' Getting out, MacMillan remembers walking around for about fifteen minutes before he 'came to': 'It was a case of being asleep with both eyes open.'[42]

In MacMillan's manuscript the contexts of rural medicine undergo alterations that edit key episodes and outcomes. The focus of the *Memoirs'* editorial tailoring suggests this project is willing to use the difficult circumstances of the narrative to create foils and challenges and add drama to a tale, but is unwilling to delve too deeply into the medical complications of a rural practice, or complicated aspects of the doctor himself. Even when the doctor is willing to admit mistakes and describe situations just as he saw them in a manuscript submitted for publication, somewhere along the publication process, it would seem, editors tried to press a diamond out of what they thought was Cape Breton coal. Who or what party actually performed this editorial task is unknown in MacMillan's case. But mining the texts upon which the autobiography was built brings this process to light, a process that includes polishing the image of a rural region as much as shaping the work of a doctor. The conflict between manuscript and *Memoirs* reveals a deeper level of MacMillan's experiences, offering more complete details of the hardships and rewards of his medical practice in 1920s and 1930s Nova Scotia.

MacMillan's original manuscript is, in fact, full of social-history gems. It is perhaps ironic that the details edited out, and the way that his *Memoirs* are rearranged for publication and sale, show not only the most human but also some of the most laudable aspects of the physician. His comfortable candour in 'Hang the Lantern on the Gate' certainly suggests a doctor–patient relationship which he relies upon, and quite clearly cherishes. His human relations are present in *Memoirs*, but are not foregrounded to the extent they are in his manuscript. In the original MacMillan organizes his material with greater attention to both chronology and relationships. Individuals and families are grouped by community, notes are made on when they came into the physician's life, and how their social connections to the doctor and to each other changed over the years. MacMillan begins each anecdote by offering details of the case, with transcripts of pertinent oral interviews interspersed with his own recollection of events. He almost always gives a full description of the call, the travel involved, the diagnosis and treatment, as well as the degree to which the individual did or did not recover, but MacMillan's interest in each 'case' does not end with a clinical and practical reconstruction. Rather, the doctor often goes on to provide copious details about the hospitality he received, the warm beds he rested in, and sometimes the more memorable meals he enjoyed at a family's home. He will also give details of the patient's life, their work, their marriages, how many children they had. If a family member or a former patient has moved away from Cape Breton, he sometimes gives details of the move and their subsequent lives as if all of these seemingly trivial elements are somehow critical to the completion of his medical autobiography. In fact, the original manuscript reads like a giant genealogy of a medical practice. The published *Memoirs* inform the reader in so many words that the doctor practised a holistic brand of family medicine, but there is more real evidence of this in the retrospective 'case notes' he fleshed out in the very personal, and even sentimental, manuscript. While the published version relies on the dramatic travel tales to carry the reader's interest and highlight the heroism of rural medicine, it is in the original that we learn just how important were the ties of friendship that sheltered him, fed him, forgave him, and sustained him along his way.

### Publishing, Readership, and Sales

The interest appears to have been reciprocal. The marketing and publishing history of MacMillan's *Memoirs* suggests that it achieved greatest popularity in MacMillan's home community and with local readerships. Two years after its publication, MacMillan's *Memoirs* was picked up by a bulk publisher in Ontario called PaperJacks Books, which attempted to market the book to a wider audience and break into the American market with a new title, *Memoirs of a Canadian Doctor*. Nonetheless, the paperback edition appears to have gone through no more than a few printings. In the mid-1980s, because of continuing local demand, *Memoirs* was re-issued by a small-press bookseller in Halifax called The Book Room, which reprinted *Memoirs* under its original *Cape Breton* title, and as a result the book is still available in the used-book trade.

Most country-doctor memoirs and biographies were published by local presses. Some of these titles were picked up by large, national publishing houses: McGraw-Hill, McClelland and Stewart, J.B. Lippincott, and Rinehart. Most examples of life writing, however, were published by small, local publishers like Virginia's Gazette Press, Brother Bill's Publishing Company of Michigan, Matrix Press in Red Deer, Alberta, or Nova Scotia's Lancelot Publishing. As figure 16.1 illustrates, the number of country-doctor stories remains fairly modest until the later decades of the twentieth century, when, in the 1970s, 1980s, and 1990s, many new titles are added to the corpus of work on rural physicians.

Figure 16.1 Rural medical life writing trends: type of publisher, 1900–2000

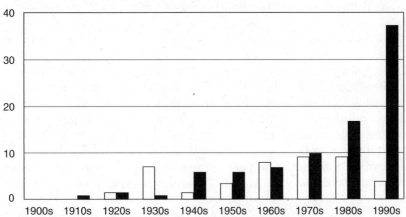

□  Major and national publishers          ■  Small, local, and regional publishers*

\*  Small, regional, and local presses include four broad categories: vanity-press publications bought by the physician her/himself or her/his family (some that are 'privately
published' in the appendix); smaller, privately owned presses that cater to local and
regional markets; titles published with funding from local civic organizations or historical groups; titles published by universities under a mandate to produce local-history or
oral-history titles.

One explanation for this phenomenon lies in the peculiar history of
local publishing. After the 1960s, North Americans witnessed the
growth of what historians have called a 'small press movement,' where
small businesses discovered they were able to compete with larger
publishing interests by catering to highly specialized group and subject categories.[43] The rapid adoption of offset printing in the 1950s and
1960s brought the cost of manufacturing books down to a scale more
easily absorbed by small businesses. These costs were further reduced
with the advent of computer typesetting. This situation is peculiar to
the book industry in marked contrast to other mass media, where
contraction of ownership has occurred. This trend has complicated the
historian's task of preparing representative bibliographies of such
sources. Unaware of this phenomenon, David J. Rothman opined in
1997 that medical autobiographies were 'a popular literary form that
has all but disappeared today.[44] Had Rothman examined the output of
small presses, however, he would have found a different story altogether. Given MacMillan's longer-standing success with a local press

after only a mediocre career with McGraw-Hill Ryerson, his autobiography certainly seems to be a part of this trend.

## The Personal Becomes Political

One final question that presents itself in this ongoing interrogation of rural medical life writing might be, What does this editorializing, and this brisk local consumption, ultimately mean? Some of these books were undoubtedly targeted to and consumed by the tourist market. But the transformation of C. Lamont MacMillan's life writing reveals a tension between the expectations and realities of rural medicine, still recognizable and important to local readerships. Through the editorial process described above, MacMillan's real-life experiences are shaped to fit a pre-existing mould. In fact, his *Memoirs* and other country-doctor life writing seem to institute a vernacular expression of a country-doctor cultural archetype such as that represented by Dafoe's 1939 biography *The Little Doc*.

The popularization of the quintuplets, and their exploitation as a symbol of youth, progress and medical science, certainly exemplifies the ways in which the boundaries between fiction and real life become difficult to discern. The same might well be said of Dafoe himself, although for the physician the process was largely affirmative. Popular response to the fictional version of Dr Dafoe in the 1936 movie, *The Country Doctor*, was certainly very positive. The response to the Dafoe-modelled character of 'Dr John Luke' was so remarkable that the actor Jean Hersholt eventually copied the avuncular style and mature kindliness to create an even more successful version of the beloved country doctor, the famous character of Dr Paul Christian. From its 1939 debut in the movie *Meet Dr. Christian*, the template was a marketing success. Dr Christian was a dedicated and beloved small-town physician with extraordinary and locally underappreciated medical gifts and technical prowess, often supplied from only the contents of his black bag. *Meet Dr. Christian* would inspire several sequels in the 1940s, all starring Hersholt.[45] These were followed by a spin-off radio series in the early 1950s, and a television series in 1956. The once extremely popular Paul Christian was in fact the rural progenitor of a long line of mid-century television medical protagonists that would include the more recognizable names of Marcus Welby and James Kildare.

The emerging country-doctor iconography was not limited to television. Journalists writing in popular magazines and writers of various descriptions regularly sought out 'country doctors' to feature by mid-century. *Life* magazine produced the most famous example of an iconic country doctor in a photo essay profiling a real-life Colorado country doctor, Ernest Ceriani.[46] The opening image of Dr Ceriani walking across a field to make a house call, with a brooding sky threatening from behind and a fatigued expression on his face, became the most recognizable doctor photograph in twentieth-century North American publishing. This non-fiction piece, shot by photo-journalist W. Eugene Smith, would be the hallmark photo essay of Smith's career. It was an intentional attempt to use the pull of the 'country doctor' to reach the American public with a political message.

This country-doctor essay was framed as an argument against socialized medicine at the end of the 1940s. As historian Glen Willumson has shown in his study of Eugene Smith's work at *Life* magazine and beyond, the editors of the popular magazine chose to use the article in order to support the American Medical Association's position against compulsory health insurance.[47] In 1948 national health care was an important political issue in the immediate post-war United States. The Truman administration felt that the medical crisis was due to an overall doctor shortage, while the American Medical Association (AMA) contended that the country's medical problems were the result of the poor distribution of physicians. *Life* endorsed the plan whereby communities should take responsibility for attracting doctors by establishing local cooperatives to offer incentives, provide housing, or even construct a hospital.[48] At the same time, articles published by the AMA urged doctors to leave their urban practices and move to the countryside, where they could be autonomous and benefit from the rewards of a rural medical vocation.[49] According to Willumson, the '*Life* magazine photo-essay became an extension of the medical association's public relations project,' because Kremmling, Colorado, represented what the AMA was calling for: a community that had raised private monies to build a small hospital and hire nurses in an effort to attract a doctor, in this case, the handsome young Ceriani.[50] Thus, the medical profession began playing a part in cultivating the iconography around country doctors for these political ends. Willumson points out this allowed the *Life* editors to, on the one hand, appeal to the romantic mythology about country doctoring while also 'updat[ing] the subject by casting him as a young, modern contemporary.'[51] The

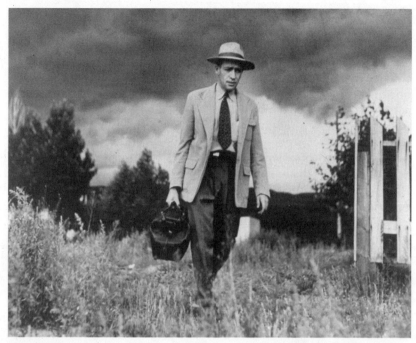

This opening photo of Ernest Ceriani is accompanied by the caption 'His end-less work has its own rewards.' W. Eugene Smith, 'The Country Doctor,' *Life Magazine*, 10 September 1948, 1. (Getty Images, Inc.)

tailoring of Ceriani's story, although more pictorial than literal, is remark-ably similar to how MacMillan's life writing was cast into publishable *Memoirs*. Certain details about Ceriani's work that could have a negative interpretation, such as his inferior income, are omitted from the published version. While one picture shows the doctor carrying a patient up some stairs, the accompanying text carefully omits the fact that he does this because the hospital is not equipped with an elevator. In a shot entitled 'After Midnight' we see a tired Ceriani slumped against a kitchen counter, staring despondently into space. The explanation of this image reads, 'After an operation which lasted until 2 a.m., Ceriani had a coffee and a cigarette in the hospital kitchen before starting home. The nurses con-stantly admonish him to relax and rest, but because they are well aware that he cannot, they keep a potful of fresh coffee simmering for him at all hours.' We do not learn in the pages of *Life* that this 'operation' is an unsuccessful Caesarean in which the mother dies.[52]

This analysis of Smith's famous photo-essay illustrates how the image of the country doctor was used by a directorial photojournalist in order to convey a political message, supported by the political position of his publishers.[3] But, as with the case of C. Lamont MacMillan, it is critically important to highlight where the truth was stretched and into what form the country-doctor archetype was manipulated – a useful exercise in that it highlights social expectations. A physician's memoirs seem to offer a 'privileged account' of medicine from the perspective of an insider, but that is largely a façade. Instead of revealing medical reality, it 'constructs a public representation of medical practice and culture.'[53] The public representations of rural medicine in MacMillan's *Memoirs* are meant, like the depictions of Ernest Ceriani in *Life* magazine, to comfort a social anxiety about the inequitable distribution of physician services in the first half of the twentieth century. This comforting quality likely explains their popularity with local readers. It is unlikely a coincidence that similar anxieties were rekindling at the time much of the rural medical life writing referenced above was going to press. When MacMillan's *Memoirs* was published in the 1970s, Canada was in the throes of another acute doctor shortage, precipitated by the post-war population boom and the advent of universal medical insurance. The editorial processing of MacMillan's life story certainly makes *Memoirs* an effective recruitment tool for a mid-century profession dealing with a critical dearth of physicians, especially in rural areas. Reading C. Lamont MacMillan's *Memoirs* leaves one feeling good about the traditional structures of rural health care. It implies that a willingness to answer every patient's call and a quick mind for medical innovation are just as effective as all the medical technology available to urban specialists. This is ironic, given that most country doctors, including MacMillan, helped to build and maintain small community hospitals, and celebrated every new mile of hard-surface road that helped them send difficult cases to the nearest hospital centre. Especially through use of the travel tale, the country doctor is painted as both autonomous and effective, even though the published version of his life must forget the death of premature infants to do so.

What can historians ultimately make of rural medical life writing? The first conclusion must be that rural physicians' memoirs are rich sources, but ones that must be well and thoroughly contextualized in order for that richness to be revealed. C. Lamont MacMillan's autobiographical renderings of country-doctor life writing contain many historically useful facts, although in order to use the material found in physician life writing, historians must be aware of the cultural projects behind the 'autobiographical act.' Only they can find the key messages that physician memoirs add to the new history of rural medicine. The cultural project underpinning MacMillan's *Memoirs* is one which denies that there is any reason to worry about access to adequate health care in rural Canada. If, as Senator Hicks's preface suggests, the Canadian nation state can be built upon the backs of such phenomenal individuals as C. Lamont MacMillan, then rural health care is in good shape. The message seems to be: despite the shortage of physician services, country doctors like MacMillan are making do every day. It is only after unpacking the black bag that we are able to read the text without being distracted by this triumphal note. In fact, the attempt to laud the exceptional individual as a panacea to systemic problems of rural health-care access is the true fiction in rural medical life writing. It does not even accurately represent what this Cape Breton physician has written about his own life and work. From reading about his life in his own unedited words, arranged so that the doctor's selection of important facts, details, and people is foremost in the text, I suggest that he would actually have argued the inverse. Especially in a far-flung practice in rural Cape Breton, the geography, the limits of service, and one's own knowledge and strength reinforce the fact that no man, and no individual doctor, is an island.

## Appendix

The following is a list of country-doctor memoirs published in the English language to the year 2000. Although the list is extensive, because the majority of country-doctor titles are either 'vanity press' publications or the products of local presses, I am reluctant to claim that it is absolutely comprehensive.

Note: In compiling this bibliography, I have decided to define 'country doctor' as a physician whose practice encompasses a rural region, who was a general practitioner for the majority of her or his professional career, and whose practice was, on a regular basis at least, peripatetic. There are exceptions to this rule. Missionary-type rural practitioners who travelled to isolated communities, such as William Grenfell, and physicians who tended rural communities solely under the auspices of a hospital-based practice, belong to a different category of physician. They are therefore are not represented in this bibliography.

Abington, E.H. *Back Roads and Bicarbonate: The Autobiography of an Arkansas Country Doctor*. New York: Vantage Press, 1955.

Adair, Fred Lyman. *The Country Doctor and the Specialist*. Maitland, FL: Adair Award Fund, 1968.

Aiken, George Russell. *The Doc Aiken Story: Memoirs of a Country Doctor*. George Aiken, 1989.

Baker-McLaglan, Eleanor Southey. *Stethoscope and Saddlebags*. Aukland: Collins, 1965.

Banks, James W. *House Calls in the Hills: Memoirs of a Country Doctor*. Charleston, SC: Mountain State Press, 1996.

Barber, Geoffrey. *Country Doctor*. Ipswich: Boydell Press, 1974.

Bauer, William. *Out of Dr. Bill's Black Bag: From Northern Wisconsin; a Country Doctor Looks Back, 1941–1991*. Rochester, MI: Brother Bill's Publishing Co., 1994.

Bede, Brandt A. *Tales of a Country Doctor: 100 Years of Health Care in Lewis County*. Gig Harbour, WA: Red Apple Publishing, 1994.

Berger, John, and Jean Mohr. *A Fortunate Man: The Story of a Country Doctor*. London: Allen Lane [published in the United States by Holt, Rinehart and Winston], 1967.

Betts, Anthony. *Green Wood and Chloroform*. Camden, ME: Down East Books, 1998.

Bishop, R.W.S. *My Moorland Patients, By a Yorkshire Doctor*. London: John Murray, 1922.

Blythe, Legette. *Mountain Doctor*. New York: William Morrow and Co., 1964.

Bolstad, Owen C. *Leslie Moren: Fifty Years an Elko County Doctor*. Reno: UNR Oral History Program, 1992.

Bradley, Ora. *The Country Doctor's Wife*. New York: House of Field, 1940.

Brasset, Edmund A. *A Doctor's Pilgrimage: An Autobiography*. Philadelphia, New York: J.B. Lippincott and Co., 1951.

Brewster, Barry, and Jeremy Mills. *The Doctor: Just Another Year*. London: BBC Books, 1992.

Brown, Marvin. *House Calls: The Memoirs of a Country Doctor*. Buffalo, NY: Prometheus Books, 1988.

Brown, Pat Rhine. *T.E. Rhine, M.D.: Recollections of an Arkansas Country Doctor*. Little Rock, AR: August House, 1985.

Browne, David Dorey. *The Wind and the Book: Memoirs of a Country Doctor*. Carlton: Melbourne University Press, 1976.

Bryson, James Gordon. *One Hundred Dollars and a Horse: The Reminiscences of a Country Doctor*. New York: Morrow Publishing, 1965.

Buck, Ruth Matheson. *The Doctor Rode Side-Saddle*. Toronto: McClelland and Stewart, 1974.

Burden, Arnold. *Fifty Years of Emergencies: The Dramatic Life of a Country Doctor.* Hantsport, NS: Lancelot Press, 1991.

Cameron, James Edwards. *Life of a Country Doctor.* Ed. Edith Cameron Blankenship. Montgomery, AL: Black Belt Press, 1996.

Cameron, Robert Bruce. *Dr. James Steven Brown, M.D.; the Country Doctor.* Hendersonville, NC: n.p., 1959.

Chatenay, Henri. *The Country Doctors.* Red Deer, AB: Mattrix Press, 1980.

Clifford, Robert. *Just Here, Doctor.* London: Pelham Books, 1978.

Coe, Urling C. *Frontier Doctor.* New York: MacMillan, 1939.

Comandini, Adele. *Doctor Kate, Angel on Snowshoes: The Story of Kate Pelham Newcomb.* New York: Rinehart, 1956.

Conger, Beach. *Bag Balm and Duct Tape: Tales of a Vermont Doctor.* Boston: Little Brown and Co., 1988.

– *It's Not My Fault: Tales of a Vermont Doctor.* Golden, CO: Fulcrum Publishing, 1995.

Cook, Hull. *Fifty Years a Country Doctor.* Lincoln: University of Nebraska Press, 1998.

Cornell, Virginia. *Doc Susie: The True Story of a Country Physician in the Colorado Rockies.* New York: Fawcett Press / Ballantine Books, 1991.

Cornish, Sid. *Country Calls: Memories of a Small-town Doctor.* Calgary: Fifth House Publishers, 1998.

Dawson, Len. *Skydoctor: Based on the Adventures and Experiences of a Flying Doctor in the 1950s.* Wingham, NSW: Gypsey Publications, 1995.

De Garis, Mary C. *Clinical Notes and Deductions of a Peripatetic: Being Fads and Fancies of a General Practitioner.* London: Balliere, Tindall and Cox, 1926.

Dewar, George. *Prescription for a Full Life.* Summerside, PEI: Williams and Crue, 1993.

Dixon, Charles D. *The Menace: An Exposition of Quackery, Nostrum, Exploitation, and Reminiscences of a Country Doctor.* San Antonio: Lodovic Print, 1914.

Doctor Anonymous. *Diary of a Country Doctor.* Johannesburg: APB Publishers, 1968.

Dole, Mary Phylinda. *Doctor in Homespun.* Privately printed, 1941.

Doyle, Helen MacNight. *A Child Went Forth: The Autobiography of Helen MacKnight Doyle.* New York: Gotham House, 1934. Reprinted as *Doctor Nellie: The Autobiography of Helen MacKnight Doyle.* Mammoth Lakes, CA: Genny Smith Books, 1983.

Dudley, Albertus T. *A Country Doctor's Daily Charge Book, 1792–1813: Dr. Benjamin Rowe, July 7, 1750–November 7, 1818, Kensington, New Hampshire.* North Barnstead: Rowe Register, 1992.

Duvall, Carol Sprague. *Our Pioneer Country Doctor: From the Journal of Jesse S. Spriggs.* Coffeyville, KS: C. Duvall, 1982.

Echols, John Wicker. *A Certain Country Doctor.* Boston: Christopher Publishing House, 1922.

Elliott, James W. *Secrets of a Country Doctor.* Johnson City, TN: Overmountain Press, 1992.

Forsyth, Victoria. *The Doctor: Hector J. Pothier, the Career and Experiences of a Country Doctor in Beaver River.* Hantsport, NS: Lancelot Press, 1982.

Fulstone, Mary Hill. *Recollections of a Country Doctor in Smith, Nevada.* Reno: UNR Oral History Project, 1980.

Geggie, H.J.G. *The Extra Mile: Medicine in Rural Quebec, 1885–1965.* H.J.G. Geggie, 1987.

Gibson, Morris. *A Doctor in the West.* Toronto: Collins, 1983.

– *A Doctor's Calling.* Toronto: Douglas and McIntyre, 1986.

Gish, Shirley. *Country Doctor: The Story of Dr. Claire Louise Caudill.* Lexington: University Press of Kentucky, 1999.

Gould, Aubrey V. *Where Does It Hurt? The Story of a New England Country Doctor.* Hancock, NH: Fieldside Press, 1990.

Gunn, Clement Bryce. *Leaves from the Life of a Country Doctor.* Ed. Rutherford Crockett, with a foreword by John Buchan. Edinburgh, London: Moray Press, 1935.

Guyther, J. Roy. *Memoirs of a Country Doctor: St. Mary's County Patients Are Special Folks.* Mechanicsville, MD: J.R. Guyther, 1999.

Harris, Robin Bellchambers. *The Life and Times of a Country Doctor, 'Dr. Fred.'* Port Huron, MI: Walkabout Ink, 1995.

Hawkins, Cora Frear. *Buggies, Blizzards and Babies.* Ames: Iowa State University Press, 1971.

Hay, Floyd B. *The Country Doctor.* Cumberland, KY: F.B. Hay, 1983.

Hertzler, Arthur. *The Horse and Buggy Doctor.* New York, London: Harper and Brothers, 1938.

Hipps, John G., and Barbara A. Smith. *The Country Doctor.* Emporium, PA: Wonderworld, 1989. Republished by Good Earth Publishing, 1999, with a new title: *The Country Doctor, Alive and Well: A Story of Love for the Land and Its People.*

Holley, James Arthur. *The Recollections of a Country Doctor.* Boston: Meador Publishing Co., 1939.

Hopkins, Arthur. *Pep, Pills and Politics: A Odyssey of Two States.* Brattleboro: Vermont Printing Co., 1944.

Hutton, Neve M. *This Mad Folly! The History of Australia's Pioneer Women Doctors.* Sydney: Library of Australian History, 1980.

Hunt, Frazier. *The Little Doc: The Story of Allan Roy Dafoe, Physician to the Quintuplets.* New York: Simon and Schuster, 1939.

Ibberson, John R. *Tales from My Little Black Bag*. Calgary: Detselig Enterprises, 1994.

Johnson, Edith E. *Leaves from a Doctor's Diary (1927–1954)*. Palo Alto, CA: Pacific Books, 1954.

Johnston, William Victor. *Before the Age of Miracles: Memoirs of a Country Doctor*. New York: P.S. Ericksson, 1972.

Kaiser, Grace. *Dr. Frau*. Intercourse, PA: Good Books, 1986.

– *Detour*. Intercourse, PA: Good Books, 1990.

Keleman, Elisabeth Zulauf. *A Horse and Buggy Doctor in Southern Indiana: 1825–1903*. Madison, IN: Historic Madison, Inc., 1973.

Kellog, David S. *A Doctor at All Hours*. Brattleboro, VT: Stephen Greene Press, 1970.

Kennison, Conrad E. *Grandma and the Doctor*. Augusta, ME: Conrad Kennison, 1956.

King, Willis Percival. *Stories of a Country Doctor*. Kansas City: Hudson-Kimberley Publishing Co., 1890.

Lacombe, Michael A. *Medicine Made Clear: House Calls from a Maine Country Doctor*. North Woodstock, ME: Dirigo Books, 1989.

Ladd, Barry. *Reflections of a Country Doctor*. Lakewood, CO: Glenbridge Publishing, 1996.

Lane, Kenneth. *Diary of a Medical Nobody*. London: Severn House, 1983.

– *West Country Doctor*. London: Severn House, 1984.

Laws, James W. *Memoirs of a Country Doctor*. Ed, Ann Buffington. Hondo, NM: Lincoln County Historical Society, 1990.

Lawson, Sidney B. *Autobiography and Reminiscences of Sidney B. Lawson, M.D., 50 Years a Mountain-country Doctor; together with Compendium of Personal Medical Observations, Theories and Advice and Some Practical Information*. Logan, WV: privately printed, 1941.

Lehn, Cornelia. *The Homemade Brass Plate: The Story of a Pioneer Doctor in Northern Alberta*. New York: Exposition Press, 1973.

Lewis, Fay Cashatt. *Doc's Wife*. New York: MacMillan and Co., 1940.

Losee, R.E. *Doc: Then and Now with a Montana Physician*. New York: Fawcett Press / Ballantine Books, 1996.

Lowery, John Robert. *Memoirs of a Country Doctor*. New York: Carlton Press, 1968.

Loxterkamp, David. *A Measure of My Days: The Journal of a Country Doctor*. Hanover, London: University Press of New England, 1997.

Macleod, Scott H. *Nova Scotia Farm Boy to Alberta M.D.* Scott H. Macleod, 1968.

MacMillan, C. Lamont. *Memoirs of a Cape Breton Doctor*. Toronto: McGraw-Hill Ryerson Ltd, 1975.

Mance, Andrew E. *Thoughts of a Country Doctor: An Immigrant's Son*. Parsons, WV: McClain Print, 1977.

Martin, Donald L. *Referees, Docs, and God: Journal of a Country Doctor*. Lima, OH: Fairway Press, 1990.

– *Tidbits for Young Doctors and Their Patients: Journal of a Country Doctor, Part II*. Lima, OH: Fairway Press, 1993.

McComb, Earl Vinton. *Doctor of the North Country*. New York: Thomas Y. Crowell, 1936.

McCue, James Westaway. *Cape Cod Doctor*. New England Book Co., 1945.

McPhee, John. *Heirs of General Practice*. New York: Farrar, Straus and Giroux, 1986.

Miller, Amy Johnson. *The Pioneer Doctor in the Ozarks White River Country; Illustrated by Photograph and Drawing*. Kansas City: Burton Publishing Co., 1947.

Mitchell, George T. *Dr. George: An Account of the Life of a Country Doctor*. Carbondale: Southern Illinois University Press, 1994.

Mooney, Charles W. *Doctor in Belle Starr Country*. Oklahoma City: Century Press, 1975.

Movius, Herbert John. *Doctor! Doctor! Incredible Stories of Medical Genius by a Country Doctor Who Became One of Hollywood's Leading Surgeons*. New York: Vantage Press, 1966.

Nay, Winfield Scott. *The Old Country Doctor*. Rutland, VT: Tuttle Publishing Co., 1937.

Oliver, Wesley B. *Country Doctor*. Raleigh, NC: Pentland Press, 1999.

Parry, Ward Hudson. *These Three – The Story of a Country Doctor in the World War*. Boston: Badger Press, 1929.

Pemberton, John. *Will Pickles of Wensleydale: The Life of a Country Doctor*. London: Bles, 1970.

Phillips, Margaret I. *Doctor of the Cotton Patch*. Margaret Phillips, 1968.

Poidevin, Leslie. *Goodbye Doctor: Stories of a Country Practice*. Leslie Poidevin, 1986.

– *Come in Doctor: Country Practice Revisited*. Leslie Poidevin, 1990.

Preston, Frances I. *Lady Doctor: Vintage Model*. Wellington, NZ: A.H. and A.W. Reed, 1974.

Reagan, Leroy Amons (Rocky). *G. P. Reagan, Country Doctor*. San Antonio: Naylor Company, 1963.

Reeves, Eleanor Baker. *A Country Doctor Goes to Town*. Galax, VA: Gazette Press, 1966.

Reimer, Mavis. *Cornelius W. Wiebe, a Beloved Physician: The Story of a Country Doctor*. Winnipeg: Hyperion Press, 1983.

Robertson, Dawn. *A Country Doctor: The Story of Dr. Isaac Bainbridge*. Kirkby Stephen, UK: Hayloft, 1999.

Rowland, Mary Canaga. *As Long as Life: The Memoirs of a Frontier Woman Doctor.* Ed. by F.A. Loomis. New York: Fawcett Press, 1994.

Schulze, Gene. *Yesterday's Seasons: Memories of a Rural Medical Practice.* New York: Hawthorn Books, 1978.

Shadduck, Louise. *Doctors with Buggies, Snowshoes and Planes.* Boise, ID: Tamarack Books, 1993.

Shastid, Thomas Hall. *A Country Doctor.* Battle Creek, MI: Thomas Hall Shastid, 1898.

Slater, Cornelius. *An Apple a Day: Adventures of a Country Doctor.* New York: Vanguard Press, 1987.

Sloop, Mary T. Martin, and Legette Blythe. *Miracle in the Hills.* New York: McGraw-Hill Book Co., 1953.

Steele, Phyllis L. *The Woman Doctor of Balcarres.* Hamilton, ON: Pathway Publications, 1984.

Strain, Samuel T. *From the Nolichucky to Memphis: Reminiscences of a Country Doctor.* Memphis: Memphis State University Press, 1979.

Stratton, Owen Tully. *Medicine Man.* Norman: University of Oklahoma Press, 1989.

Thane, P.T. *The Reminiscences of an Australian Country Doctor.* Glebe, NSW: Wild and Wooley, 1998.

Townshend, John Wilson. 'A Country Doctor of the Blue Grass.' In *Three Kentucky Gentlemen of the Old Order.* Frankfort, KY: Roberts Printing Co., 1946.

Trent, Bill. *Northwoods Doctor.* Philadelphia: J.B. Lippincott, 1962.

Turner, Richard B. *Once Upon a Country Doctor.* San Francisco, CA: [privately printed,] 1994.

Tyre, Robert. *Saddlebag Surgeon: The Story of Murrough O'Brien, M.D.* Toronto: J.M. Dent and Sons, 1954.

Washburn, Benjamin Earle. *A Country Doctor in the South Mountains.* Asheville, NC: Stephens Press, 1955.

Weiss, Harry B. *Country Doctor: Cornelius Wilson Larison of Ringoes, Hunterdon County, New Jersey, 1837–1910, Physician, Farmer, Educator, Author, Editor, Publisher, and Exponent of Phonetic Spelling.* Trenton: New Jersey Agricultural Society, 1953.

Welch, G. Kemble. *Doctor Smith Hokianga's 'King of the North.'* Wellington, NZ: Blackwood and Janet Paul, 1965.

Welch, James K. *The Country Doctor: A Collection of Favourite newspaper columns by a Spoon River Rural Physician.* Ed. LaVonne A. Straub. Macomb: Western Illinois University, 1996.

Wilson, Dorothy Clark. *The Big-Little World of Doc Pritham.* New York: McGraw-Hill, 1971.

Wilson, Gaines L. *Descendants of Dr. Isaac Alvis Wilson, Country Doctor, Union County, Tennessee*. Topeka, KS: Jostens Publishing, 1993.

Windell, Roland. *The Brush of Angel's Wings: The Story of the Country Doctor*. San Antonio: Naylor, 1952.

Wisewood, Gweneth. *Outpost: A Doctor on the Divide*. Kilmore, AU: Lowden Publishing, 1971.

Wood, Voilet. *So Sure of Life: A Mountain Doctor's Story*. New York: Friendship Press, 1965.

NOTES

This article is part of a larger manuscript project on the history of rural medicine in Canada and the United States, entitled *Unpacking the Black Bag*. I would like to recognize the generous support of Associated Medical Services, Inc., formerly the Hannah Institute for the History of Medicine, whose doctoral scholarships allowed me to pursue this research. I have benefited from the insights, comments, and constructive criticism of many scholars, in particular Kathryn McPherson, Ian Radforth, and J.T.H. Connor, who served on my thesis/defence committees. And of course, Michael Bliss deserves special thanks, and not only for being a good and patient supervisor. It was his work on William Osler, another potent medical icon, that inspired the approach taken in this piece and my other work on rural medicine.

1 Jan Coombs, 'Rural Medical Practice in the 1880s: A View from Central Wisconsin,' *Bulletin of the History of Medicine* 64 (1990): 35–62.

2 Jacalyn Duffin, *Langstaff: A Nineteenth Century Medical Life* (Toronto: University of Toronto Press, 1993).

3 Judith Walzer Leavitt, '"A Worrying Profession": The Domestic Environment of Medical Practice in Nineteenth Century America,' *Bulletin of the History of Medicine* 69 (1995): 1–29.

4 Sandra Barney, *Authorized to Heal: Gender, Class and the Transformation of Medicine in Appalachia* (Chapel Hill: University of North Carolina Press, 2000).

5 These are listed in the appendix.

6 Although there is a country-doctor tradition in other literatures and media, for example, the phenomenon of the 'bare-foot doctor' in China, this article focuses on those published in the English language, depicting an Anglo-Canadian/Anglo-American experience of rural general practice and the lives of 'country doctors.'

7  S.E.D. Shortt, 'Before the Age of Miracles: The Rise, Fall and Rebirth of General Practice in Canada, 1890–1940,' in *Health, Disease, and Medicine: Essays in Canadian History,* ed. Charles G. Roland (Toronto: Hannah Institute for the History of Medicine, 1984), 123–52. The majority of the autobiographies he cites are based on rural practices.

8  Although he does acknowledge that his work will, for the most part, 'consider the non-urban practitioner,' he does not believe rural practice altered doctors' attitudes towards practice, that is, their opinions about the quality and efficacy of medical training and medical skills. I will argue these opinions were indelibly shaped by the practical problems associated with their geographic location, as well as the 'country doctor' ideal. Ibid., 124–5.

9  This nostalgia for an authoritarian physician role, Pollock argues, must be at least to some degree shared with the wider reading public, as they consume the books. Donald Pollock, 'Training Tales: U.S. Medical Autobiography,' *Cultural Anthropology* 11 (1996): 339–61.

10  Donald Pollock, 'Physician Autobiography: Narrative and the Social History of Medicine,' in Cheryl Mattingly and Linda Garro, eds, *Narrative and the Cultural Construction of Illness and Healing* (Berkeley: University of California Press, 2001), 108–27. Although his analysis of narratives in rural medical history is insightful, Pollock cites only five rural autobiographies in this project. His theoretical framework also does not allow for an overlap among these genres, which include those of women physicians challenging patriarchy in medicine, the story of the 'wounded healer' who uses traumatic experience to better understand medical practice, and the medical missionary.

11  See A.O.J. Cockshut, *The Art of Autobiography in Nineteenth and Twentieth Century England* (New Haven: Yale University Press, 1984); Thomas Cooly, *Educated Lives: The Rise of Autobiography in America* (Columbus: University of Ohio Press, 1976); John Paul Eakin, *American Autobiography: Retrospect and Prospect* (Madison: University of Wisconsin Press, 1991); Jane Verner Gunn, *Autobiography: Toward a Poetics of Experience* (Philadelphia: University of Pennsylvania Press, 1982); Estelle Jelinek, ed., *Women's Autobiography: Essays in Criticism* (Bloomington: University of Indiana Press, 1980); William C. Spengemann, *The Forms of Autobiography: Episodes in the History of a Literary Genre* (New Haven: Yale University Press, 1980); and Karl J. Weintraub, *The Value of the Individual: Self and Circumstance in Autobiography* (Chicago: University of Chicago Press, 1978).

12  Willis Percival King, *Stories of a Country Doctor.* Kansas City: Hudson-Kimberley Publishing Co., 1890; Thomas Hall Shastid, *A Country Doctor* (Battle Creek, MI: Thomas Hall Shastid, 1898).

13  Arthur Hertzler, *Horse and Buggy Doctor* (New York: Harper and Brothers, 1938; repr. Lincoln: University of Nebraska Press, 1970).

14 His autobiography was preceded by a large body of work on surgery beginning with *A Treatise on Tumors* (New York and Philadelphia: Lea and Gebiger, 1912), followed by many works on surgical pathology, including *Surgery of a General Practice* (St Louis: C.V. Mosby Co., 1934).

15 The autobiography signalled a change in the physician's publishing career from scientific explorations to more political and philosophical writings, such as *The Doctor and His Patients: The American Domestic Scene as Viewed by the Family Doctor* (New York: Harper and Brothers, 1940); *The Grounds of an Old Surgeon's Faith* (Halstead, KS: A.E. Hertzler, 1944); *Ventures in Science of a Country Surgeon* (Halstead, KS: A.E. Hertzler, 1944); *Always the Child* (Wichita, MS: Wichita Eagle Press, 1946). After *Horse and Buggy Doctor,* he published only one more scientific title: *Diseases of the Thyroid Gland, Presenting the Experience of More than Forty Years* (New York: P.B. Hoeber, 1941).

16 Frazier Hunt, *The Little Doc: The Story of Allan Roy Dafoe, Physician to the Quintuplets* (New York: Simon and Schuster, 1939).

17 *The Country Doctor,* dir. Henry King, with the Dionne Quintuplets and Jean Hersholt, Twentieth Century Fox, 1936. See also Willis Thornton, *The Country Doctor* [a novelization of the Twentieth Century Fox film 'The Country Doctor,' 1936] (Grosset and Dunlap, 1936). The storyline follows the movie version faithfully, and all illustrations are taken from the film. The first photo that greets the reader is a snapshot of Jean Hersholdt, the actor who came to epitomize the cinematic version of the country doctor, and Dr Dafoe pouring over a book and 'sharing a hobby.'

18 Leavitt, '"A Worrying Profession."'

19 C. Lamont, MacMillan, *Memoirs of a Cape Breton Doctor* (Toronto: McGraw-Hill Ryerson, 1975), foreword.

20 Ibid.

21 C. Lamont MacMillan, 'Hang the Lantern on the Gate,' unpublished manuscript, Nova Scotia Archives and Records Management [microfilm collection, reel 3859], Halifax, Nova Scotia.

22 Ibid., 2.

23 Ibid., 19.

24 These are meant as humourous reprints of the historical sketches offered by a Dr Morrison, past president of the Nova Scotia Medical Society. Ibid., 7–8. Although the midwives are called a 'noble body,' the depictions of their various types range from the 'tea-drinking, thin-visaged, philosophical midwife' fond of 'incantations,' to the 'motherly woman with the nursing instinct' fond of all poultices and 'disagreeable concoctions,' to the 'large, beaming optimistic, rosy-faced woman with expansive waist and expansive smile' whose cheerful presence calmed fears. The portrayals of superstitious, instinctual

mothering do not acknowledge any actual skill on the part of women healers. Despite the humourous intent, these depictions beg comparison to Morrison's portrayals of nineteenth-century rural physicians of rural Nova Scotia as 'strong characters ... cultured gentlemen and well-informed outside of their own professional work.' Ibid., 7.

25 Ibid., 24.

26 MacMillan, *Memoirs*, xiv.

27 MacMillan, 'Hang the Lantern on the Gate,' 6.

28 Ibid., 67.

29 Ibid., 49.

30 The laments are referenced only on the first edition's dust jacket. 'The islanders, who had been accustomed to having medical attention perhaps twice in their lives, only slowly ... gave up their folk remedies. The result was a swing in the other extreme: every pain became an emergency requiring the doctor's presence.'

31 MacMillan 'Hang the Lantern on the Gate,' 96–7.

32 Ibid.; MacMillan, *Memoirs*, 113.

33 MacMillan, *Memoirs*, 115–16.

34 MacMillan, 'Hang the Lantern on the Gate,' 213.

35 Ibid., 106, 108–9.

36 MacMillan, *Memoirs*, 107.

37 Ibid., 63.

38 MacMillan, 'Hang the Lantern on the Gate,' 247.

39 Pollock, 'Physician Autobiography,' 113.

40 MacMillan, 'Hang the Lantern on the Gate,' 240.

41 MacMillan, *Memoirs*, 83.

42 'Hang the Lantern on the Gate,' 86.

43 Michael R. Gabriel, 'The Astonishing Growth of Small Publishers, 1958–1988,' *Journal of Popular Culture* 24 (1990): 61–8. His analysis of small presses listed in *Publisher's Weekly* shows an increase from 1000 in 1958 to 12,000 in 1985. Ibid., 63.

44 Editor's preface to David M. Hughes, 'Twenty-Five Years in Country Practice,' in David J. Rothman, ed., *Beginnings Count: The Technological Imperative in American Health Care* (New York: Oxford University Press, 1997), 3.

45 These include *The Courageous Dr. Christian* (1940), *Dr. Christian Meets the Women* (1940), *Remedy for Riches* (1940), *Melody for Three* (1941), and *They Meet Again* (1941).

46 Eugene Smith, 'The Country Doctor,' *Life Magazine*, 10 September 1948, 1. The caption for this opening page reads: 'His Endless Work Has Its Own Rewards.' This was actually *Life*'s second article on rural physicians praising

the work of family doctors in the United States. See 'Old Doctors,' *Life*, 23 June 1947, 81–4.

47 Glen G. Willumson, *W. Eugene Smith and the Photographic Essay* (London: Cambridge University Press, 1992), 53. Willumson shows how support for the AMA position was widespread in post-war journalism by highlighting, for instance, Verne E. Edwards, Jr, 'The American Medical Association as Reported in Six U.S. Dailies,' *Journalism Quarterly* 26 (1949): 417–23. See also 'Shortages of Medical Men: Dispute Whether Lack Is Fundamental or Due to Uneven Distribution,' *U.S. News*, 5 September 1947, 20–1.

48 See, for example, *Medicine and the Changing Order: Report of the New York Academy of Medicine* (New York: Commonwealth Fund, 1947). The AMA thought that an encouragement of individual initiative would be enough, along with an improvement of existing health programs. They engaged radio broadcasts, organized a speaker's bureau, and created leaflets bearing the Luke Fildes painting *The Doctor*, accompanied by the question, Do you want the government in this picture?' Ibid., 53.

49 The Colorado State Medical Association's former president, Dr Arthur Sudan, who had been voted 'Family Doctor of the Year' in 1948, engaged in a vigourous public-relations campaign to push against public opinion, which favoured socialized medicine. He went about 'talking to young doctors, showing them that by putting their social consciousness to work they'll avoid socialized medicine.' Qtd. in Willumson, *W. Eugene Smith*, 55. He is shown in some *Life* photo montages posing with Dr Ceriani, who had taken over his practice in Kremmling. As Willumson has shown, these photos did not make the cut for the essay piece in *Life*.

50 *Collier's* and *Look* magazines had directed their reporting on the national doctor shortage by focusing on the need to train more physicians. Ibid.

51 Ibid., 57.

52 Smith, 'The Country Doctor,' 5.

53 Pollock, 'Physician Autobiography,' 108.

# Bibliography of Michael Bliss

## Scholarly Books

*A Living Profit: Studies in the Social History of Canadian Business, 1883–1911.* Toronto: McClelland and Stewart, 1974.

*A Canadian Millionaire: The Life and Business Times of Sir Joseph Flavelle, Bart., 1858–1939.* Toronto, Macmillan, 1978; 2nd ed. with new preface, University of Toronto Press, 1992.

*The Discovery of Insulin:* Toronto: McClelland and Stewart, 1982; Chicago: University of Chicago Press, 1983; Edinburgh: Paul Harris, 1983; London: Macmillan, 1987; trans. into French, Japanese, Greek, Polish; 2nd Canadian ed., McClelland and Stewart, 1996; 3rd Canadian ed., University of Toronto Press, 1999; rev. 25th anniversary ed., Chicago and Toronto, 2007.

*Banting: A Biography.* Toronto: McClelland and Stewart, 1984; 2nd ed., with new preface, University of Toronto Press, 1992.

*Northern Enterprise: Five Centuries of Canadian Business.* Toronto: McClelland and Stewart, 1987; Oxford University Press 1996.

*Plague: A Story of Smallpox in Montreal.* Toronto: HarperCollins, 1991; reissued with a new preface as *Plague: How Smallpox Devastated Montreal*, Harper-Collins, 2003. Trans. as *Montréal au Temps du Grand Fléau.* Montreal: Éditions Libre Expression, 1993.

*Right Honourable Men: The Descent of Canadian Politics from Macdonald to Mulroney.* Toronto: HarperCollins, 1994, Revised ed.: *Right Honourable Men: The Descent of Canadian Politics from Macdonald to Chrétien.* Toronto: HarperCollins, 2004.

*William Osler: A Life in Medicine.* Toronto, University of Toronto Press; New York, Oxford University Press, 1999.

*Harvey Cushing: A Life in Surgery.* Toronto: University of Toronto Press; New York: Oxford University Press, 2005.

## Books, Texts, Editions

Bliss, ed., *Canadian History in Documents, 1763–1966*. Toronto: Ryerson Press, 1966.
– with L.M. Grayson. *The Wretched of Canada: Letters to R.B. Bennett, 1930–1935*. Toronto: University of Toronto Press, 1971.
*Confederation 1867*. New York: Franklin Watt, 1975.
*Confederation: A New Nationality.* Toronto: Grolier, 1981.
*Years of Change, 1967–1985*. Toronto: Grolier, Century of Canada Series, 1986.

## Scholarly Articles, Chapters, etc.

'The Methodist Church and World War I. *Canadian Historical Review*, 49, 3 (September 1968), 213–33; reprinted in C.C. Berger, ed., *Conscription 1917* (Toronto: University of Toronto Press, 1969).
'Searching for Canadian History.' *Queen's Quarterly* 75 (1968); reprinted in G. Milburn, ed., *Teaching History in Canada* (Toronto: McGraw-Hill Ryerson, 1972).
'Canadianizing American Business: The Roots of the Branch Plant.' In I. Lumsden, ed., *Close the 49th Parallel, etc.: The Americanization of Canada*, 27–42. Toronto: University of Toronto Press, 1970.
'"Pure Books on Avoided Subjects": Pre-Freudian Sexual Ideas in Canada,' Canadian Historical Association, *Historical Papers*, 1970, 89–108; reprinted in Michiel Horn and Ronald Sabourin, eds, *Studies in Canadian Social History* (Toronto: McClelland and Stewart, 1974); reprinted in S.E.D. Shortt, ed., *Medicine in Canadian Society, Historical Perspectives* (Montreal: McGill-Queen's University Press, 1981).
'A Canadian Businessman and World War I: The Case of Joseph Flavelle.' In J.L. Granatstein and R. Cuff, eds, *War and Society in North America*, 20–36. Toronto: Nelson, 1971.
'Cultural Tariffs and Canadian Universities.' In John Redekop, ed., *The Star-Spangled Beaver*, 80–88. Toronto: Peter Martin Associates, 1971.
'"Dyspepsia of the Mind": The Canadian Businessman and His Enemies, 1880–1914.' In David S. Macmillan, ed., *Canadian Business History: Selected Studies, 1497–1971*, 175–91. Toronto: McClelland and Stewart, 1972.,
'Introduction' to Alan Sullivan, *The Rapids*, vii–xx. Reprinted, Toronto: University of Toronto Press, 1972.
'The Protective Impulse: An Approach to the Social History of Oliver Mowat's Ontario.' In D. Swainson, ed., *Oliver Mowat's Ontario*, 174–88. Toronto: Macmillan, 1972.

'Another Anti-trust Tradition: Canadian Anti-combines Policy, 1889–1910.' *Business History Review*, 47, 2 (1973): 177–88; repr. in Glenn Porter and Robert Cuff, eds, *Enterprise and National Development: Essays in Canadian Business and Economic History.* Toronto: Hakkert, 1973.

'Economic and Business History.' In J.L. Granatstein and Paul Stevens, eds, *Canada since 1867: A Bibliographical Guide*, 57–74. Toronto: Hakkert, 1974; rev. ed., 64–84. Toronto: Samuel Stevens, 1977; 3rd ed., *A Reader's Guide to Canadian History*, vol. 2, *Confederation to the Present*, 76–95. Toronto: University of Toronto Press, 1983.

With William Dendy. 'Holwood.' *Canadian Collector*, 20 (November–December 1975): 17–21.

'The Ideology of Domination: An Eastern Big-Shot Businessman Looks at Western Canada.' In Henry C. Klassen, ed., *The Canadian West: Social Change and Economic Development*, 181–96. Calgary: University of Calgary, 1977.

'"Rich by Nature, Poor by Policy": The State and Economic Life in Canada.' In R. Kenneth Carty and W. Peter Ward, eds, *Entering the Eighties: Canada in Crisis*, 78–90. Toronto: Oxford University Press, 1980.

'War Business as Usual: Canadian Munitions Production, 1914–1918.' In N.F. Dreisziger, ed., *Mobilization for Total War: The Canadian, American and British Experience 1914–1918, 1939–1945*, 43–56. Waterloo: Wilfrid Laurier University Press, 1981.

'The Evolution of Industrial Policies in Canada: An Historical Survey.' Background paper. Economic Council of Canada, 1982.

'Banting's, Best's, and Collip's Accounts of the Discovery of Insulin.' *Bulletin of the History of Medicine* 56, 4 (Winter, 1982): 554–68.

'A Sudden Reprive Called Insulin.' Originally published in *Saturday Night*, ca. 1982; republished in David Jackel and Maurice R. Legris, eds, *Essential Essays: Canadian, American & British*, 70–6. Toronto: Oxford University Press, 1990.

With E. Cukerman, O.V. Sirek, and A. Sirek. 'The Cost and Other Aspects of the Discovery of Insulin: What Were They in 1921 and What Would They Be in 1981.' In *Paediatric and Adolescent Endocrinology* 11 (1983): 156–60.

'The Aetiology of the Discovery of Insulin.' In Charles G. Roland, ed., *Health, Disease and Medicine: Essays in Canadian History* 333–46. Toronto: Clarke, Irwin, 1984.

'Founding F.I.R.A.: The Historical Background.' In J.M. Spence and W. Rosenfeld, eds, *Foreign Investment Review Law in Canada*, 11–12. Toronto: Butterworths, 1984; reprinted in *Partners Nevertheless*, Toronto: Copp Clark Pitman, 1989.

'Resurrections in Toronto: Fact and Myth in the Discovery of Insulin.' American Academy of Arts and Sciences *Bulletin* 38, 3 (December 1984): 15–36.

'Forcing the Pace: A Reappraisal of Business-Government Relations in Canadian History.' In *Theories of Business-Government Relations in Canada*, 36–54. Proceedings of the Max Bell Conference in Business-Government Relations, Faculty of Administrative Studies, York University, 1985.

'The Discovery of Insulin: How It Really Happened.' In Morley Hollenberg, ed., *Insulin, Its Receptor and Diabetes*, 7–20. New York: Marcel Dekker, 1985.

'Who Discovered Insulin?' *News in Physiological Sciences* 1 (February 1986): 31–6; reprinted in *Chem 13 News* 164 (March/April 1986); reprinted in *Australian Chemistry Resource Book* 8 (1989); responses, *NIPS* 1: 143, 211.

*Enterprise in a Cold Climate: Reflections on the History of Canadian Business*. Pamphlet. J.J. Carson Lecture Series, Faculty of Administration, University of Ottawa, 1987.

'J.B. Collip: A Forgotten Member of the Insulin Team.' In Wendy Mitchinson and Janice Dickin McGinnis, eds, *Essays in the History of Canadian Medicine*, 110–25. Toronto: McClelland and Stewart, 1988.

'Conducted Tour' (Alexander Mackenzie's Journey to the Arctic Ocean in the Year 1789). *The Beaver* 69, 2 (April/May 1989): 16–24.

'J.J.R. Macleod and the Discovery of Insulin.' *Quarterly Journal of Experimental Physiology* 74 (1989): 87–96; reprinted in *The Endocrinologist* 4, 2 (March 1994): 85–91.

'The Discovery of Insulin.' In John C. Pickup and Gareth Williams, eds, *Textbook of Diabetes*, 10–14. Oxford: Blackwell, 1991.

'"The Yolk of the Trusts": A Comparison of Canada's Competitive Environment in 1889 and 1989.' In R.S. Khemani and W.T. Stanbury, eds, *Historical Perspectives on Canadian Competition Policy*, 239–51. Halifax: Institute for Research on Public Policy, 1991.

'"Something Terrible": The Odour of Contagion, Montreal 1885.' *The Beaver* 71, 6 (December 1991/January 1992): 6–13.

'Privatizing the Mind: The Sundering of Canadian History, the Sundering of Canada' (Creighton Lecture). *Journal of Canadian Studies* 26, 4 (Winter 1991–2): 5–17; excerpts reprinted in *Rapport: The Journal of the Ontario History and Social Science Teachers' Association* 13, 3 (Spring 1992): 18–21.

'History Fragmented' (abbreviation of Creighton Lecture). *University of Toronto Magazine* 19, 2 (Winter 1991): 7–11.

'Canadian Business History at the Crossroads.' *Business Quarterly* 56, 3 (Winter 1992): 33–7.

'Foreword' to paperback edition of Georgette Gagnon and Dan Rath, *Not without Cause: David Peterson's Fall from Grace*. Toronto: HarperCollins, 1992.

'Foreword' to Patrick Boyer, *Direct Democracy in Canada: The History and Future of Referendums*. Toronto: Dundurn, 1993.

'Rewriting Medical History: Charles Best and the Banting and Best Myth.' *Journal of the History of Medicine and Allied Sciences* 48 (July 1993): 253–74.

'Sisters on the South Shore: The Diaries of Lucy Palmer and Lilly Palmer Inman, 1883–1887.' *The Island Magazine* 34 (Fall–Winter 1993): 15–19.

'The History of Insulin.' *Diabetes Care* 16, supp. 3 (December 1993): 4–7.

'Research Methods and the Discovery of Insulin.' *Research Methodologies in Human Diabetes – Part 1*, 1–10. Berlin, New York: Walter de Gruyter, 1994.

'Party Time in Malpeque: The Social Life of Lucy Palmer, Schoolteacher, 1887–1890.' *The Island Magazine* 36 (Fall–Winter 1994): 13–19.

'Northern Wealth: Economic Life in the Twentieth Century.' *The Beaver* 74, 6 (December–January 1994–5): 4–16.

'Rights and the Flowering of Assertive Individualism.' *University of New Brunswick Law Journal* 44 (1995): 75–7.

'A Farmer Takes a Wife: The Courtship of Lucy Palmer and George Haslam.' *The Island Magazine* 38 (Fall–Winter 1995): 1–6.

'The Discovery of Insulin.' In *The Discovery of Insulin at the University of Toronto: An Exhibition Commemorating the 75th Anniversary*, 13–38. Toronto: Thomas Fisher Library, 1996.

'Life Writing in Medical History.' Interview, in company with J. Duffin. *Canadian Bulletin of the History of Medicine* 13 (1996): 123–37.

'Canada in the Age of the Visible Hand.' In Tom Kent, ed., *In Pursuit of the Public Good: Essays in Honour of Allan J. McEachen*, 21–34. Montreal, Kingston: McGill-Queen's University Press, 1997.

'The Discovery of Insulin: The Inside Story.' In Gregory J. Higby and Elaine C. Stroud, eds, *The Inside Story of Medicines: A Symposium*, 93–100. Madison, WI: American Institute of the History of Pharmacy, 1997.

'Guarding a Most Famous Stream: Trudeau and the Canadian Political Tradition.' In Andrew Cohen and Jack Granatstein, eds, *Trudeau's Shadow: The Life and Legacy of Pierre Elliott Trudeau*, 9–19. Toronto: Random House, 1998.

'Discovering the Insulin Documents: An Archival Adventure.' *The Watermark* (Newsletter of the Archivists and Librarians in the History of the Health Sciences) 21, 3 (Summer 1998): 60–6.

'William Osler at 150.' Canadian Medical Association *Journal* 161, 7 (October 1999): 831–4.

'A Long View of Pierre Trudeau's Legacy.' *Cité Libre* 27, 1 (Winter 1999): 85–9. (Remarks to the York University conference on the Trudeau era, October 1998.)

'Lessons of Kosovo.' Interview with Janice Stein. *Policy Options*, October 1999: 7–17.

'Hugh Hood, Canada, and History: A Historian's View.' Paper delivered to the Visionary Arts Conference, Guelph, November 1999. Published in

*Literary Review of Canada* 8, 2 (March 2000): 3–5; to be anthologized in a
volume of essays edited by Tim Struthers on Hugh Hood.
'Beyond the Granting Agency: The Medical Research Council in the 1990s.'
Pamphlet. Ottawa: Medical Research Council of Canada, 2000.
'The Whole Great Gang: The Passion for History.' *Queen's Quarterly* 107, 1
(Spring 2000): 22–3.
'Integrity, Professionalism and the Cultural Marketplace.' The Carol
Sprachman Memorial Lecture. *Muse* 18, 4 (2000): 24–7.
'A Response to the Commentaries.' Contribution to 'Constructing History in
Biography: A Symposium on *William Osler: A Life in Medicine.*' *Bulletin of the
History of Medicine* 75, 4 (Winter 2001): 740–70.
'Health Care without Hindrance: Medicare and the Canadian Identity.' In
David Gratzer, ed., *Better Medicine: Reforming Canada's Health Care*, 31–43.
Toronto: ECW Press, 2002.
'New News from Norham Gardens: The Osler Letters to Kate Cushing.' In
Charles Roland and Jeremiah Bardondess, eds, *The Persisting Osler III:
Selected Transactions of the American Osler Society, 1991–2000*, 43–8. Malabar,
FL: Krieger, 2002.
'Growth, Progress, and the Quest for Salvation: Confessions of a Medical His-
torian.' *Ars Medica: A Journal of Medicine, the Arts, and Humanities* 1, 1 (Fall
2004): 4–14.
'Resurrections in Toronto: The Emergence of Insulin.' *Hormone Research* 64, S2
(2005) (Proceedings of the 16th Novo Nordisk Symposium on Growth Hor-
mone and Endocrinology), 98–102.
'Has Canada Failed? National Dreams That Have Not Come True.' *Literary
Review of Canada* 14, 2 (March 2006): 3–5.
With Charles F. Wooley. 'William Osler: Slow Pulse, Stokes-Adams Disease, and
Sudden Death in Families.' *American Heart Hospital Journal* 4 (2006): 60–5.
'Fathers and Sons: The Lost Age of Medical Heroism.' Foreword to James
Goodwin, *'Our Gallant Doctor' Enigma and Tragedy: Surgeon Lieutenant George
Hendry and HMCS Ottawa, 1942.* Toronto: Dundurn, 2007.

## Biographical articles

*American National Biography*: 'Charles Best.'
*The Canadian Encyclopaedia* (1985): 'Frederick Banting,' 'Charles Best,'
'J.B. Collip,' 'J.J.R. Macleod.'
*Dictionary of Canadian Biography*: 'Daniel Massey,' vol 8; 'John Harris,' 'John
Macdonald,' vol. 11; 'George Cox,' vol. 14; 'William Davies,' vol. 15; forth-
coming: Sir Joseph Flavelle, Sir Frederick Banting.
*Dictionary of Scientific Biography*, supplement 2 (New York: Scribner's, 1990):
'Charles Best'; with Suzanne Zeller, 'Oskar Minkowski.'

*New Dictionary of National Biography*: 'Sir Joseph Flavelle,' 'Sir Frederick Banting.'

## Book Reviews

### Major

'Beaverbrook: The Canadian Adventuress.' *Acadiensis* 3, 1 (Autumn 1973), 109–13.
Review of T. Naylor, *The History of Canadian Business*. In *Social History / Histoire Sociale* 9, 18 (November 1976): 446–9;  exchange with Naylor, ibid., 10, 19
Review of the *Report* and *Studies* of the Royal Commission on Corporate Concentration. *Canadian Historical Review* 60 (December, 1979).

### Minor

*Canadian Historical Review,* September 1968, 288–9; June 1970, 195–6; June 1972, 205; September 1974, 323–5; June 1980, 227; September 1981, 338–9; March 1983, 77; *Histoire Sociale / Social History,* May 1975, 212–13; *Business History Review,* Summer 1978, 000–0; Summer 1980, 227–9; *Ontario History,* March 1979, 53–4; *Revue d'histoire de l'Amérique française* June 1979, 269–70; *Bulletin of the Committee on Canadian Labour History,* Spring 1979, 16–17; *Journal of Historical Geography,* April 1980, 220–1;  *Journal of the Canadian Church Historical Society,* April 1982, 52–5; *Bulletin of the History of Medicine,* Spring 1985, 139–41; *American Historical Review,* October 1986, 889–90; *Medical History,* Winter 1988–9, 137–8; April 1992, 230–1; *Pharmacy in History,* 1990, 83–4; *The Beaver,* December 1991 / January 1992, 60–2; February–March 1998, 42; February–March 2007, 48;  *Canadian Children's Literature* 1993, 85–6; 2000–1, 175–7; *Literary Review of Canada,* April 2004, 15; *The Lancet,* 367, 24 June 2006, 2051–2.

## Journalism

Several hundred articles and book reviews in various Canadian newspapers and magazines, including *Saturday Night* (esp. 1981–3, 1988–9), *Report on Business Magazine,* (esp. 1985–6, 1989–92), *Maclean's, Canadian Business* (esp. 1992–4), the *Financial Post,* the *Globe and Mail,* the *Toronto Star* (esp. 1992–7), and the *National Post.*

## Fiction

With Jack Batten. 'Sherlock Holmes' Great Canadian Adventure.' *Weekend Magazine,* ca. March 1977; reprinted as 'The Adventure of the Annexationist Conspiracy,' in J.R. Colombo, *Colombo's Book of Canada* (Toronto: Hurtig,

1978); reprinted in Michael Richardson, ed., *Maddened by Mystery: A Casebook of Canadian Detective Fiction* (Toronto: Penguin, 1982), and several other anthologies.

## Various media

Consultant for four-hour, two-part television movie 'Glory Enough for All,' based on *The Discovery of Insulin* and *Banting: A Biography*; produced by Gemstone Productions Ltd for Thames Television and the CBC.

Historical consultant to CBC / Mark Blandford for series *Empire Inc.*, and *Chasing Rainbows*.

Consultant to ExCITE project, Simon Fraser University, 1995–96, for preparation of CD-ROM, the Prime Ministers of Canada.

Consultant to Public Broadcasting Corporation (WGBH, Boston) for Medicine segment of their eight-hour *Evolution of Science* series, 1997–8.

# Contributors

**Gene Allen** teaches in the journalism program at Ryerson University after an extensive career in television news, documentary production, and newspaper reporting. From 1997 to 2001 he was director of research and a senior producer of the CBC/Radio-Canada television series *Canada: A People's History*. His current research projects include a history of the Canadian Press news agency and a study of the relation between news coverage and national identity in Canada from 1890 to 1930.

**Michael Bliss** retired from the University of Toronto in 2006 and holds the rank of University Professor Emeritus. He lives in Toronto and continues to write.

**Barbara Clow** is executive director of the Atlantic Centre of Excellence for Women's Health, a centre for research and policy advice on women's health at Dalhousie University and the IWK Health Centre. She is the author of *Negotiating Disease: Power and Cancer Care, 1900–1950* (2001).

**Ben Forster** is chair of the Department of History at the University of Western Ontario. He is the author of *A Conjunction of Interests: Business, Politics, and Tariffs, 1825–1879* (1986).

**John Fraser** is an award-winning journalist, author, and scholar with numerous publications including *Eminent Canadians: Candid Tales of Then and Now* (2001). He is Master of Massey College at the University of Toronto and a member of the Order of Canada.

**Elsbeth Heaman** holds a Canada Research Chair in Early Canadian History at McGill University. She is the author of *The Inglorious Arts of Peace: Exhibitions in Canadian Society during the 19th Century* (1999) and *St Mary's: The History of a London Teaching Hospital* (2003).

**Brian F. Hogan** was ordained a Roman Catholic priest in the congregation of St Basil in 1975. He has taught at the University of Saskatchewan and the University of Toronto, where he recently retired as dean of the Faculty of Theology, St Michael's College. He is completing a *Bibliography of Canadian Religious History, 1964–2007*, 2nd ed.

**Alison Li** is an Associate Scholar at the Institute for the History and Philosophy of Science and Technology, University of Toronto. She is the author of *J.B. Collip and the Development of Medical Research in Canada* (2003) as well as co-editor and contributor of *Women, Health and Nation* (2003).

**Elizabeth MacCallum** is an award-winning former broadcaster with the CBC-TV's *The Nature of Things* and was for many years the children's book reviewer for both the *Globe and Mail* and the *National Post*. She is co-author with her husband John Fraser of *Mad About the Bay* (2004).

**David B. Marshall** is Associate Professor of History at the University of Calgary. He is the author of *Secularizing the Faith: Canadian Protestant Clergy and the Crisis of Belief* (1992). He is now working on a full-length biography of Charles W. Gordon.

**Shelley McKellar** is Associate Professor of History at the University of Western Ontario. She is the author of *Surgical Limits: The Life of Gordon Murray* (2003).

**Sasha Mullally** is a Hannah Postdoctoral Fellow at the Gorsebrook Research Institute, Saint Mary's University. She is currently preparing a manuscript on rural physicians in Canada and the United States for publication.

**Geoffrey Reaume** is Associate Professor in the Critical Disability Studies, Graduate Program, and School of Health Policy and Management, Faculty of Health, at York University. He is also co-founder of the Psychiatric Survivor Archives, Toronto. His publications include *Remembrance of*

*Patients Past: Patient Life at the Toronto Hospital for the Insane, 1870–1940* (2000) and *Lyndhurst: Canada's First Rehabilitation Centre for People with Spinal Cord Injuries, 1945–1998* (2007).

**Christopher J. Rutty** is founder of Health Heritage Research Services and conducts research on various medical-history topics. He is the author of *A Circle of Care: St. Mary's General Hospital: 75 Years of Caring* (1999) as well as a forthcoming book on the history of poliomyelitis in Canada.

**Veronica Strong-Boag** is the author of numerous publications on Canadian women's history including *Finding Families, Finding Ourselves: English Canada Confronts Adoption from the 19th Century to the 1990s* (2006), *Rethinking Canada: The Promise of Women's History* (4th ed., 2003), *Paddling Her Own Canoe: The Times and Texts of E. Pauline Johnson [Tekahionwake]* (2000), and *New Day Recalled: Lives of Girls and Women in English Canada, 1919–1939* (1987), among others. She is Professor in Women's Studies and Educational Studies at the University of British Columbia, and a Fellow of the Royal Society of Canada.

**James Struthers** is Professor in the Department of Canadian Studies at Trent University. His publications include *The Limits of Affluence: Welfare in Ontario, 1920–1970* (1994) and *No Fault of Their Own: Unemployment and the Canadian Welfare State, 1914–1941* (1983).

**John Turley-Ewart** completed a PhD in Canadian political and business history under the supervision of Michael Bliss in 2000. He is a member of the *National Post*'s editorial board and its deputy comment editor, and writes on political and banking issues. Turley-Ewart also appears regularly on television and radio as a political commentator.

**Richard White** remains associated with the University of Toronto as a regular lecturer in Canadian history (at the University of Toronto Mississauga) and as a Research Associate. He is currently researching and writing the history of Toronto's urban and regional planning, with support from the Neptis Foundation. He is the author of *Gentlemen Engineers: The Working Lives of Frank and Walter Shanly* (1999) and *The Skule Story: The University of Toronto Faculty of Applied Science and Engineering, 1873–2000* (2000).